Multiagency Approach to Disaster Management, Focusing on Triage, Treatment and Transport

Multiagency Approach to Disaster Management, Focusing on Triage, Treatment and Transport

Editors

Amir Khorram-Manesh
Krzysztof Goniewicz

MDPI • Basel • Beijing • Wuhan • Barcelona • Belgrade • Manchester • Tokyo • Cluj • Tianjin

Editors
Amir Khorram-Manesh
University of Gothenburg
Sweden

Krzysztof Goniewicz
Polish Air Force University
Poland

Editorial Office
MDPI
St. Alban-Anlage 66
4052 Basel, Switzerland

This is a reprint of articles from the Topic published online in the open access journal *International Journal of Environmental Research and Public Health* (ISSN 1660-4601), *Safety* (ISSN 2313-576X), *Sustainability* (ISSN 2071-1050), and *Healthcare* (ISSN 2227-9032) (available at: https://www.mdpi.com/topics/Multiagency_Approach_Disaster_Management).

For citation purposes, cite each article independently as indicated on the article page online and as indicated below:

LastName, A.A.; LastName, B.B.; LastName, C.C. Article Title. *Journal Name* **Year**, *Volume Number*, Page Range.

ISBN 978-3-0365-7706-7 (Hbk)
ISBN 978-3-0365-7707-4 (PDF)

Cover image courtesy of Camilo Jimenez

Contents

Preface to "Multiagency Approach to Disaster Management, Focusing on Triage, Treatment and Transport"

The Multiagency Approach to Disaster Management topic collection, published by MDPI, brings together a diverse array of research articles that delve into the intricacies of multiagency collaboration in the context of disaster management. This compilation of studies provides valuable insights into interagency cooperation's benefits, challenges, and opportunities and offers innovative solutions to enhance disaster resilience and preparedness.

Disaster management has evolved beyond traditional response and recovery measures in recent years. The focus has shifted towards proactive planning, prevention, and preparedness. Recognizing the complexities associated with modern-day disasters, this collection emphasizes the importance of a multiagency approach to address these challenges effectively. The collaboration between government agencies, non-governmental organizations, private sector entities, and local communities is crucial to achieving a comprehensive and coordinated response to disasters.

This topic collection comprises research articles that cover a wide range of subjects related to multiagency disaster management, including:

- Theoretical frameworks and models for interagency collaboration.
- The role of communication, coordination, and information sharing in effective disaster management.
- Case studies of successful multiagency collaborations in various disaster scenarios.
- The impact of technology and innovation in fostering cooperation among agencie.s
- The role of local communities and social networks in disaster management efforts.
- Best practices and lessons learned from international experiences in multiagency collaboration.
- Challenges and barriers to effective collaboration, along with potential solutions.

The articles in this collection contribute to the body of knowledge on multiagency approaches in disaster management by addressing the gaps and challenges that often hinder effective cooperation. Moreover, the collection highlights the importance of adaptive, flexible, and inclusive strategies that consider the unique needs and capacities of various stakeholders involved in disaster management.

The Multiagency Approach to Disaster Management topic collection is a valuable resource for researchers, practitioners, policymakers, and other stakeholders in the disaster management field. The shared knowledge and experiences found in these articles not only promote a deeper understanding of the benefits of collaboration but also provide practical guidance for implementing multiagency approaches to improve disaster resilience and preparedness.

Amir Khorram-Manesh and Krzysztof Goniewicz
Editors

safety

MDPI

Article

Gender and Public Perception of Disasters: A Multiple Hazards Exploratory Study of EU Citizens

Arturo Cuesta [1,*], Daniel Alvear [1], Antonio Carnevale [2] and Francine Amon [3]

1 Department of Transports Projects and Processes, University of Cantabria, Ave. Los Castros, s/n, 39005 Santander, Spain
2 CyberEthics Lab., Via Giuseppe Vasi 18/A, 00187 Rome, Italy
3 RISE Research Institutes of Sweden, P.O. Box 857, 50115 Borås, Sweden
* Correspondence: arturo.cuesta@unican.es

Abstract: Aim: To explore gender influence on individual risk perception of multiple hazards and personal attitudes towards disaster preparedness across EU citizens. **Method:** An online survey was distributed to 2485 participants from Spain, France, Poland, Sweden and Italy. The survey was divided into two parts. The first part examined perceived likelihood (L), perceived personal impact (I) and perceived self-efficacy (E) towards disasters due to extreme weather conditions (flood, landslide and storm), fire, earthquake, hazardous materials accidents, and terrorist attacks. The overall risk rating for each specific hazard was measured through the following equation $R = (L \times I)/E$ and the resulting scores were brought into the range between 0 and 1. The second part explored people's reactions to the Pros and Cons of preparedness to compute the overall attitudes of respondents towards preparation (expressed as a ratio between −1 and 1). **Results:** Although we found gender variations on concerns expressed as the likelihood of the occurrence, personal consequences and self-efficacy, the overall risks were judged significantly higher by females in all hazards ($p < 0.01$). We also found that, in general, most respondents (both males and females) were in favour of preparedness. More importantly, despite the gender differences in risk perception, there were no significant differences in the attitudes towards preparedness. We found weak correlations between risks perceived and attitudes towards preparedness (rho < 0.20). The intersectional analysis showed that young and adult females perceived higher risks than their gender counterparts at the same age. There were also gender differences in preparedness, i.e., females in higher age ranges are more motivated for preparedness than men in lower age ranges. We also found that risk perception for all hazards in females was significantly higher than in males at the same education level. We found no significant differences between sub-groups in the pros and cons of getting ready for disasters. However, females at a higher level of education have more positive attitudes towards preparedness. **Conclusions:** This study suggests that gender along with other intersecting factors (e.g., age and education) still shape differences in risk perception and attitudes towards disasters across the EU population. Overall, the presented results policy actions focus on promoting specific DRR policies and practices (bottom-up participatory and learning processes) through interventions oriented to specific target groups from a gender perspective.

Keywords: gender; public perception; multiple hazards; risk perception; preparedness

Citation: Cuesta, A.; Alvear, D.; Carnevale, A.; Amon, F. Gender and Public Perception of Disasters: A Multiple Hazards Exploratory Study of EU Citizens. *Safety* **2022**, *8*, 59. https://doi.org/10.3390/safety8030059

Academic Editor: Raphael Grzebieta

Received: 17 May 2022
Accepted: 2 August 2022
Published: 5 August 2022

1. Introduction

Between 2000 and 2021 in total 14.189 disasters have occurred worldwide causing around 1.5 million casualties. Of these, 1.633 disasters have occurred in Europe with 169.402 reported casualties [1]. The role people play before, during and after a disaster is of crucial importance. In fact, the active participation of individuals and communities is a principle of the Sendai Framework for Disaster Risk Reduction 2015-2030 (SFDRR) [2]. Bottom-up participatory and learning processes in which citizens can act by themselves and/or together with emergency services are the suggested mechanisms to improve Disaster Resilience and Response (DRR) [3,4]. The Sendai Framework also recognizes the importance of integrating a gender perspective into all DRR policies and practices. Hence, for effective bottom-up implementation of DRR policies and practices, we need first to understand the differences/similarities of the risks perceived by both women and men and their subsequent attitudes toward preparedness (as a behavioural precursor).

Although disasters affect whole communities, they are not gender neutral as they impact women and men differently. Gender issues (economic, social, and political inequalities) can create specific vulnerabilities for women in disasters [5,6]. Moreover, gender structures shape the roles, experiences, and responsibilities of individuals in disasters [6,7]. The typical gender roles in disasters are described by Enarson [8] and Fothergill [9].

Gender can also be related to risk judgments and attitudes towards safety [10–13]. In this sense, risk perception and preparedness have been the central investigated issues. Some studies directly address gender influence on these subjects and others include gender among other predictors/variables by simply reporting gender "differences". Regardless of the method used, the literature indicates that women in general perceive hazards as being more serious and riskier than men [8,14–17] and that men express more confidence to face disasters [13,18,19]. Researchers have also focused on preparedness by exploring gender among other factors (e.g., race/ethnicity, age, education, etc.). Some studies showed that gender acts as a predictor of preparedness with women being less likely to be prepared than men for specific hazards [20–23] but other studies were not conclusive (e.g., [24,25]).

Risk perception is usually conceptualised as a logical predictor of preparedness. However, the link between these constructs is still not clear [26,27]. Whereas some studies found that risk perception is associated with or predicts preparedness [23,28,29], others did not [30–32]. Furthermore, most previous studies concentrated on unique disasters (past and/or potential) in specific geographical regions with distinct degrees of gender relations/inequalities, or they were conducted for specific communities or groups of people living in the affected areas. Hence most research findings, although useful for regional and local authorities, are context dependent and difficult to generalize to other hazards and areas. For instance, for an EU policy implementation. Another aspect not fully addressed in the literature is the analysis of gender along with intersectional factors (intersectional approach) (Gendered Innovations: http://genderedinnovations.stanford.edu/terms/intersectionality.html, accessed on 10 May 2022) in the context of disaster response as gender identities, norms, relations and attitudes both shape and are shaped by other social attributes.

The aim of this study is to investigate gender influence on risk perception for multiple hazards and attitudes toward preparedness from a regional perspective, i.e., across the EU population. The first question to investigate is, since women are likely to perceive higher risks than men, is it reasonable to think that they are also more motivated for preparedness? Otherwise (i.e., if there is no positive association between risk and preparedness in gender groups) is it reasonable to infer that gender, among other intersectional factors, contributes to shaping people's attitudes towards disasters? Therefore, the present study aims at contributing to current knowledge by analysing datasets from a multinational survey. The collected responses provided the opportunity to explore gender differences/similarities of EU citizens (from Spain, Poland, Sweden, France and Italy).

The main objectives of the current study are listed below:

- To find gender differences/similarities in risk perception and attitudes toward disaster preparedness;
- To investigate whether risk perception is associated with the intent to prepare for disasters in different genders;
- To explore subgroup differences among males and females according to age and educational background.

Datasets produced here not only have scientific value but also have the potential to inform policymakers and first responders for developing risk management policies and training and communication campaigns, thus improving disaster response and resilience of society as viewed using a gender perspective in Europe.

2. Method

The Checklist for Reporting Results of Internet E-Surveys (CHERRIES) was used as a reference to provide exhaustive information on the survey and to facilitate reproducibility [33].

Design.—The survey was designed to cover people's risk perceptions and attitudes towards preparedness for disasters. The questions used to investigate these factors are listed in Table 1. To analyze risk perception we focused on three main factors inspired by the Protection Motivation Theory developed by Rogers [34,35] and also applied to disaster research [36,37]. These three factors are: (1) the likelihood of disasters to occur (L), (2) the personally relevant impact if disasters occur nearby (I) and (3) the perceived self-efficacy to face the disasters (E). Each question was asked in relation to extreme weather conditions, fires, earthquakes, hazardous material accidents and terrorist attacks. The rationale for the selection of these hazards was their global relevance in Europe (Table 1): meteorological (storms, extreme temperatures, floods), climatological (wildfires), geophysical (earthquakes), technological (industrial accidents) [1] and terrorism (terror attacks) [38,39].

Table 1. Human consequences of selected disasters for the last 20 years in Europe. Sources: EM-DAT [1] and GTD [40].

Hazard	People Affected	Injuries	Casualties
Extreme weather conditions	11,540,045	35,918	154,864
Extreme temperature	688,787	23,350	151,884
Flood	6,852,496	8847	2134
Storm	3,998,762	3721	846
Wildfire	1,287,245	3981	538
Earthquake	594,175	4402	782
Industrial accident	18,564	4264	1323
Terrorist attack *		4547	642

* Bomb and shooting attacks in Western Europe.

In addition, 9-item questions were included to explore the attitudes of males and females towards disaster preparedness: 4 statements for the Pros and 5 statements for the Cons. For simplicity, the statements are expressed as Resilience, Information, Confidence, Assistance for the Pros and Uselessness, Buck-passing, Avoidance, Denial and Cost for the Cons (Table 2).

Table 2. Survey questions and the related available answers. * Extreme weather conditions, Fire, Earthquake, Hazardous materials accidents, and Terrorist attacks. ^ words in parentheses were not included in the questionnaire but are included here to remind the reader of the survey design.

	Variable	Question	Available Answers
Risk Perception	Likelihood	*How likely do you consider that * will occur nearby?*	On a scale from 1 "Highly unlikely" to 4 "Highly likely"
	Impact	*If * occur in your vicinity, what in your view is the impact for you and your family?*	On a scale from 1 "Very low" to 4 "Very high".
	Self-efficacy	*Which statement best represents your ability to deal with *.*	On a scale from 1 "I don't know what to do" to 3 "I know what to do"

Table 2. *Cont.*

	Variable	Question	Available Answers
Attitudes towards preparedness	*Pros*	*Getting ready is worthwhile because:* • *It is easier to get back to normal (Resilience)* ^ • *I can have information about what to do (Information)* • *Acting makes me worry less (Confidence)* • *If I am ready, I can help others (Assistance)*	On a scale from 1 "Strongly disagree" to 5 "Strongly agree"
	Cons	*Getting ready is not worthwhile because:* • *It won't make a difference (Uselessness)* • *It is not my responsibility* • *(Buck-passing)* • *I would rather not think about bad things happening (Avoidance)* • *It doesn't matter; disasters don't happen where I live (Denial)* • *It takes too much time and effort (Cost)*	

Ethics.—The questionnaire was anonymous, and the privacy policy of the individual's posted information was noted (e.g., the purpose of the study, length of time to complete the survey, personal data and data protection, withdrawal rights, etc.). Due to the nature of this study written informed consent was not required. However, respondents were informed about the purpose of the study, and their rights and gave consent to participate by filling in the agreement part of the survey form. This study was approved by the Ethical Committee of the University of Cantabria.

Development.—A pilot was conducted involving 56 participants, allowing us the possibility to know whether a designed questionnaire fulfilled the purpose of the study (i.e., the respondents were asked whether the questions were clear and if they interpreted them as expected). The English version of the questionnaire was reviewed by two external experts and then translated into the target languages by native speakers. During the translation process, we paid special attention to achieving semantic, idiomatic, experiential, and conceptual equivalence to the original version. The initial translation into each target language was made by two independent translators per language to detect and resolve subtle differences/discrepancies. Also, the resulting versions were back-translated to ensure the accuracy of the translation. Then, the online prefinal versions were sent again to the translators for checking and final approval. Check-box answers were provided in the questionnaire to reduce the time to answer each item. Different scales were used. We considered a standard 5-point Likert scale (with a neutral option) for the Pros and Cons of preparedness as we wanted to collect enough granularity in opinions and attitudes. For self-efficacy, we reduced the response options using a 3-point Likert scale forcing the respondents to provide two pieces of information (two polar points along with a neutral option) based on the assumption that collapsing data from a longer scale into three-point scales does not diminish the reliability or validity of the resulting scores while enabling to collect clear responses about perceptions of self-efficacy to face disasters. For likelihood and impact, we used a 4-point Likert with no neutral option thus participants were required to form a judgment while reporting the intensity of the direction. Place of residence (village/town/city), education (no studies/primary/secondary/university), age, occupation (self-employed/employee/unemployed/retired/student) and gender (male/female/binary/other) were gathered at the starting section of the questionnaire.

Survey administration.—The usability and functionality of the electronic questionnaires were tested before fielding the final versions. A hired survey company sent an email invitation to individuals 2.485 living in the targeted countries. In total, we received 1.047 responses (response rate of 41.13%). Respondents belonged to validated databases and were given a monetary incentive for their participation. The company ensured a level of quality control, before and during the data collection.

The questionnaire had in total of 26 items in addition to the sociodemographic information on the first screen. Items were randomized to prevent biases in responses. Overall, the questionnaire took approximately 10–15 min to complete. The responses (only one per participant) were automatically captured and checked through the online survey system. The timeframe for the data collection was from 1 to 14 November 2020.

Participants.—Out of the 1.047 responses 1.2% identified as "non-binary" or "other" rather than "man" or "woman". This "non-binary" group comprised a very small sample size for statistical testing. Therefore, the population sample for the study involved 1.014 respondents (510 who identified as men and 504 who identified as women) from five countries representative of northern (Sweden), southern (Italy and Spain), eastern (Poland) and western (France) regions of Europe. Table 3 displays the characteristics of the surveyed participants. We compared our sample and the sociodemographic characteristics of those surveyed with the Eurostat census data [41]. The Eurostat for adults (aged 20 years and over) shows that 52% of females gave a 2.27% point (pp) difference between our data and the EU population. The age of respondents (20–69 years) was quite representative with an average difference of 4.69% (pp). Yet, there was an over-representation from respondents <29 years (absolute difference of 9.93%) and an under-representation from respondents >60 years (absolute difference of 7.68%). The dwelling type of our sample had absolute differences of 8.8% for cities, 0.3% for towns and 9.2% for rural areas when compared with Eurostat data. Education level (Secondary and University: sample = 91.4% vs. EU population = 79.50%) and occupation (people in the labour force; sample = 69% vs. EU population = 77.10%) had differences but reasonably represented in our study.

Table 3. Baseline characteristics of study participants. Significant *p*-values in bold.

Variable	Overall (n = 1.014)	Male (n = 510, 50.3%)	Female (n = 504, 49.7%)	*p*-Value
Age, years (Mean ± SD)	41 ± 22.7	45 ± 15.7	37 ± 13.3	**<0.001**
Dwelling type [*n* (%)]				0.23
City	480 (47.34)	248 (24.46)	232 (22.88)	
Town	348 (34.32)	179 (17.65)	169 (16.67)	
Rural areas	186 (18.34)	83 (8.19)	103 (10.16)	
Country [*n* (%)]				0.99
France	207 (20.41)	107 (10.55)	100 (9.86)	
Italy	202 (19.92)	100 (9.86)	102 (10.06)	
Poland	201 (19.82)	100 (9.86)	101 (9.96)	
Spain	203 (20.02)	103 (10.16)	100 (9.86)	
Sweden	201 (19.82)	100 (9.86)	101 (9.96)	
Education level [*n* (%)]				0.23
No studies	11 (1.08)	7 (0.69)	4 (0.34)	
Primary	76 (7.5)	41 (4.04)	35 (3.45)	
Secondary	437 (43.10)	231 (22.78)	206 (20.32)	
University	490 (48.32)	231 (22.78)	259 (25.54)	
Occupation [*n* (%)]				**<0.001**
Self-employed	95 (9.37)	56 (5.52)	39 (3.85)	
Employee	535 (52.76)	270 (26.63)	265 (26.13)	
Unemployed	146 (14.40)	43 (4.24)	103 (10.16)	
Retired	109 (10.75)	77 (7.59)	32 (3.16)	
Student	65 (12.72)	64 (6.31)	65 (6.41)	

Analysis.—Descriptive statistics are presented as absolute counts and/or percentages for ordinal variables while interval variables are expressed by means (with SD). To measure an individual's risk rating (R) for each of the five hazards we computed the likelihood (L), the personal impact (I) and the perceived self-efficacy (E) through the following equation $R = (L \times I)/E$ based on [16]. We assumed that the perceived self-efficacy affects the risk perceived rather than simply considering the perceived likelihood and impact to measure risk ratings [17]. Hence, the perceived risk is minimized/reduced (or not) by the perceived self-efficacy here assumed as a value between 1 and 3 where 1 is "I don't know what to do", 2 is "I might know what to do" and 3 is "I know what to do". In the first case, self-efficacy does not change the perceived likelihood and impact. In the second case likelihood and impact are reduced by half. In the third case likelihood and impact are reduced by three times. The resulting scores were brought into the range between 0 and 1 for better understanding and further comparison with other datasets. To measure the attitudes toward preparedness, the responses to each item were summed to create composite scores (of Pros and Cons) for each respondent. The resulting scores were also normalized, and the overall attitudes were expressed as a ratio between −1 and 1 that resulted from subtracting the Pros score from the Cons score. Non-parametric methods were used to assess differences between groups: cross-tabulation and Pearson's chi-square for relative frequencies, Wilcoxon rank sum test and Kruskal-Wallis (Dunn's test) for ordinal and interval scales. The JASP statistical program v0.15 was used for statistical tests throughout the entire study (JASP Team, 2021). For all analyses performed in our study, p-values < 0.05 were considered statistically significant.

3. Results

Risk perception.—The variables related to likelihood (L), impact (I) and self-efficacy (E) for multiple hazards are listed in Table 4. There were gender differences when anticipating the occurrence of extreme weather (W =137,559, $p = 0.03$) and fire (W = 138,582, $p = 0.01$) considered less likely by males than females. We also found that gender is associated with the perceived impact of extreme weather (W = 139,124, $p = 0.01$), fire (W = 137,607, $p = 0.03$) and earthquake (W = 141,289, $p < 0.01$) if it occurs nearby. Nevertheless, the item score distributions of the perceived impacts for hazardous materials accidents (W=133,452, $p = 0.27$) and terrorist attacks (W = 131,533, $p = 0.50$) did not differ significantly between males and females. Our results also suggest that males expressed higher perception of their coping abilities than females to face potential hazards: extreme weather conditions ($\chi^2 = 20.4$, $p < 0.01$), fire ($\chi^2 = 22.45$, $p < 0.01$), earthquake ($\chi^2 = 12.18$, $p < 0.01$), hazardous materials accident ($\chi^2 = 36.60$, $p < 0.01$) and terrorist attack ($\chi^2 = 47.93$, $p < 0.01$). Importantly, gender differences were found to be statistically significant ($p < 0.01$) in the overall risk perception with higher scores in females than in males (Table 5).

Table 4. Absolute counts of respondents in the perceived likelihood (from 1 = highly unlikely to 4 = highly likely), impact (from 1 = very low to 4 = very high) and self-efficacy (1 = I do not know what to do; 2 = I fairly know what to do; 3 = I know what to do) for extreme weather conditions, fire, earthquake, hazardous material accidents and terrorist attack. p-values of the two-sided Wilcoxon rank sum test for likelihood and impact and Chi-Square test for self-efficacy. The significant p-value is in bold.

	Likelihood (L)				Impact (I)				S-Efficacy (E)		
	1	2	3	4	1	2	3	4	1	2	3
Extreme weather											
Female (*n*)	49	131	241	83	51	246	163	44	174	286	44
Male (*n*)	67	144	228	71	91	231	147	41	113	332	65
p-value	**0.03**				**0.01**				**<0.001**		
Fire											
Female (*n*)	31	105	270	98	50	231	165	58	111	309	84
Male (*n*)	46	130	245	89	73	228	174	35	71	300	139
p-value	**0.01**				**<0.01**				**<0.001**		

Table 4. *Cont.*

	Likelihood (L)				Impact (I)				S-Efficacy (E)		
	1	2	3	4	1	2	3	4	1	2	3
Earthquake											
Female (*n*)	170	181	123	30	121	193	136	54	218	244	42
Male (*n*)	187	173	114	36	168	176	125	41	175	266	69
p-value		0.50				**<0.01**				**<0.01**	
Hazardous material accident											
Female (*n*)	146	208	128	22	106	185	140	73	366	119	19
Male (*n*)	148	205	129	28	140	151	152	67	278	192	40
p-value		0.77				0.27				**<0.001**	
Terrorist attack											
Female (*n*)	126	195	143	40	117	189	131	67	331	155	18
Male (*n*)	138	175	134	63	136	177	127	70	236	214	60
p-value		0.59				0.50				**<0.001**	

Table 5. Differences in overall risk perception according to gender. Normalized Mean scores, SD standard deviation [0, 1]. *p*-values of the two-sided Wilcoxon rank sum test. The significant *p*-value is in bold.

Hazards/Disasters	Male Mean ± SD	Female Mean ± SD	W	*p*-Value
Extreme weather	0.21 ± 0.17	0.26 ± 0.19	150,839	**<0.001**
Fire	0.20 ± 0.15	0.24 ± 0.16	152,388	**<0.001**
Earthquake	0.15 ± 0.15	0.19 ± 0.16	144,860	**<0.001**
Hazardous Materials Accident	0.22 ± 0.19	0.25 ± 0.19	143,337	**<0.01**
Terrorist attack	0.23 ± 0.22	0.26 ± 0.22	143,289	**<0.01**

Attitudes towards preparedness.—Most respondents were in favour of getting prepared for disasters (Table 6). There were no statistically significant gender differences for Resilience "it is easier to get back to normal", Information "people have information about what to do" and Confidence "taking action makes me worry less" as Pros of preparedness. Interestingly, the importance of preparedness for helping others (i.e., Assistance) was significantly higher for females than males ($W = 138{,}204$, $p = 0.02$). Around one-fourth of respondents did not form an opinion on the Cons of preparedness and chose the neutral option "undecided" for Avoidance (28% females; 25% males), Denial (23% females; 25% males) and Cost (22% females; 24% males). No significant gender differences were found for Uselessness "getting ready won't make a difference", Buck-passing "It is not my responsibility", and Cost "It takes too much time, effort, or money". Yet, differences were statistically significant for Avoidance "I would rather not think about bad things happening" ($W = 138{,}848.5$, $p = 0.02$) and Denial "It doesn't matter; disasters don't happen where I live" ($W = 119{,}186$, $p = 0.03$). However, one of the interesting results that emerged from the data was that gender differences in the composite scores for Pros and Cons of getting ready and the overall attitudes toward preparedness were not statistically significant (Table 7).

Table 6. Respondents' reactions to the Pros and Cons of disaster preparedness (from 1 = strongly disagree to 5 = strongly agree). *p*-values of the two-sided Wilcoxon rank sum test. The significant *p*-value is in bold.

Pros	Score					Cons	Score				
	1	2	3	4	5		1	2	3	4	5
Resilience						Uselessness					
Female (%)	3	5	20	48	25	Female (%)	43	32	13	10	2
Male (%)	1	6	22	46	26	Male (%)	38	32	17	11	2
p-value			0.95			*p*-value			0.05		
Information						Responsibility					
Female (%)	5	12	17	32	34	Female (%)	38	30	19	10	3
Male (%)	5	10	19	41	25	Male (%)	34	28	22	13	2
p-value			0.09			*p*-value			0.07		
Confidence						Avoidance					
Female (%)	3	6	18	46	28	Female (%)	22	21	28	23	6
Male (%)	1	7	23	44	25	Male (%)	25	25	25	19	5
p-value			0.18			*p*-value			**0.02**		
Assistance						Denial					
Female (%)	1	4	11	40	44	Female (%)	32	32	23	11	2
Male (%)	1	3	17	41	38	Male (%)	27	31	25	14	3
p-value			**0.02**			*p*-value			**0.03**		
						Cost					
						Female (%)	31	29	22	14	4
						Male (%)	27	29	24	15	5
						p-value			0.10		

Table 7. Two-sided Wilcoxon rank sum test results for the attitudes of males and females towards preparedness. Pros and Cons [0, 1]. Overall attitude [−1, 1].

	Male Mean ± SD	Female Mean ± SD	W	*p*-Value
Pros *"Getting ready is worthwhile"*	0.72 ± 0.18	0.73 ± 0.19	135,463.5	0.13
Cons *"Getting ready is not worthwhile"*	0.33 ± 0.23	0.31 ± 0.21	123,049.5	0.23
Overall attitude (Pros-Cons)	0.39 ± 0.32	0.42 ± 0.33	135,673.5	0.12

Risk perception and preparedness.—A question directly addressed in this study was whether the perceived risk can motivate preparedness. We computed Spearman's rank correlation to assess the relationship between our risk perception results (likelihood, impact, self-efficacy and overall risk perception) for each of the reported hazards and the overall attitudes towards preparedness. We found weak correlations for the gender groups in all cases (rho < 0.20) suggesting that in our study the considered risk factors have a very low association with motivations for preparedness.

Gender and intersectional factors.—While gender is important it is shaped by other factors likely to reveal subgroup differences among males and females. We conducted an additional intersectional analysis considering gender related to age and educational background. This analysis revealed interesting findings that emerged during the process of the investigation.

Gender and age: We defined six categories for the comparison: YF (young female < 30 years), AF (adult female 30–50 years), OF (Older female > 50 years), YM (young male < 30 years), AM (adult male 30–50 years), OM (older male > 50 years). The mean and standard deviation of risk scores produced by each subgroup are displayed in Table 8. Kruskal-Wallis tests showed statistically significant differences in risk perception between subgroups (Table 8). Pairwise comparisons using Dunn's test indicated that several subgroups were observed to be significantly different (Table 9). Interestingly, risk perception for all hazards in females was significantly higher than in males in the same range of age (AF vs. AM and YF vs. YM). We only found significant differences between the same gender in males > 50 years (OM) who perceived higher risks in all hazards than males 30–50 years (AM).

Table 8. Mean and standard deviation of risk scores [0, 1] by gender and age and *p*-values from the Kruskal-Wallis test (α = 0.05).

Group	Gender	Age (Years)	Extreme Weather	Fire	Earthquake	Hazard. Mate Accident	Terrorist Attack
AF	Female	30–50	0.25 ± 0.19	0.24 ± 0.16	0.18 ± 0.16	0.22 ± 0.18	0.25 ± 0.21
OF	Female	>50	0.26 ± 0.18	0.22 ± 0.15	0.21 ± 0.17	0.29 ± 0.22	0.29 ± 0.24
YF	Female	<30	0.26 ± 0.19	0.25 ± 0.17	0.18 ± 0.16	0.25 ± 0.19	0.25 ± 0.20
AM	Male	30–50	0.20 ± 0.16	0.18 ± 0.13	0.13 ± 0.12	0.20 ± 0.17	0.21 ± 0.22
OM	Male	>50	0.23 ± 0.18	0.22 ± 0.15	0.19 ± 0.18	0.24 ± 0.21	0.25 ± 0.22
YM	Male	<30	0.19 ± 0.16	0.18 ± 0.16	0.13 ± 0.13	0.20 ± 0.19	0.20 ± 0.22
	p-value		<0.001	<0.001	<0.001	<0.001	<0.001

Table 9. Results of pairwise comparison using Dunn's test (z-statistic and *p*-values) for risk perception according to gender and age (α = 0.05). Grey cells indicate significant differences between subgroups for all hazards.

	Extreme Weather	Fire	Earthquake	Hazard. Mate Accident	Terrorist Attack
AF vs. OF	−0.52	0.71	−1.57	−2.13 *	−1.51
AF vs. YF	−0.56	−0.50	−0.13	−1.39	−0.30
AF vs. AM	3.43 ***	4.08 ***	3.07 **	1.90 *	2.19 *
AF vs. OM	1.46	1.35	−0.40	−0.12	−0.18
AF vs. YM	3.38 ***	4.58 ***	3.03 **	1.37	2.96 **
OF vs. YF	0.05	−1.07	1.40	0.93	1.21
OF vs. AM	3.19 *	2.51 **	3.93 ***	3.57 ***	3.19 ***
OF vs. OM	1.65 *	0.37	1.21	1.97 *	1.33
OF vs. YM	3.24 **	3.14 ***	3.89 ***	3.02 **	3.79 ***
YF vs. AM	3.74 **	4.28 ***	2.98 **	3.11 ***	2.33 *
YF vs. OM	1.90 *	1.74 *	−0.25	1.22	0.12
YF vs. YM	3.68 **	4.76 ***	2.98 **	2.47 **	3.06 **
AM vs. OM	−1.87 *	−2.60 **	−3.31 ***	−1.93 *	−2.26 *
AM vs. YM	0.38	1.00	0.35	−0.28	1.03
OM vs. YM	2.02 *	3.28 ***	3.26 ***	1.42	3.01 **

* $p < 0.05$; ** $p < 0.01$; *** $p < 0.001$.

Table 10 displays the mean and standard deviation of preparedness scores and the results of the Kruskal-Wallis test showing significant differences between subgroups (Table 10). Results of the pairwise comparisons by Dunn's test (Table 11) revealed significant intergender differences in the overall measures between adult females (AF) and young males (YM), older females (OF) and adult males (AM), older females (OF) and young males and (YM). We also found differences in the overall measures between the same genders: adult vs. older in females (AF vs. OF), adult vs. older males (AM vs. OM) and older vs. young males (OM vs. YM).

Table 10. Mean and standard deviation of preparedness scores by gender and age and p-values from the Kruskal-Wallis test ($\alpha = 0.05$). Pros [0, 1] = in favour of preparedness; Cons [0, 1] = against preparedness; Overall [−1, 1] = Overall attitude toward pre-preparedness.

Group	Gender	Age (Years)	Pros	Cons	Overall
AF	Female	30–50	0.73 ± 0.19	0.33 ± 0.23	0.40 ± 0.34
OF	Female	>50	0.77 ± 0.19	0.27 ± 0.21	0.50 ± 0.34
YF	Female	<30	0.72 ± 0.18	0.31 ± 0.20	0.41 ± 0.31
AM	Male	30–50	0.72 ± 0.18	0.34 ± 0.23	0.38 ± 0.32
OM	Male	>50	0.75 ± 0.18	0.30 ± 0.22	0.45 ± 0.31
YM	Male	<30	0.69 ± 0.18	0.37 ± 0.22	0.32 ± 0.32
	p-value		**<0.01**	**0.012**	**<0.001**

Table 11. Results of pairwise comparison using Dunn's test (z-statistic and p-values) for attitudes towards preparedness ($\alpha = 0.05$). Grey cells indicate significant differences between subgroups for all the measures.

	Pros	Cons	Overall
AF vs. OF	−1.92 *	1.99 *	−2.52 **
AF vs. YF	0.00	0.76	−0.39
AF vs. AM	0.98	−0.37	0.63
AF vs. OM	−1.15	1.60	−1.70 *
AF vs. YM	2.05 *	−1.69 *	2.33 **
OF vs. YF	1.83 *	−1.29	2.09 *
OF vs. AM	2.64 **	−2.23 *	2.95 **
OF vs. OM	0.95	−0.67	1.11
OF vs. YM	3.40 ***	−3.16 ***	4.16 ***
YF vs. AM	0.91	−1.08	0.96
YF vs. OM	−1.08	0.76	−1.21
YF vs. YM	1.94 *	−2.25 *	2.54 **
AM vs. OM	−2.04 *	1.89 *	−2.23 *
AM vs. YM	1.16	−1.32	1.73 *
OM vs. YM	2.95 **	−2.98 **	3.68 ***

* $p < 0.05$; ** $p < 0.01$; *** $p < 0.001$.

***Gender and Education*:** We categorized the sample into six subgroups according to gender and education background: PF (primary female), SF (secondary female), UF (university female), PM (primary male), SM (secondary male), UM (university male). There were significant differences between the subgroups (Tables 12 and 13). We found that risk perception for all hazards in females was significantly higher than in males at the same education level, i.e., secondary (SF vs. SM) and university (UF vs. UM). We also found that females with secondary education (SF) perceived risk to be significantly higher than their gender counterparts with university education (UM).

The Kruskal-Wallis test showed significant differences only between subgroups by gender and education for the overall attitudes toward preparedness (Table 14). Pairwise comparisons showed significant intergender differences for UM vs. PF ($p = 0.012$), UF vs. PM ($p = 0.018$) and UF vs. SM ($p < 0.01$). We also found differences between subgroups of the same gender: SF vs. PF ($p = 0.012$), and UF vs. PF ($p < 0.01$).

Table 12. Mean and standard deviation of risk scores [0, 1] by gender and education and p-values from the Kruskal-Wallis test ($\alpha = 0.05$).

Group	Gender	Education	Extreme Weather	Fire	Earthquake	Hazard. Mate Accident	Terrorist Attack
PF	Female	Primary	0.22 ± 0.21	0.25 ± 0.16	0.20 ± 0.16	0.24 ± 0.17	0.23 ± 0.19
FS	Female	Secondary	0.25 ± 0.18	0.22 ± 0.15	0.18 ± 0.17	0.23 ± 0.17	0.24 ± 0.20
FU	Female	University	0.26 ± 0.18	0.25 ± 0.17	0.17 ± 0.15	0.25 ± 0.20	0.26 ± 0.22
PM	Male	Primary	0.18 ± 0.14	0.16 ± 0.09	0.15 ± 0.12	0.19 ± 0.17	0.20 ± 0.20
SM	Male	Secondary	0.19 ± 0.15	0.19 ± 0.14	0.15 ± 0.15	0.21 ± 0.19	0.21 ± 0.22
UM	Male	University	0.22 ± 0.18	0.20 ± 0.16	0.15 ± 0.15	0.22 ± 0.19	0.23 ± 0.22
	p-value		<0.001	<0.001	0.013	0.034	0.038

Table 13. Results of pairwise comparison using Dunn's test (z-statistic and p-values) for risk perception according to gender and education background ($\alpha = 0.05$).

	Extreme Weather	Fire	Earthquake	Hazard. Mate Accident	Terrorist Attack
PF vs. SF	−1.97 *	0.93	0.64	0.27	−0.22
PF vs. UF	−2.08 *	0.34	0.69	−0.00	0.34
PF vs. PM	0.33	2.81 **	0.81	1.47	1.02
PF vs. SM	0.40	2.48 **	1.93 *	1.48	1.15
PF vs. UM	−0.71	2.19 *	2.05 *	0.96	0.57
SF vs. UF	−0.14	−1.10 **	0.06	−0.52	−0.22
SF vs. PM	2.60 **	2.76 **	0.39	1.68 *	1.61
SF vs. SM	4.27 ***	2.76 **	2.30 *	2.16 *	2.45 **
SF vs. UM	2.33 **	2.27 *	2.55 **	1.25	1.45
UF vs. PM	2.73 **	3.47 ***	0.35	2.02 *	1.78 *
UF vs. SM	4.66 ***	4.05 ***	2.36 **	2.82 **	2.83 **
UF vs. UM	2.62 **	3.56 ***	2.63 **	1.87 *	1.77 *
PM vs. SM	−0.02	−1.10	1.00	−0.37	−0.13
PM vs. UM	−1.23	−1.44	1.13	−0.95	−0.76
SM vs. UM	−2.06 *	−0.56	0.20	−0.97	−1.07

* $p < 0.05$; ** $p < 0.01$; *** $p < 0.001$.

Table 14. Mean and standard deviation of preparedness scores by gender and education and p-values from the Kruskal-Wallis test ($\alpha = 0.05$). Pros [0, 1] = in favor of preparedness; Cons [0, 1] = against preparedness; Overall [−1, 1] = Overall attitude toward preparedness. The significant p-value is in bold.

Group	Gender	Education	Pros	Cons	Overall
PF	Female	Primary	0.64 ± 0.26	0.37 ± 0.23	0.27 ± 0.41
FS	Female	Secondary	0.73 ± 0.18	0.32 ± 0.22	0.41 ± 0.32
FU	Female	University	0.74 ± 0.17	0.29 ± 0.20	0.44 ± 0.31
PM	Male	Primary	0.70 ± 0.19	0.35 ± 0.21	0.35 ± 0.31
SM	Male	Secondary	0.72 ± 0.19	0.34 ±0.23	0.37 ± 0.33
UM	Male	University	0.72 ± 0.16	0.31 ± 0.21	0.41 ± 0.30
	p-value		0.106	0.083	**0.019**

4. Discussion

This exploratory study looks at gender differences in two central aspects (1) risk perception of multiple hazards and (2) attitudes towards disaster preparedness. People (n = 1.014) from different countries (Italy, Sweden, Poland, France and Spain) were included in this study.

Risk perception.—Our results indicate gender differences in concerns about hazards expressed as the likelihood of the occurrence, personal consequences and self-efficacy. Females were more aware of the occurrence of disasters resulting from extreme weather and fire. Females also exhibited a higher perception of the potential consequences of extreme weather, fire and earthquake than males. These results are in line with previous findings confirming that women are more worried about natural hazards than men, especially if family members are threatened [10,42]. It is important to note that items did not necessarily have the same meaning for females and males as they may give priority to different hazards and/or show different concerns about the same hazards [43]. The questions of this section included "what in your view is the impact for you and your family?" Female respondents perhaps felt more oriented towards home and family when they thought about the presented hazards. Following this type of interpretation would yield an explanation as to why female respondents showed higher concerns. Our results reinforce a recent finding that reports no gender effects in the perceived vulnerability regarding terrorist attacks [44].

Self-efficacy has been identified as an important variable that should be considered within the context of hazards research, since it may be linked to the perceived risk and the adoption of hazard adjustments [45]. Our study confirms that gender is an important factor in the perceived self-coping abilities to deal with disasters. Males reported higher self-efficacies for all the presented hazards (i.e., extreme weather, fire, earthquake, hazardous accident and terrorist attack). A possible explanation suggests that women may be less confident than men, but this conceivably denotes a more realistic view of their own self-capacities [13].

To measure the overall risk perception (R) for the five hazards we computed the three subjective factors, namely: the likelihood of a disaster to occur (L), the impact if a disaster occurs nearby (I) and the perceived self-efficacy to cope with the disaster (E) through the following equation $R = (L \times I)/E$. The resulting scores of males and females were compared. Our results showed that the risks were judged significantly higher by females in all hazards. The main reason that explains these results may be associated with the incorporation of self-efficacy (E) by assuming that this factor affects the risk perceived rather than simply considering the perceived likelihood (L) and impact (I) to measure risk ratings [17]. Additionally, we computed this approach (i.e., $R = L \times I$) and the differences were also statistically significant (females scored higher risk than males) when applying two-sided Wilcoxon rank sum test for extreme weather conditions (W = 140,553.5, $p < 0.001$), fire (W = 141,096, $p < 0.001$) and earthquake (W = 138,242, $p = 0.03$). But the differences were not significant for hazardous materials accidents (W = 131,362, $p = 0.53$) and terrorist attacks (W = 129,487, $p = 0.83$). Overall, this finding emphasises gender differences in risk perception for natural hazards. But this might not be the case for man-made hazards, thus warranting further research to explore the factors that may account for it.

Attitudes towards preparedness.—Participants were also asked about the Pros and Cons of preparedness to measure their individual interest in getting prepared. Responses to some items differed between males and females. The importance of being prepared to help others (Assistance) was significantly higher in female respondents. This result was in line with previous studies attesting that women tend to be more altruistic than men (see for some references [46–49]. The statement that disasters "don't happen where I live" (Denial) had significantly higher scores in male respondents denoting differences in judgments based upon such events [43] and optimistic bias [50]. The 'It will not happen to me' belief is a very important aspect of preparedness that has already been reported [51] since overconfidence can keep individuals from realizing how little they know and how much information they may need to be ready. By contrast, females were significantly more likely to "not think about bad things happening" (Avoidance) than males. This result supports previous studies attesting that gender is a significant predictor of coping through avoidance [52,53]. Avoidance here can be associated with information avoidance leading to misinformation which has been recently analysed in the context of the COVID 19 pandemic [54,55]. More research is needed to explore gender influence on this aspect of behaviour in the context of disasters.

Risk perception and preparedness.—A question addressed in this study was whether the perceived risk can motivate preparedness. Risk perception has been considered a predictor or correlates of preparedness behaviour. While some studies found that risk perception predicted or was associated with preparedness others found no effects [27]. Overall, results showed that most respondents (both males and females) were in favour of preparedness. More importantly, despite the gender differences in risk perception, there were no significant differences in attitudes towards preparedness. We found weak correlations for the gender groups in all cases (rho < 0.20) suggesting that in our study the considered risk factors have a very low association with motivations to seek preparedness.

Gender and intersectional factors.—Previous results open a new question addressed in this study. There are differences/similarities between women and men but which women? and which men? An intersectional approach was used to analyze the multiplicative impact of gender when combined with age and educational background which also shapes the identity, perceptions, and attitudes of individuals towards disasters. This analysis produced more detailed information showing the differences between different but interdependent categories and factors. We compared six subgroups categorized by gender (male; female) and age (<30 years; 30–50 years; >50 years). The subgroups were observed to be significantly different, especially between subgroups of different genders. Young and adult females perceived higher risks than their gender counterparts of the same age. There were also gender differences in preparedness between subgroups of different ages denoting that age is also a contributing factor to people's attitudes (e.g., females in a higher age range are more motivated for preparedness than men in a lower age range). We defined six subgroups according to gender (male; female) and education (primary; secondary; university). We found that risk perception for all hazards in females was significantly higher than in males at the same education level (e.g., secondary and university education background). Furthermore, females with secondary education (SF) perceived risks to be significantly higher than their gender counterparts with university education (UM). When it comes to the attitudes towards preparedness, we found no significant differences between subgroups in the reported scores for the pros and cons of getting ready for disasters. However, females at a higher level of education have more positive attitudes towards preparedness.

The current study has several strengths. First, it contributes to the literature by providing a general approach to exploring gender on public perception of multiple hazards/disasters, which predominantly has been concerned with specific disasters and affected communities. Second, the datasets generated in this study are available allowing third parties to conduct further research. Third, this study proposes a new approach to computing the subjective factors (likelihood, impact and self-efficacy) of risk perception and personal attitudes toward preparedness (Pros and Cons). Fourth, the resulting scores were presented in more analytical forms, i.e., [0, 1] and [−1, 1] for better understanding and further comparison with other datasets. Fifth, the intersectional analysis presented here (combining gender age and education) will allow policy-makers and first responders to better identify subgroups and factors among the population to implement DRR policies and practices. Finally, as mentioned the results produced here not only have scientific value but also have the potential to inform EU policymakers and first responders. The current study also has its limitations. First, compared with other studies a "small" sample size was employed (n = 1.014). However, we believe that the subset of the population used was representative thus providing a sufficient amount of information to conclude the EU population. Second, the study is limited in scope, i.e., whether or not gender is "significant" along with other two factors (i.e., age and education level). Third, the association between risk perception and preparedness was not found, perhaps due to the design of the items in the questionnaire as this was not the initial purpose of the study. Fourth, non-parametric methods were conducted for the statistical analysis potentially leading to less powered results. Finally, the results presented here are rather indicative than definitive.

5. Conclusions

Results presented in this study constitute the first process of gender analysis (e.g., data collection, data processing, and analysis) and advocate to conduct of the second process which is interpretative in nature [56]. The gender discrepancies may reveal the underlying mechanisms apart from biological and physiological differences such as everyday life behaviours and beliefs as well as stereotypes derived from gender norms [57]. Conceivably, socioeconomic and cultural differences between men and women are more evident in lower-income countries leading to a higher exposure of women to risks in case of a disaster [5]. The present results suggest that gender differences in relation to risk perception of multiple hazards might still be present in European societies. The different social roles and activities of men and women within the household and community are examples of how gender norms and ideals manifest. The role of nurturer and caregiver primarily played by women has been associated with greater concern about the risk of potential disasters and the well-being of others [58]. Also, different gender roles can be reinforced in disasters because expectations for men and women are usually based on stereotypes. For instance, a recent study focused on actions during a large Swedish forest fire, indicated that women were praised when they followed the traditional norms but denigrated when they performed what was perceived as male-coded tasks [59].

Our results suggest the same predisposition of females and males to seek preparedness. Women are slightly present in emergency planning and disaster management programs but more involved in household and community care in practice [57,60,61] and often ignored in official evaluations after disasters [5]. It is argued here that gender skills may benefit the prevention and mitigation of hazard situations.

Although limited to risk perception and preparedness, the outcomes of this study can provide insights into the integration of gender-sensitive practices in disaster preparedness and response. First, conducting more qualitative and quantitative research to better understand gender-based roles and responsibilities is highly desirable. For studying a complex area such as gender constructs and roles, multi-disciplinary research could be beneficial. Second, improving women's capacities and knowledge (training and education) can increase individual and community resilience. Third, promoting policies and actions to involve women in official emergency management programs and decision-making is essential to minimize gender gaps in disaster planning and response. Much work remains to be done to systematically integrate gender analysis into relevant domains of safety science and technology—from strategic considerations for establishing research priorities to guidelines for establishing best practices in formulating research questions, designing methodologies and interpreting data.

The practical implications of this study can be summarized as follows:

- Datasets produced here are available to practitioners, policymakers and first responders to conduct further analyses on gender in DRR across the EU population.
- The present study has gone one step beyond gender analysis by providing information on risk perception and motivation for disaster preparedness across different population subgroups (individual-level categories while considering gender). Therefore, the interested parties will be able to focus on promoting specific DRR policies and practices (bottom-up participatory and learning processes) through interventions oriented to specific target groups.

Author Contributions: Conceptualization, A.C. (Arturo Cuesta), D.A. and A.C. (Antonio Carnevale); data curation, A.C. (Arturo Cuesta); Formal analysis, A.C. (Arturo Cuesta); Funding acquisition, all authors; investigation, A.C. (Arturo Cuesta); methodology, A.C. (Arturo Cuesta), D.A. and A.C. (Antonio Carnevale); Project administration, D.A.; supervision, A.C. (Arturo Cuesta) and D.A.; writing—original draft, A.C. (Arturo Cuesta); writing—review & editing, F.A. All authors have read and agreed to the published version of the manuscript.

Funding: This project has received funding from the European Union's Horizon 2020 research and innovation programme under grant agreement No 832576.

Institutional Review Board Statement: The study was conducted in accordance with the Declaration of Helsinki and approved by the Ethics Committee of the University of Cantabria (CE Proyecto 06/2019).

Informed Consent Statement: Informed consent was obtained from all subjects involved in the study.

Data Availability Statement: The datasets in this study are available from the corresponding author upon request.

Acknowledgments: The authors would like to thank the European Commission and the members of the ASSISTANCE consortium for their collaboration and support to this study. We would like to express our very great appreciation to the team members involved in the translation of the questionnaire into Italian (CYBERETHICS LAB SRLS), Swedish (RISE RESEARCH INSTITUTES OF SWEDEN AB), Polish (PRZEMYSLOWY INSTYTUT AUTOMATYKI I POMIAROW PIAP), French (THALES SA) and Spanish (UNIVERSIDAD DE CANTABRIA).

Conflicts of Interest: The authors declare no conflict of interest. The funders had no role in the design of the study; in the collection, analyses, or interpretation of data; in the writing of the manuscript, or in the decision to publish the results.

References

1. Guha-Sapir, D.; Below, R.; Hoyois, P. EM-DAT: The CRED/OFDA International Disaster Database. Université Catholique de Louvain, Brussels, Belgium. Available online: https://public.emdat.be/ (accessed on 5 February 2020).
2. Sendai Framework for Disaster Risk Reduction 2015–2030. United Nations. Available online: https://www.undrr.org/publication/sendai-framework-disaster-risk-reduction-2015-2030 (accessed on 18 July 2021).
3. Nkombi, Z.; Wentink, G.J. The role of public participation in disaster risk reduction initiatives: The case of Katlehong township. *Jàmbá J. Disaster Risk Stud.* **2022**, *14*, a1203. [CrossRef]
4. National Disaster Risk Assessment. UNISDR (United Nations Office for Disaster Risk Reduction). Words in Action Guidelines. 2017. Available online: https://www.unisdr.org/files/52828_nationaldisasterriskassessmentpart1.pdf (accessed on 20 April 2022).
5. Neumayer, E.; Plümper, T. The Gendered Nature of Natural Disasters: The Impact of Catastrophic Events on the Gender Gap in Life Expectancy, 1981–2002. *Ann. Assoc. Am. Geogr.* **2007**, *97*, 551–566. [CrossRef]
6. Ashraf, M.A.; Azad, A.K. Gender Issues in Disaster: Understanding the relationships of vulnerability, preparedness and Capacity. *Environ. Ecol. Res.* **2015**, *3*, 136–142. [CrossRef]
7. Enarson, E.; Scanlon, J. Gender Patterns in Flood Evacuation: A case study of couples in Canada's Red River Valley. *Appl. Behav. Sci. Rev.* **1999**, *7*, 103–124. [CrossRef]
8. Enarson, E. SWS Fact Sheet: Women and Disaster. 2006. Available online: http://nhma.info/uploads/resources/gender/SWS%20G%26D%20Fact%20Sheet.pdf (accessed on 2 February 2020).
9. Fothergill, A. Gender, risk, and disaster. *Int. J. Mass Emergencies Disasters* **1996**, *14*, 33–56. Available online: http://ijmed.org/articles/96/ (accessed on 2 February 2020).
10. Enarson, E.; Morrow, B.H. A Gendered Perspective: The voices of women. In *Hurricane Andrew: Ethnicity, Gender, and the Sociology of Disasters*; Peacock, W.G., Morrow, B.H., Gladwin, H., Eds.; Routledge: New York, NY, USA, 1997; pp. 116–140.
11. Ho, M.-C.; Haw, D.; Lin, S.; Chiu, Y.-C. How Disaster Characteristics Influence Risk Perception? *Risk Anal.* **2008**, *28*, 635–643. [CrossRef]
12. Khan, A.A.; Rana, I.A.; Nawaz, A. Gender-based approach for assessing risk perception in a multi-hazard environment: A study of high schools of Gilgit, Pakistan. *J. Disaster Risk Reduct.* **2020**, *44*, 101427. [CrossRef]
13. Cvetkovic, V.M.; Rober, G.; Öcal, A.; Dragicevic, S. The Role of Gender in Prepared-ness and Response Behaviors towards Flood Risk in Serbia. *Int. J. Environ. Res. Public Health* **2018**, *15*, 2761. [CrossRef] [PubMed]
14. Flynn, J.; Slovic, P.; Mertz, C.K. Gender, race, and perception of environmental health risks. *Risk Anal.* **1994**, *14*, 1101–1108. [CrossRef]
15. Finucane, M.; Slovic, P.; Mertz, C.K.; Flynn, J.; Satterfiled, T.A. Gender, race, and perceived risk: The e 'white male' effect. *Health Risk Soc.* **2020**, *2*, 159–172. [CrossRef]
16. O'Neill, E.; Brereton, F.; Shahumyan, H.; Clinch, J.P. The Impact of Perceived Flood Exposure on Flood-Risk Perception: The Role of Distance. *Risk Anal.* **2016**, *36*, 2158–2186. [CrossRef] [PubMed]

17. Brown, G.V.; Largey, A.; McMullan, C. The impact of gender on risk perception: Implications for EU member states' national risk assessment processes. *Int. J. Disaster Risk Reduct.* **2021**, *63*, 102452. [CrossRef]
18. Barberi, F.; Davis, M.S.; Isaia, R.; Nave, R.; Ricci, T. Volcanic risk perception in the Vesuvius population. *J. Volcanol. Geotherm. Res.* **2008**, *172*, 244–258. [CrossRef]
19. Armas, I.; Avram, E. Perception of flood risk in Danube Delta, Romania. *Nat. Hazards* **2009**, *50*, 269–287. [CrossRef]
20. Eisenman, D.P.; Wold, C.; Fielding, J.; Long, A.; Setodji, C.; Hickey, S.; Gelberg, L. Differences in individual-level terrorism preparedness in Los Angeles County. *Am. J. Prev. Med.* **2006**, *30*, 1–6. [CrossRef] [PubMed]
21. Boscarino, J.A.; Adams, R.E.; Figley, C.R.; Galea, S.; Foa, E.B. Fear of terrorism and preparedness in New York City 2 years after the attacks: Implications for disaster planning and research. *J. Public Health Manag. Pract.* **2006**, *12*, 505–513. [CrossRef]
22. Blessman, J.; Skupski, J.; Jamil, M.; Jamil, H.; Bassett, D.; Wabeke, R.; Arnetz, B. Barriers to at-home preparedness in public health employees: Implications for disaster preparedness training. *J. Occup. Environ. Med.* **2007**, *49*, 318–326. [CrossRef]
23. Ablah, E.; Konda, K.; Kelley, C.L. Factors predicting individual emergency preparedness: A multi-state analysis of 2006 BRFSS data. *Biosecurity Bioterrorism Biodefense Strategy Pract. Sci.* **2009**, *7*, 317–330. [CrossRef]
24. Miceli, R.; Sotgiu, I.; Settanni, M. Disaster preparedness and perception of flood risk: A study in an alpine valley in Italy. *J. Environ. Psychol.* **2008**, *28*, 164–173. [CrossRef]
25. Baker, E.J. Household preparedness for the Aftermath of Hurricanes in Florida. *Appl. Geogr.* **2011**, *31*, 46–52. [CrossRef]
26. Domingues, R.B.; de Jesus, S.N.; Ferreira, Ó. Place attachment, risk perception, and preparedness in a population exposed to coastal hazards: A case study in Faro Beach, southern Portugal. *Int. J. Disaster Risk Reduct.* **2021**, *60*, 102288. [CrossRef]
27. Bourque, L.B.; Regan, R.; Kelly, M.M.; Wood, M.M.; Kano, M.; Mileti, D.S. An Examination of the Effect of Perceived Risk on Preparedness Behavior. *Environ. Behav.* **2012**, *45*, 615–649. [CrossRef]
28. Kim, Y.C.; Kang, J. Communication, neighbourhood belonging and household hurricane preparedness. *Disasters* **2010**, *34*, 470–488. [CrossRef]
29. Spittal, M.J.; McClure, J.; Siegert, R.J.; Walkey, F.H. Predictors of two types of earthquake preparation: Survival activities and mitigation activities. *Environ. Behav.* **2008**, *40*, 798–817. [CrossRef]
30. Basolo, V.; Steinberg, L.J.; Burby, R.J.; Levine, J.; Cruz, A.M.; Huang, C. The effects of confidence in government and information on perceived and actual preparedness for disasters. *Environ. Behav.* **2009**, *41*, 338–364. [CrossRef]
31. Tekeli-Yeşil, S.; Dedeoğlu, N.; Braun-Fahrlaender, C.; Tanner, M. Factors motivating individuals to take precautionary action for an expected earthquake in Istanbul. *Risk Anal.* **2010**, *30*, 1181–1195. [CrossRef]
32. Mishra, S.; Suar, D. Do lessons people learn determine disaster cognition and preparedness? *Psychol. Dev. Soc.* **2007**, *2*, 143–159. [CrossRef]
33. Eysenbach, G. Improving the Quality of Web Surveys: The Checklist for Reporting Results of Internet E-Surveys (CHERRIES). *J. Med. Internet Res.* **2004**, *6*, e34. [CrossRef]
34. Rogers, R.W. A protection motivation theory of fear appeals and attitude change. *J. Psychol.* **1975**, *91*, 93–114. [CrossRef]
35. Rogers, R.W. Cognitive and physiological processes in fear appeals and attitude change: A Revised theory of protection motivation. In *Social Psychophysiology*; Cacioppo, J., Petty, R., Eds.; Guilford Press: New York, NY, USA, 1983.
36. Grothmann, T.; Reusswig, F. People at risk of flooding: Why some residents take precautionary action while others do not. *Nat. Hazards* **2006**, *38*, 101–120. [CrossRef]
37. Westcott, R.; Ronan, K.; Bambrick, H.; Taylor, M. Expanding protection motivation theory: Investigating an application to animal owners and emergency responders in bushfire emergencies. *BMC Psychol.* **2017**, *5*, 13. [CrossRef] [PubMed]
38. European Commission. Communication From the Commission to the European Parliament, the Council, the European Economic and Social Committee and the Committee of the Regions. Action Plan to Support the Protection of Public Spaces. Brussels, 18 October 2017. COM (2017) 612 Final. 2017. Available online: https://eur-lex.europa.eu/legal-content/EN/TXT/PDF/?uri=CELEX:52017DC0612&from=EN (accessed on 10 June 2021).
39. Karlos, V.; Larcher, M. *Guideline: A Guide to Key Information on the Protection of Public Spaces*; EUR 30744 EN; Publications Office of the European Union: Luxembourg, 2021.
40. START (National Consortium for the Study of Terrorism and Responses to Terrorism). Global Terrorism Database 1970–2020. 2022. Available online: https://www.start.umd.edu/gtd (accessed on 6 August 2021).
41. Eurostat Database. Population Demographic Info 2021. *European Commission*. 2021. Available online: https://ec.europa.eu/eurostat/data/database (accessed on 22 March 2022).
42. Asian Disasters Reduction Centre (ADRC). Living with Risk—A Global Review of Living with Risk–A Global Review of Disaster Reduction. Chapter 2. Risk Awareness and Assessment. 2022. Available online: https://www.adrc.asia/publications/LWR/LWR_abridged/contents.php (accessed on 3 February 2021).
43. Slovic, P. Perception of risk: Reflections on the psychometric paradigm. In *Social Theories of Risk*; Krimsky, S., Golding, D., Eds.; Praeger: Weastpost, CT, USA, 1990; pp. 117–152. Available online: https://scholarsbank.uoregon.edu/xmlui/bitstream/handle/1794/22510/slovic_289.pdf?sequence=1 (accessed on 26 March 2020).
44. Cohen-Louck, K.; Levy, I. Risk perception of a chronic threat of terrorism: Differences based on coping types, gender and exposure. *Int. J. Psychol.* **2018**, *55*, 115–122. [CrossRef] [PubMed]
45. Paton, D. Disaster preparedness: A social-cognitive perspective. *Disaster Prev. Manag.* **2003**, *12*, 210–216. [CrossRef]
46. Croson, R.; Gneezy, U. Gender differences in preferences. *J. Econ. Lit.* **2009**, *47*, 448–474. [CrossRef]

47. Rand, D.G. Social dilemma cooperation (unlike dictator game giving) is intuitive for men as well as women. *J. Exp. Soc. Psychol.* **2017**, *73*, 164–168. [CrossRef] [PubMed]
48. Rand, D.G.; Brescoll, V.L.; Everett, J.A.; Capraro, V.; Barcelo, H. Social heuristics and social roles: Intuition favors altruism for women but not for men. *J. Exp. Psychol. Gen.* **2016**, *145*, 389–396. [CrossRef] [PubMed]
49. Soutschek, A.; Burke, C.J.; Raja Beharelle, A.; Schreiber, R.; Weber, S.C.; Karipidis, I.I.; Ten Velden, J.; Weber, B.; Haker, H.; Kalenscher, T.; et al. The dopaminergic reward system underpins gender differences in social preferences. *Nat. Hum. Behav.* **2017**, *1*, 819–827. [CrossRef] [PubMed]
50. Helweg-Larsen, M.; Shepperd, J.A. Do moderators of the optimistic bias affect personal or target risk estimates? A review of the literature. *Personal. Soc. Psychol. Rev.* **2001**, *5*, 74–95. [CrossRef]
51. Kunreuther, H. Disaster Mitigation and Insurance: Learning from Katrina. *Ann. Am. Acad. Political Soc. Sci.* **2006**, *604*, 208–227. [CrossRef]
52. Foa, E.B.; Kozak, M.J. Emotional processing of fear. Exposure to corrective information. *Psychol. Bull.* **1986**, *99*, 20–35. [CrossRef] [PubMed]
53. Panayiotou, G.; Karekla, M.; Leonidou, C. Coping through avoidance may explain gender disparities in anxiety. *J. Contextual Behav. Sci.* **2017**, *6*, 215–220. [CrossRef]
54. Taylor, S.; Landry, C.A.; Paluszek, M.M.; Rachor, G.S.; Asmundson, G.J. Worry, avoidance, and coping during the COVID-19 pandemic: A comprehensive network analysis. *J. Anxiety Disord.* **2020**, *76*, 102327. [CrossRef]
55. Kim, H.K.; Ahn, J.; Atkinson, L.; Kahlor, L.A. Effects of COVID-19 Misinformation on Information Seeking, Avoidance, and Processing: A Multicountry Comparative Study. *Sci. Commun.* **2020**, *42*, 586–615. [CrossRef]
56. Tannenbaum, C.; Ellis, R.P.; Eyssel, F.; Zou, J.; Schiebinger, L. Sex and gender analysis improves science and engineering. *Nature* **2019**, *575*, 137–146. [CrossRef] [PubMed]
57. Ariyabandu, M. Sex, gender and gender relations in disasters. In *Women, Gender and Disaster: Global Issues and Initiatives*; Enarson, E., Chakrabarti, P.D., Eds.; SAGE Publications India Pvt Ltd.: Delhi, India, 2009; pp. 5–17.
58. Davidson, D.J.; Freudenburg, W.R. Gender and Environmental Concerns: A Review and Analysis of Available Research. *Environ. Behav.* **1996**, *28*, 302–339. [CrossRef]
59. Danielsson, E.; Eriksson, K. Women's invisible work in disaster contexts: Gender norms in speech on women's work after a forest fire in Sweden. *Disasters* **2020**, *46*, 141–161. [CrossRef] [PubMed]
60. Gustafson, P.E. Gender differences in risk perception: Theoretical and methodological perspectives. *Risk Anal.* **1998**, *18*, 805–811. [CrossRef]
61. Galvankova, B.; Freizer, S.; Sadasivam, B.; Kim, S.; Bozrikova, T. *Gender and Disaster Risk Reduction in Europe and Central Asia*; Workshop Guide for Facilitators. United Nations Entity for Gender Equality and the Empowerment of Women (UN Women); United Nations Development Programme (UNDP): New York, NY, USA, 2018.

International Journal of
Environmental Research and Public Health

MDPI

Article

The Need for a Preparedness Training Model on Disaster Risk Reduction Based on Culturally Sensitive Public Health Nursing (PHN)

Haris Sofyana [1,*], Kusman Ibrahim [2,*], Irvan Afriandi [1], Erna Herawati [3] and Heru Santoso Wahito Nugroho [4]

1 Doctoral Program, Faculty of Medicine, Padjadjaran University, Bandung 45363, Indonesia
2 Department of Medical and Surgical Nursing, Faculty of Nursing, Padjadjaran University, Bandung 45363, Indonesia
3 Department of Anthropology, Faculty of Social and Political Sciences, Padjadjaran University, Bandung 45363, Indonesia
4 Department of Health, Poltekkes Kemenkes Surabaya, Surabaya 60282, Indonesia
* Correspondence: haris20003@mail.unpad.ac.id (H.S.); k.ibrahim@unpad.ac.id (K.I.)

Abstract: The Indonesian Disaster Risk Index (IRBI) in 2018 found that 52.33% of districts or cities in Indonesia were at high risk of natural disasters and the others were at moderate risk. The World Risk Index places Indonesia at number 33 in the very high-risk category. The policy direction of the Implementation of Disaster Management in Indonesia in 2020–2024 is to increase disaster resilience toward sustainable prosperity for sustainable development. Purpose: This study aims to identify the various needs for a culturally sensitive PHN-based disaster risk-reduction preparedness training model. Methods: This study used a descriptive qualitative research design. Data collection was done through in-depth interviews, Focus Group Discussions (FGDs), and expert panel stages in the Indonesian language. Samples involved in the research included 4 experts and 11 informants. Results: There were 10 themes generated from the results. The analysis results revealed that the level of knowledge, attitudes, and skills of the community is still low. Almost all of the people of Mekar Mukti Village stated that they had never received community-based disaster management training. Conclusions: The study findings highlighted the importance of the Disaster Risk-Reduction Preparedness Model Based on Culturally Sensitive Public Health Nursing for the community.

Keywords: preparedness training; disaster risk reduction; public health nursing; culturally sensitive

Citation: Sofyana, H.; Ibrahim, K.; Afriandi, I.; Herawati, E.; Wahito Nugroho, H.S. The Need for a Preparedness Training Model on Disaster Risk Reduction Based on Culturally Sensitive Public Health Nursing (PHN). *IJERPH* **2022**, *19*, 16467. https://doi.org/10.3390/ijerph192416467

Academic Editors: Amir Khorram-Manesh and Krzysztof Goniewicz

Received: 23 September 2022
Accepted: 10 November 2022
Published: 8 December 2022

1. Introduction

Indonesia is an archipelago prone to disasters. It is located in the path of major earthquake sources such as the megathrust–plate subduction zone and active faults on the mainland. Based on the BNBP report, 295 faults have been identified to be active fault segments that have the potential to produce earthquakes above 6.5 magnitude [1]. Thus, Indonesia's natural disaster risk is high. The Indonesian Disaster Risk Index (IRBI) in 2018 found that 52.33% of districts or cities in Indonesia were at high risk of natural disasters while the others were at moderate risk. These conditions place Indonesia as one of the countries with the highest rates of natural disasters in the world. Indonesia's Natural Disaster Risk Index (IRB) statistical data in 2021 for tsunamis, floods, landslides, droughts, and forest fires are also relatively high compared to other countries [2].

In 2021, there were 5400 natural disasters in Indonesia, which was an increase from 2500 natural disasters in 2018. This illustrates the very high rate of natural disasters in Indonesia. Floods (1310 incidents), tornadoes (814 incidents), and landslides (633 incidents) are the dominating natural disasters. Natural disasters in 2021 caused more than 8.6 million people to suffer and be displaced, along with the deaths of 676 people. Furthermore, more than 142,000 houses and 3700 education, health, office, road, and bridge facilities were impacted by the natural disasters [3].

In addition to natural disasters, Indonesia is also still trying to control the spread of COVID-19 that caused the loss of 100,000 people and has been labeled as a National Non-Natural Disaster [4]. National data on COVID-19 cases, as of 17 March 2022, recorded 153,411 deaths with new confirmed cases of 9528 people, increasing to 5,958,610 people. The COVID-19 pandemic in Indonesia has had an impact on almost all development sectors. One of these development sectors is the Reform (Strengthening) of the Disaster Resilience System, developed to be able to overcome non-natural disasters on a national scale without reducing resilience to handle natural disasters occurring at the same time as non-natural disasters [3]. Data from the Centre For Research On The Epidemiology Of Disasters (CRED) for 2008–2018, revealed that every year Indonesia occupies the top 10 in the world as the country most frequently affected by natural disasters and the country with the highest number of deaths from natural disasters [5]

West Java is one of the areas in Indonesia with a high frequency of natural disasters. 4465 of 5957 villages were included in the category of high-level disaster-prone villages [6]. Additionally, there are numerous active volcanoes in West Java, including Mount Salak, Mount Gede, Mount Tangkuban Parahu, Mount Papandayan, Mount Guntur, Mount Galunggung, and Mount Ciremai. The complex geographical conditions of the West Java region paired with the largest population in Indonesia make this province's natural disaster risk high. Based on the 2020 Indonesian Disaster Risk Index (IRBI), West Java Province has a risk index of 145.81 (high) [4].

This further pushes the direction of the policy for the Implementation of Disaster Management in Indonesia for 2020–2024, which aims to improve disaster resilience toward sustainable prosperity for sustainable development [7].

Strengthening the paradigm shift in disaster management from conventional emergency response to disaster risk reduction is one strategy to accomplish this. According to the Disaster Risk Reduction Paradigm (DRR), the community is an active participant in disaster management, thus it must have the necessary knowledge, attitudes, and abilities [8]. This means that in order to effectively manage disasters, the paradigm of disaster risk reduction also calls for community empowerment, which may be accomplished through a variety of community socialization, education, and training programs.

The study by Setiawan et al. (2017) recommend the importance of training to empower rural communities living in disaster-prone areas to normalize the physical and psychological problems of natural disaster victims [9]. This is in line with the study conducted by Salasa et al. (2017) that identified community preparedness as an important key to minimizing health problems resulting from natural disasters. These results also show that the empowerment process through a contingency planning approach is able to increase youth preparedness against life threatening situations due to disasters. It is advised for all disaster activists to empower youth with contingency planning to increase their readiness to face life threatening situations [10]. In addition, it is necessary to adjust communication strategies to the sociocultural aspects of the local community to effectively emphasize the importance of community empowerment as it would be more easily accepted and relevant to the needs of the people. Culture has become one of the factors for a community's ability to survive during disasters [11].

Other studies have linked this cultural aspect approach with approaches to nursing care for communities affected by disasters. The concept of nursing actions based on cultural considerations provides strong evidence that in a disaster, community nurses must take advantage of cultural forms such as bonds and relationships by providing information and supplements, respecting culture such as local rules and characters as well as healing and comforting the affected residents [12]. In line with this, nurses need to consider the socio-cultural scope of the community and long-term care in order to respond effectively to disasters. This can start from planning, noting positive and negative consequences of assistance, and individual planning in the community [13]. This is in accordance with Senday's disaster risk reduction framework, which is establishing a national platform for disaster risk reduction. This becomes a general term used as a national policy for coordination and as a policy guide on multisectoral and interdisciplinary disaster risk reduction that involves all relevant entities in a country, whether public or private. Disaster risk reduction requires knowledge, capacity and input from various sectors and organizations, including UN agencies present at the national level. National platforms provide the means to enhance national action to reduce disaster risk, and they represent national mechanisms for the International Disaster Reduction Strategy [14]. Facilitating the community's ability to anticipate, prepare for and recover from disasters is an important component of the UNISDR strategy for disaster risk reduction [15].

One of the theories in nursing that is closely related to community empowerment and cultural care is the theory of the Transcultural Nursing model, published by Madeleine Leininger in 1978. The theory requires an awareness and appreciation of cultural differences that influence providing nursing care with approaches to respecting individual cultural values [16]. Therefore, nurses are required to have knowledge of and engage in a practice that is based conceptually on culture [17]. Transcultural nursing is an area of community and cultural science in the field of nursing that focuses on the differences and similarities between cultures by respecting care, health and illness based on cultural values, beliefs and actions. Thus, several aspects of culture can be studied in an effort to provide nursing care [18]. Based on the background, the research problem is how to create a culturally sensitive disaster risk-reduction model in disaster-prone areas. Therefore, this study aimed to identify the various needs for a culturally sensitive Public Health Nursing (PHN)-based disaster risk-reduction preparedness training model. This study is imperative to explore the need for community preparedness in disaster management based on local culture.

2. Materials and Methods

2.1. Study Design

This study used descriptive qualitative research design to identify the various needs for a culturally sensitive Public Health Nursing (PHN)-based disaster risk-reduction preparedness training model.

The initial quantitative survey had already been conducted in order to identify the model's demands for training and testing, and to evaluate the model's effectiveness using a small sample, track its development, and alter the procedure in response to input that would be seen throughout model training. Sixty respondents from the Pasir Jambu subdistrict, Bandung district, and Sugih Mukti village community participated in this survey, with 22 women (38.3%) and 37 males (61.7%) being the majority. The composition of the initial respondents consisted of the following elements: government/village officials, community leaders, health cadres, and youth organizations. According to the survey results, earthquakes (80%), landslides (11.7%), and high winds (8.3%) are the top three disaster hazards that the residents of Sugih Mukti Village feel most at risk from. The examination of knowledge and attitudes about disasters and disaster management produced very unsatisfactory results, with the average knowledge score being 58.75 (SD 12.54) and the average attitude score being 59.31 (SD 10.57). None of the responders could show that they had the necessary abilities or fundamental rescue techniques for catastrophe victims, which were self-performed by the community.

2.2. Settings and Participants

The study setting was Marga Mukti Village, Pasir Jambu District, Bandung Regency, West Java, Indonesia. The study was conducted from April to August 2022. The participants were divided into key informants and general informants, with the following inclusion criteria: academics, experts chosen by researchers as conceptual reference materials, indigenous people of the local community who serve as community leaders and have experienced disasters, and traditional stakeholders who are used as reference figures and experts. A total of 4 experts and 11 informants from the defense forces, government officials, community leaders, BNPB, business owners, and professional nurses were selected through a purposive sampling technique.

2.3. Data Collection

Data collection was done through in-depth interviews, Focus Group Discussions (FGDs), and expert panel stages in the Indonesian language. In-depth interviews were conducted for 30–60 min, and FGDs were conducted for 60–90 min. Each respondent's responses were calcified until data saturation was reached. The protocol for preventing the spread of COVID-19 is carried out by the standards established by the Indonesian government, including the use of masks and face shields, establishing a minimum distance of one meter between participants, washing hands with disinfectant before entering and leaving the room, and measuring body temperatures before participants enter the room. The expert panel stages were held virtually by using Zoom for 60 min.

Field notes are made by writing down everything significant that happened while conducting the research, including taking photos of significant areas. The study team conducted the interviews with the aid of two administrative officers who supported the interview procedure. Data saturation was accomplished after the researcher identified repeated answers from research informants with meanings (themes) that lead to the same topic.

2.4. Data Analysis

Data analysis is carried out in four stages of analysis, as described by Leininger (2002). The first stage is collecting, describing, and documenting raw data. At this stage, researchers collect data, followed by explaining and documenting the raw data obtained from interviews, FGDs, surveys, and documentation studies. The second stage is the identification and categorization of descriptors and components, specifically, selecting and classifying descriptors and data elements that are the primary study topic. At this point, the emphasis is on identifying the contributing elements and impediments that hinder the creation of a community-based disaster risk-reduction model with a culturally sensitive strategy to enhance community preparedness. The third stage is the pattern and contextual analysis, which identifies patterns of interactions, values, beliefs, and practices when they are related to informants and data gathered through field observations. Identifying the key themes, research findings, and patterns of community engagement in disaster risk-reduction strategies in the community are covered in the fourth stage, which is titled "major themes, research findings, theoretical formulations, and recommendations". The steps of interpretation and synthesis of results form the foundation at this level.

2.5. Ethical Considerations

Ethical approval for this study was granted by the Health Research Ethics Committee of the Ministry of Health, Republic of Indonesia, Bandung Polytechnic of Health (ref. No. 01/KEKP/EC/II/2022). Permission to conduct the study was also obtained from the community leader of Marga Mukti Village, Pasir Jambu District, Bandung Regency, West Java, Indonesia. The voluntary and confidential nature of the study was explained to participants before each interview, Focus Group Discussions (FGDs), and expert panel stages process. To enhance confidentiality, pseudonyms were used in the study.

2.6. Trustworthiness

Trustworthiness was completed by identifying research findings evaluated through a process including credibility, confirmability, meaning in context, recurrent patterning, saturation, and transferability. Credibility was established by participating in the daily lives of informants, ongoing observation, triangulation, peer debriefing, and community support groups, community leaders, and social organizations that promote DRR. Confirmability was clarified by stating ideas or findings that were heard, seen, or experienced with key informants and several general informants. In order to interpret and grasp the significance of meaning in context, researchers incorporated the information from interviews, observations, and documents. All key informants and some general informants then corroborated regarding the interpretation. All information was based on contextual reality and the environment. Recurrent patterning was carried out with researchers who used informants' repeated experiences, expressions, events, or activities in relation to community-based disaster risk reduction. Transferability and saturation were met when the data collected reveal duplication of content related to ideas, meanings, experiences, descriptions, and other similar expressions from the informants or repeated observations. Further research findings were reported in a rich language style, including quotes, comments, and stories that added to the richness of the report and provided for understanding the context of the experience in which it all took place. Researchers attempted to facilitate transferability by providing detailed documentation across all phases of research.

3. Results

3.1. Document Analysis

Based on the document analysis, Sugihmukti Village is located in Pasir Jambu District, Bandung Regency, West Java Province. This village located in a mountainous highland, with an area of 1767.96 km^2, at 107.407795 east longitude and −7.19077 south latitude. The distance from the village to the subdistrict capital is as far as 7000 km. Sugih Mukti Village is a disaster-prone village due to its unstable soil structure and is located in an area adjacent to an active volcano and geothermal mining activities in the Patuha Mountains. Previous research was conducted on community representatives involving 60 respondents from two disaster-prone areas in the village of Sugih Mukti. The results reveal that the priority disaster risks that are most experienced by the people of Sugih Mukti Village are earthquakes (80%), landslides (11.7%), and strong winds (8.3%), while the others are fire disasters and conflicts between communities. The results of measuring the level of knowledge, attitude and skill of the community about disaster, are obtained: knowledge, 58.75% (SD 12.54); attitude, 59.31% (SD 10.57); and skills in providing basic health assistance, 0%, indicating the inability to take action. Based on these results, this research was developed.

3.2. Expert Discussions and National Seminar

The initial stage of the research began with expert discussions and national seminars with four key informants from BNPB, PPKK-Kemenkes, PPNI, and academics of disaster nursing experts. The results of expert discussions and seminars were identified as central themes in the development of a culturally sensitive Public Health Nursing (PHN)-based disaster risk-reduction preparedness training model. The resulting research themes are as follows.

1. The implementation of the global target achievement of the Sendai Framework in Indonesia is carried out using the Disaster Risk Reduction (DRR) paradigm for the Disaster Resilient Village program.
2. DRR is operated in the form of community empowerment.
3. The steps for community empowerment in disaster management are identical to the community nursing process: assessment, diagnosis, planning, implementation, and evaluation.
4. The PPNI Professional Organization believes that there is a need for community empowerment through guiding community nurses with structured disaster management training.
5. Community-integrated training in disaster preparedness is needed as a DRR effort.

3.3. Focus Group Discussions (FGDs)

The next stage was FGDs and in-depth interviews with 11 informants from the defense forces, government officials, community leaders, BNPB, business owners, and professional nurses. The results of FGDs and in-depth interview are us follow (Table 1):

Table 1. Qualitative data of the FGD results.

Data	Subthemes	Theme
" . . . The people of Sugih Mukti Village often experience disasters. Especially landslides and tropical cyclones" (Respondents: 1, 2, 4, 5, 10) "Well, we're used to it, sir. Happens very often. Especially if you've heard the roar from the Geo Dipa Gas Production" (Respondents: 4, 5, 6) "The location is indeed close to the drilling center, not the production process itself but very close to Patuha Mountain, which makes small earthquakes and has volcanic activity" (Respondents: 1, 2, 3, 10) " . . . South Bandung Regency is prone to disasters because of geological and geographical factors . . . " (Respondents: 1, 2, 6, 10) "often sir, even though I'm new, we're already used to the vibrations, not because of Geodipa, . . . Geodipa wants to help" (Respondents: 6, 7, 11) "We know the risks, but we just do not care, the government has thought of us, if we move where will we go?" (Respondents: 5, 11) "Once, sir, there was a hurricane, there were people whose houses were partially damaged, but most often there were landslides" (Respondents: 5, 11) "The hardest thing, sir, was a flash flood, sir, there were many victims, there were 13. Wow, at that time it was like the end of the world, I was not yet a village official, but I was bewildered, sir, the people were suffering" (Respondents: 4, 11)	1. Disasters that often happen: constant landslides; 2. A big flash flood in 2013; 3. Whirlwinds and volcanic earthquakes all the time; 4. The location is close to the Patuha volcano and Geodipa Ltd., a natural gas production center.	Geographically, the Sugih Mukti area is prone to natural disasters
"I don't know what to do if there is a landslide or flood, maybe because my house is far away, but other people also don't know yet. Those who know if an earthquake is happening run away" (Resp: 4, 5, 11) "As government officials, we are always ready for orders, instructions from commanders, there are 'babinsa' (army officers) and village police who monitor general security, but if we are needed, we often go down " (Resp: 1, 2, 3, 4, 6, 10) "The residents are only focused on finding a way to get food, sir, they don't understand how to fight a disaster, if there's a flood we flee, if there we hear rumbling noises we just let it go, the most important thing is to pray" (Resp: 4, 5, 11) "The government has tried to explain to villages, maybe not sugih mukti village, but other parties have done it, we will help and support" (Respondents: 4, 6, 10) "There are difficulties, sir, in educating the public like money, methods and government support, as well as those who have money . . . well the company. In order for them to want to help, they must be given consumption, food, transportation, etc." (Respondents: 4, 5, 6, 9, 10) "As I see it, it's not optimal yet. We are only limited to the health sector through cadres. As for disasters, we haven't been able to do it" (Resp: 7, 8, 10) "it's very important, sir, we are even ready to learn, to help, after all I guide this area"(Resp: 1, 2, 7, 8) "It's time to do more. For example, COVID, sir. For the residents, it's normal. If you get a fever, well you just compress your forehead with cloth, you lose your sense of smell, ah, just take village medicine, we give them bandrek, or a potion, no one wears a mask, so there's no need, the most important thing is if you are able to eat" (Respondents: 6, 11) "The government officials are the ones who are the most responsible, the people are the citizens, we just follow the government's advice" (Respondents: 5, 11) "We will support, we know that the community must be involved, that's why I like coordinating with villages, MSMEs, clinics, and treatments at the public health center, we will help" (Respondents: 7, 8)	1. People do not think there is a problem in terms of disaster; 2. Sectoral support has not been managed properly; 3. The government's efforts have been carried out but have not been effective; 4. Lack of coordination in disaster management involving the community and industry; 5. The readiness of the industry to assist and support disaster prevention and management through CSR.	PRB efforts have not been optimal

Table 1. *Cont.*

Data	Subthemes	Theme
"As health workers in the community, we certainly need things like this, to train the community with disaster management, in particular" (Respondents: 7, 10) "In the community, it is very necessary. In our hospital there is a Hospital Disaster Plan (HDP) for nurses and all health workers, so they can contribute. We don't know the HDP training method or model at the hospital yet" (Respondents: 10) "Don't know how, need to be told how to do it or be trained, sir. So that people know. The village is ready to support . . . " (Respondents: 4, 5, 6, 11) "Someone has to start sir. We are ready to help. We don't know the models and methods of training our society. Especially in the health sector. There should be guidelines so that people can be educated " (Respondents: 7, 8, 6, 11) "In the army, there is training for soldiers, sir. If we train people, we don't know the method yet. If using the military route is not suitable, we are ready to help and cooperate with the public health center and other health care providers" (Respondents: 1, 2, 6) "If BPBD often conducts community training, it is only selective, not for all groups, just certain villages. It's about the budget too. Those who have been trained are in Cicalengka and Majalya. South Bandung has not been done. Every year there are only enough for 2 villages. The name of the program is Destana" (Respondents: 3, 7) "As far as the health sector is concerned, there is no such thing, I haven't heard of it" (Respondents: 3, 7, 8, 9, 10) "Nurses are not optimal, sir, because they have a lot of activities. Those who participate in the training are also limited, there are none in the community health centers yet, we have not participated in the community development training in the field of disaster, we still have to continue with other programs" (Respondents: 9, 10) "Community Nurses are too busy with administrative work, sir, this disaster problem has not been addressed, there must be training first, so that we know how far we can train the community" (Respondents: 9, 10)	1. Health workers have not received information related to disaster care in the community; 2. There is no model that can be used as a guide in educating the public; 3. Cross-sectoral coordination is not yet optimal—(TNI/Polri/Government) do not know the guidelines for community development in the field of disaster management planning; 4. The community needs guidance for disaster management from a health worker.	There needs to be a model of community development in disaster management
"The government's efforts have not gone well, for example the need for heavy equipment for landslides, it is difficult and takes time if needed" (Respondents: 1, 2, 3, 11) "The government has been good. The Health Office has coordinated to meet the needs, it just needs more organization. For example, referrals to hospitals have not been optimal, difficulty in costs, treatment requirements. Because of this, there are victims who are rejected" (Respondents: 9, 10, 7) "People usually struggle when there is a disaster. Help is lacking and late and we are the ones who are blamed, sir. Especially if there are health problems that we don't know what to do" (Respondents: 4, 5, 11) "I'm not sure about the government, but us as community partners are responsible. We will help if there is an institution that will develop the community, like now. we are ready to cooperate if needed" (Respondents: 7, 8, 11) "The government has tried, there are many programs for disasters. For example, for COVID 19. This is a disaster too; it just can't be solved as fast as turning the palm of the hand. Moreover, the community has different characters, now the government has tried very hard, the sub-district always coordinates with BPBD to map if there are locations that are threatened with landslides" (Respondents: 3, 6) "For the wider community, it has not been felt, sir, the government likes to be unfair, in other places it is fast, while in our place it takes a long time. I don't know why, the fast ones are the army, sir. Maybe it's because there are noncommissioned law enforcement officers, huh . . . And the police take action if there is a report" (Respondents: 4, 5, 11) "At BPBD, we try to maximize our efforts, sir, but it's only limited to human resources. For example, if there is a health problem, we coordinate with the service, we cannot handle it directly. BPBD can only coordinate. That's right, sir, we can't do it all, especially human resources. We don't have all professions, so we really need cooperation" (Respondents: 3)	1. Need cooperation and coordination; 2. Health coordination model should be developed; 3. People have not fully felt the presence of the government; 4. The program exists, but it is not yet operational.	Government efforts have not been effective

Table 1. *Cont.*

Data	Subthemes	Theme
"I have never participated in any training, and indeed there has never been any in the village for our community, especially those related to the health sector" (Respondents: 4, 5, 6, 7, 10, 11) "If we have not participated in disaster management training, and in the Army, the training is the same as military training. If you want to go to the area there has to be a special course on how to approach the community. Just not specialized in disaster management training" (Respondents: 1, 2) "As a BPBD extension worker, I have often participated in training, but I have never attended training in the community that was held by health workers. The most frequent, yes.. training with 'PT" (a company), but the materials are usually trauma healing, soup kitchens, rarely about health . . . " (Respondents: 3) "To my knowledge in our area there has never been any special disaster management training for community members, including by BPBD. I feel like it's never been done. So if the Polytechnic of Health wants to hold it, we will support and help" (Respondents: 7, 8, 6) "I was once invited by the Geodipa representative for disaster counseling in Ring 1, our area, only so far it has not been held, but I heard that Geodipa held it themselves without coordination with us. That we don't know for sure" (Respondents: 4) "If it is true that there will be training in our area, we have been waiting for this, actually this is included in our program too, especially in villages that are in direct contact with the mountain and gas production center, indeed there has been compensation, but there has never been training and counseling about disasters" (Respondents: 5, 6) "In our area, there is no cadre training for nurses, let alone for the community. So we have never guided the community for disaster management, in the future, if God wills it, we will program it" (Respondents: 7, 10) "I work at the hospital and the Disaster Hospital Plan training had been done, specifically with the emergency room team and the disaster team in each hospital, but for the surrounding community, we at the hospital have never held it" (Respondents: 9)	1. The community has not been involved in integrative disaster training; 2. BPBD, TNI, Polri, village, and subdistrict governments do not know the integrated disaster training model for the community.	No involvement yet in an integrated disaster training program in the health sector

Based on Table 1, five themes are generated which become the basis for developing a preparedness training model for Public Health Nursing. The five themes are:

1. The Sugih Mukti area is prone to disasters due to its geographical structure.
2. No one in the community or its officials have participated in integrated disaster training in the health sector based on community needs.
3. Government efforts have not been effective in community disaster management.
4. A community development model in integrated disaster management that involves all components of society is needed.
5. DRR efforts are not yet optimal

4. Discussion

4.1. Description of Model Requirements

Figure 1 describes the results found through investigating the need for a Public Health Nursing (PHN) disaster risk-reduction preparedness training model as a guide for community nurses. The model is an integrated implementation of community care and empowerment stages in disaster-prone areas. The thematic exploration results from all community members show that a disaster risk-reduction preparedness training model that is integrated with community empowerment is very much needed.

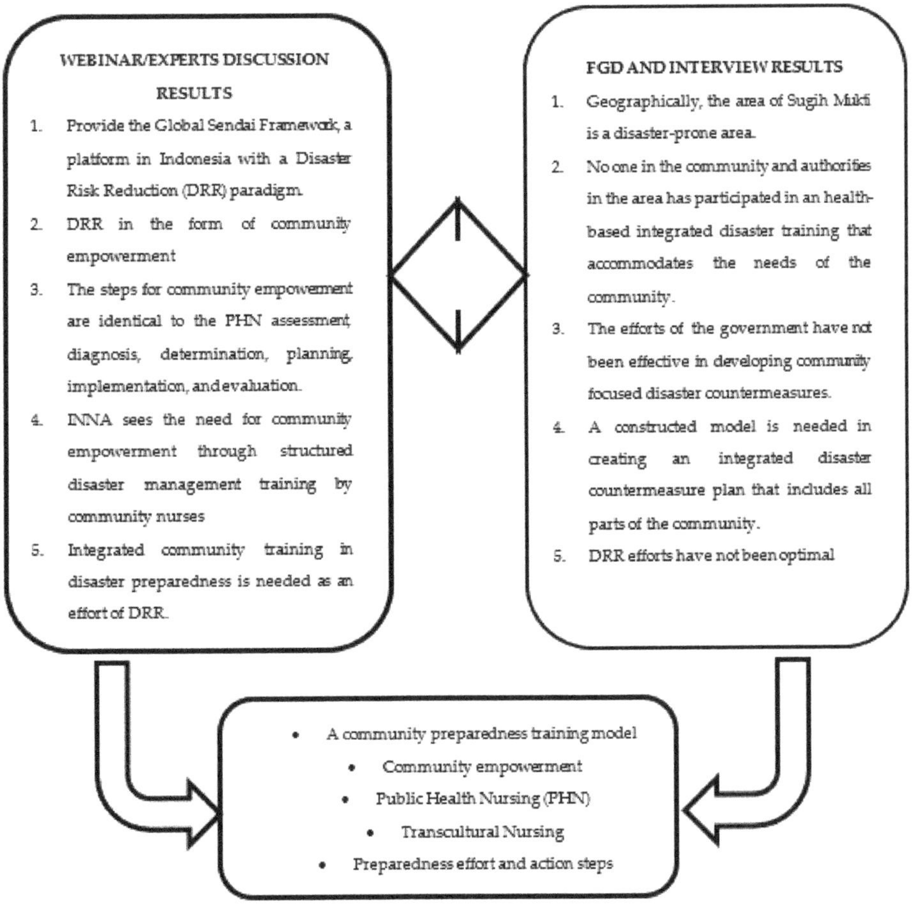

Figure 1. Thematic description of Disaster Risk Reduction (DRR) needs in community nursing.

This need is in line with BNPB's values, which are preparedness and level of community independence as the most important aspects for disaster management, followed by the help of family members, friends, SAR team, health team, and surrounding components [19]. To strengthen this opinion, the community becomes the focus of studies in disaster risk reduction, which starts from groups of school children and adolescents, health cadres, and community leaders as targets for empowerment in disaster risk reduction. Community empowerment in disaster risk reduction requires a community-centered, interprofessional socialization approach that is systematic, culturally informed, and focuses on modeling the role of trainers, caring for officers as well as attention to the needs of participants [20].

Involving the community in disaster risk-reduction studies will increase the awareness of the community. Research on public health recommended the need for a stronger emphasis on public health in managing disasters. For example, the Reserve Corps provides civil medical training to improve public health infrastructure and provides greater opportunities to collaborate with communities in disaster management [21] Lebowitz (2015). In order to make these various components effective, a model is needed that can accommodate the increasing capacity of the community. According to Paton (2019), facilitating the community's ability to anticipate, prepare, and recover from disasters is an important component of the UNISDR strategy [15]. Pourvakhshoori et al.'s (2017) research provides clarity that nurses are part of the health profession which has a very important role [22].

Understanding the experience of nurses in disasters can help identify problems in the disaster nursing services field, which can be resolved by better planning and preparation [22]. One of the major problems in the disaster management system is the lack of planning to employ and organize volunteers in the health sector during a disaster [23]. The nursing process approach, using the concept of the Transcultural Nursing model, is used as an effort to accelerate the Public Health Nursing (PHN) program, which is in accordance with the government program.

The integrated implementation program of Public Health Nursing in Disaster Risk Reduction (DRR) and the transcultural nursing approach is very relevant to community groups that are socioculturally heterogeneous. In the context of providing holistic service, services with a culturally sensitive approach are needed; nurses must adapt to the system, norms, and culture that apply in a community.

This is in line with the anthropological view, which believes that cultural factors influence human behavior. When faced with danger, people not only consider the dangers they can face, but also prioritize factors such as social values, religious beliefs, traditions, and attachments to a particular place or location. Culture has the power to increase or decrease a society's vulnerability to disasters. Lack of consideration of the cultural aspects of the affected communities can hinder effective DRR strategies, thereby increasing the vulnerabilities of the affected communities rather than reducing them. Therefore, culture has the power to increase or reduce community vulnerability to disasters [11] Kulatunga (2010). Research by Kertamuda and Chris (2012) explains that the culture of resignation and patience in the three largest ethnic groups on the island of Java (Betawi, Sundanese, and Javanese) is still very dominant in responding to disasters [24].

4.2. *Constructed Model Requirements*

Figure 2 shows the structure of the model that was built based on the thematic analysis of the need for disaster risk-reduction preparedness training. The training model is constructed from the concept of community nursing theory (PHN) as well as the strengthening of the transcultural nursing model. The steps of community empowerment in disaster management are in line with the steps of the community nursing process, which are assessment, planning, intervention, implementation, and evaluation.

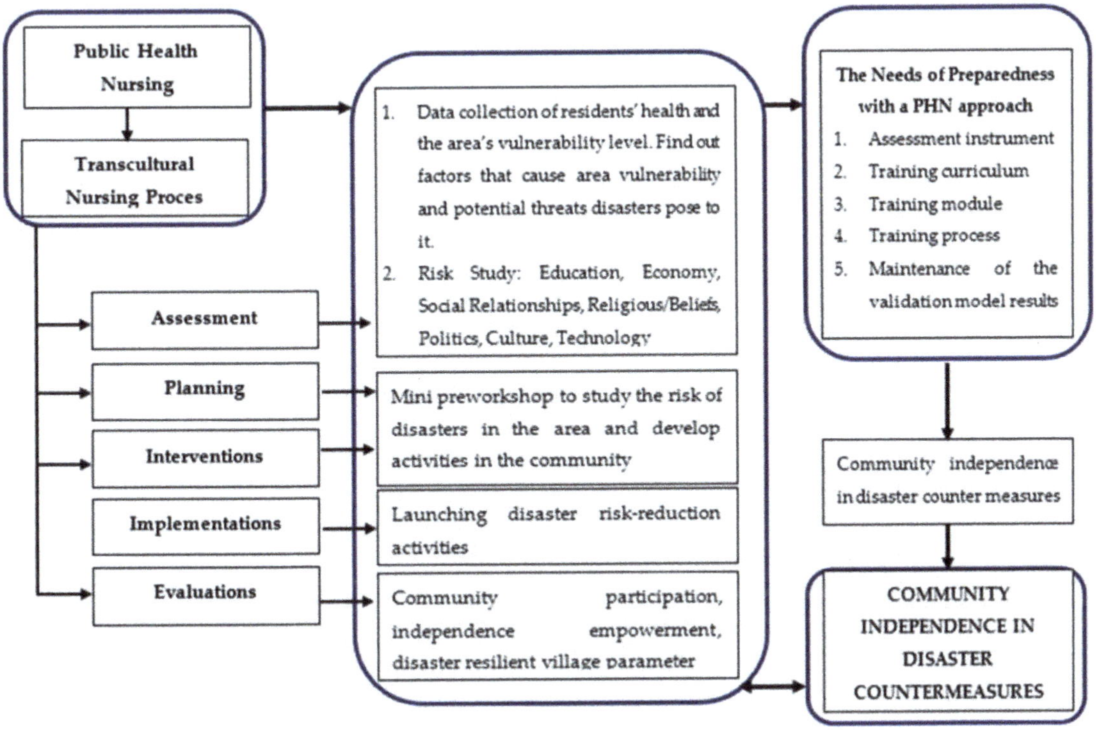

Figure 2. Constructed requirements for the Public Health Care-Based Disaster Preparedness Training integration model.

The three types of priority disasters that the people of Sugih Mukti frequently experience are earthquakes, landslides, and hurricanes. This result is similar to the Bandung Regency BPBD report, which identifies the types of priority disasters in Bandung Regency: floods, landslides, cyclones, droughts, and earthquakes. Sugih Mukti Village, Pasir Jambu District, Bandung Regency, is included in the list of areas prone to landslides and earthquakes [25]. This is due to the geographical location of Sugih Mukti Village. It is located within a geothermal exploration area, also known as the Geothermal Patuha Mountain in Bandung district. The activity of the Geodipa Energi project is a leading factor that increases Sugih Mukti Village's vulnerability to landslides and volcanic earthquakes [26]. Research conducted on the residents reveals that the level of knowledge, attitudes, and skills of the community are still low. Almost all of the people of Mekar Mukti Village stated that they had never received community-based disaster management training. These results are in line with research conducted by Setiawan et al. (2017), which emphasizes the importance of training to empower rural communities living in disaster-prone areas that will normalize the physical and psychological problems of natural disaster victims [9].

The role of the community nurse becomes very important in this situation. Research by Walsh et al. (2012) explains that effective disaster preparedness, response, and recovery requires a well-planned, concerted effort by experienced professionals who can apply specific knowledge and skills in critical situations. The results can provide a useful starting point to identify the level of competence expected of health professionals in disaster medicine and public health [27]. A study by Gulzar et al. (2012) provides results that support this. The intervention, collaboratively chosen by the CHN, was shaped by a planning framework that fits the nursing process. It is a method used to take a holistic approach in the earthquake-affected area. Such a framework includes four phases; assessment, planning, implementation, and evaluation. The framework provides systematic and specific directions for healthcare providers while promoting public health [28].

Communities in disaster-prone areas must have the ability, strength, and independence in managing disasters at every stage. Results from a study link cultural factors with Disaster Reduction Risk (DRR) activities and highlight how culture has influenced DRR activities. In some ways, culture has become one of the factors of community survival from disasters. Therefore, it can be said that culture has the power to increase or decrease people's vulnerability to disasters [11]. An expert opinion, Rush et al. (2019), explain that disasters can occur in any community at any time. Such an opinion becomes true in any disaster. Nurses have a central role in managing and preparing for medical care during these catastrophic episodes [29]. Study results from Salmani et al. (2019) show the importance of having working management. It is necessary to have complete legislation, NGOs, and sociocultural factors, preparedness, response, retention, relocation, termination, and follow-up in each nurse's role in disaster-prone areas [23].

However, not all nursing roles can be easily implemented in disaster situations. A study by Ahmadi et al. (2018) found that the elders of a community that went through a disaster faced various challenges in their everyday life, which means that more efforts were needed to help them reach the stage of recovery. Taking into account these conditions, the need for community empowerment during the disaster period must not be postponed. Training the community to be independent must be done constantly by taking into account local cultural conditions [30]. The results of research in China show several conditions that push the need for community empowerment in disaster locations, which follow [20]. The behavior of the trainers influences the participants through their interactions during the training process. A mental health training program is needed to identify the needs of disaster workers and victims. Building a systematic interprofessional education strategy is required. Systematic interprofessional education can assist in responding to complex local problems due to a collaborative approach because it bridges the gap between theory and practice, and solves local needs and international guidelines.

Training regulations are needed to maintain and monitor the quality of the content, standards, ethics, and codes of conduct at all levels. A community-centered interprofessional education approach is required. It focuses on modeling the role of trainers, caring for staff, attending to the needs of trainees, and building a systematic, culturally informed, and informed interprofessional education strategy.

The results of the study by Lebowitz (2015) supported this opinion, regarding the need for a stronger emphasis on public health workers in managing disasters. For example, civil medical training for reserve corps can be done to improve public health infrastructure and provide greater opportunities to collaborate with the community in handling disasters [21].

Raising awareness through disaster education and socialization is very necessary. By doing so, everyone can understand risks, be able to manage threats, and, in turn, contribute to encouraging community resilience from the threat of disaster. Additionally, social cohesion, collaboration, and mutual trust are the adhesive values of the society that have been nurtured, both individually and collectively by the community, to prepare for, respond to, and rise from adversity caused by disasters.

5. Limitation

This research is limited since the model has not been tested or used in this study, and its effectiveness has not been determined. During the following stage of the research, the model will be tested and used. Additionally, obtaining data relating to culturally sensitive features and local strengths has not been thoroughly investigated, and requires a more thorough investigation in future research.

6. Conclusions

The study findings highlight the importance to the community of the Disaster Risk-Reduction Preparedness Model Based on Culturally Sensitive Public Health Nursing.

The community is approached using a combination of the Public Health Nursing (PHN) and Transcultural Nursing principles. An integrated model for disaster preparedness training based on public healthcare as a solution to empower communities in managing disaster risk is validated, constructed, and designed. This model consists of five main components: nursing care assessment instruments and introductory surveys for disaster-prone communities; public health nursing-based disaster preparedness training integration curriculum; public health nursing-based disaster preparedness training module integration training process; public health nursing-based disaster preparedness training process; and maintenance of training results.

Author Contributions: Conceptualization, H.S., K.I., E.H. and I.A.; methodology, H.S., K.I., E.H. and I.A.; software, H.S. and H.S.W.N.; validation, H.S. and K.I.; formal analysis, H.S., E.H. and H.S.W.N.; investigation, H.S. and K.I.; resources, H.S., I.A. and H.S.W.N.; data curation, H.S. and E.H.; writing—original draft preparation, H.S., K.I., E.H., I.A. and H.S.W.N.; writing—review and editing, H.S., K.I., E.H., I.A. and H.S.W.N.; visualization, H.S., K.I. and I.A.; supervision, K.I., E.H. and I.A.; project administration, H.S. and H.S.W.N.; funding acquisition, H.S. All authors have read and agreed to the published version of the manuscript.

Funding: This research received no external funding.

Institutional Review Board Statement: Ethical clearance: this research paper has passed the ethical clearance test and received approval from the Institute for Ethics Studies, Polytechnic of Health Ministry of Health, Bandung (No. 01/KEPK/EC/II/2022).

Informed Consent Statement: Informed consent was obtained from all subjects involved in the study. Written informed consent has been obtained from the subject(s) to publish this paper.

Data Availability Statement: Not applicable.

Acknowledgments: The acknowledgment of support was obtained from Dean of the Faculty of Medicine Padjajaran University, Dean of the Faculty of Nursing Padjajaran University and Dean of the Faculty of Social and Political Sciences, Padjadjaran University.

Conflicts of Interest: The authors declare no conflict of interest.

References

1. BNPB. *Rencana Nasional Penanggulangan Bencana 2020–2024*; BNPB: Jakarta, Indonesia, 2019; pp. 1–115. Available online: https://bnpb.go.id/buku/rencana-nasional-penanggulangan-bencana-20202024 (accessed on 9 January 2022).
2. BNPB. *Indeks Risiko Bencana Indonesia (IRBI) Tahun 2020*; BNPB: Jakarta, Indonesia, 2021; p. 199. Available online: https://inarisk.bnpb.go.id/pdf/BUKUIRBI2020KP.pdf (accessed on 5 March 2022).
3. Suryotomo, P. *Webinar "Peran Perawat dalam Kesiapsiagaan Bencana" oleh Persatuan Perawat Nasional Indonesia (PPNI) Tahun 2022 Kesiapsiagaan dan Peran Perawat dalam Menghadapi Bencana*; PPNI: Jakarta, Indonesia, 2022.
4. Adi, A.; Shalih, O.; Shabrina Fathia Rizqi, A.; Putra, A. *Indeks Resiko Bencana Indonesia (IRBI) Tahun 2021*; Yunus, R., Ed.; Pusat Data, Informasi dan Komunikasi Kebencanaan Badan Nasional Penanggulangan Bencana 1: Jakarta, Indonesia, 2021; Volume 1, pp. 8–11. Available online: https://inarisk.bnpb.go.id/pdf/BUKU%20IRBI%202021%20(PDF).pdf (accessed on 22 September 2022).
5. Mcdonald, A.; Wilcox, T.; Aslam, P.; Pannawadee, S.; Janne, P.; Animesh, K.; Calle, I.T.; Amach, O. *Disaster Risk Reduction in Indonesia*; Spring: Berlin/Heidelberg, Germany, 2020; p. 40.
6. Supriyanto Melilano, I.; Budianto, A.; Andreas, H.; Mariany, A.; Novianto, B. *Jabar Resilience Culture Province (JRCP) Cetak Biru: Jawa barat Berbudaya Tangguh Bencana*; JRCP: Bandung, Indonesia, 2021.
7. BNPB. *Kajian Risiko Bencana Nasional Provinsi Jawa Barat 2022–2026*; BNPB: Jakarta, Indonesia, 2021.
8. Badan Nasional Penanggulangan Bencana (BNPB). *Rencana Nasional Penanggulangan Bencana 2015-2019 RINGKASAN EKSEKUTIF*; BNPB: Jakarta, Indonesia, 2014; pp. 1–115. Available online: https://www.bnpb.go.id/documents/buku-renas-pb.pdf (accessed on 13 April 2022).
9. Setiawan, A.; Sofyana, H.; Suhanda, P. *Health Notions, Volume 1 Issue 1 (January–March 2017) ISSN 2580-4936 Empowering Village Cluster as Task Force in The Normalization of Disaster Victims ' Physical Problems 22*; Humanistic Network for Science and Technology Health Notions: Ponorogo, Indonesia, 2017; Volume 1, pp. 22–28. ISSN 2580-4936.
10. Salasa, S.; Murni, T.W.; Emaliyawati, E. Pemberdayaan pada Kelompok Remaja melalui Pendekatan Contingency Planning dalam Meningkatkan Kesiapsiagaan terhadap Ancaman Kematian Akibat Bencana. *J. Pendidik Keperawatan Indones.* **2017**, *3*, 154–166. [CrossRef]
11. Kulatunga, U. Impact of culture towards disaster risk reduction. *Int. J. Strateg. Prop. Manag.* **2010**, *14*, 304–313. [CrossRef]

12. Marutani, M.; Kodama, S.; Harada, N. Japanese public health nurses' culturally sensitive disaster nursing for small island communities. *Isl. Stud. J.* **2020**, *15*, 371–386. [CrossRef]
13. Covan, E.K.; Fugate-Whitlock, E. Emergency planning and long-term care: Least paid, least powerful, most responsible. *Health Care Women Int.* **2010**, *31*, 1028–1043. [CrossRef] [PubMed]
14. United Nations. 2009 UNISDR Terminologi on Disaster Risk Reductions. In *Handbook of Rural Aging*; Routledge: Oxfordshire, UK, 2021; pp. 111–115.
15. Paton, D. Disaster risk reduction: Psychological perspectives on preparedness. *Aust. J. Psychol.* **2019**, *71*, 327–341. [CrossRef]
16. Gonzalo, A. Madeleine Leininger: Transcultural Nursing Theory. 20191–26. Available online: https://nurseslabs.com/madeleine-leininger-transcultural-nursing-theory/ (accessed on 13 April 2022).
17. Murdiyanti, D. *Keperawatan Transkultural Pengetahuan Praktik Berdasarkan Budaya [Internet]*, 1st ed.; Elzha, E., Dianawati, L., Eds.; Keperawatan Transkultural; Pustaka Baru Press: Yogyakarta, Indonesia, 2017; pp. 285–287. Available online: http://repository.akperykyjogja.ac.id/102/1/BukuKeperawatanTranskulturalLengkap.pdf (accessed on 13 April 2022).
18. Badriah, S. Model Keperawatan Keluarga Peka Budaya Sunda dalam meningkatkan Pengetahuan Keluarga dan menurunkan Kadar Hula darah Pada Diabetisi Lansia. *J. Keperawatan Silampari* **2021**, *4*, 6. [CrossRef]
19. Amri, M.R.; Yulianti, G.; Yunus, R.; Wiguna, S.; Adi, A.W.; Ichwana, A.N.; Septian, R.T. *Risiko Bencana Indonesia (Disasters Risk of Indonesia)*; Badan Nasional Penanggulangan Bencana: Jakarta, Indonesia, 2016; pp. 9–140.
20. Ren, Z.J.; Wang, H.T.; Zhang, W. Experiences in disaster-related mental health relief work: An exploratory model for the interprofessional training of psychological relief workers. *J. Interprof. Care* **2017**, *31*, 35–42. [CrossRef] [PubMed]
21. Lebowitz, A.J. Community Collaboration as a Disaster Mental Health Competency: A Systematic Literature Review. *Community Ment. Health J.* **2015**, *51*, 125–131. [CrossRef] [PubMed]
22. Pourvakhshoori, N.; Norouzi, K.; Ahmadi, F.; Hosseini, M.; Khankeh, H. Nurse in limbo: A qualitative study of nursing in disasters in Iranian context. *PLoS ONE* **2017**, *12*, e0181314. [CrossRef] [PubMed]
23. Salmani, I.; Seyedin, H.; Ardalan, A.; Farajkhoda, T. Correction: Conceptual model of managing health care volunteers in disasters: A mixed method study. *BMC Health Serv. Res.* **2019**, *19*, 241. [CrossRef] [PubMed]
24. Kertamuda, F.E.; Chris, H. Pasrah (Surrender) and Sabar (Patience) Among Indonesia Ethnics (Javanese, Sundanese, Betawi) Through Disaster: An Indigenous Psychological Analysis. In Proceedings of the HKICEPS 2012: 2012 Hong Kong International Conference on Education, Psychology and Society, Hong Kong, China, 14–16 December 2012.
25. BPBD Kab Bandung. Profil BPBD Kabupaten Bandung. 2017. Available online: https://bpbd.jabarprov.go.id/bpbd-kabupaten-dan-kota/ (accessed on 13 April 2022).
26. Geodipa, P.T. *Profile PT Geodipa Enenrgi*, 1st ed; Bandung, Indonesia, 2020; Available online: https://www.geodipa.co.id/ (accessed on 13 April 2022).
27. Walsh, L.; Subbarao, I.; Gebbie, K.; Schor, K.W.; Lyznicki, J.; Strauss-Riggs, K.; Cooper, A.; Hsu, E.B.; King, R.V.; Mitas, J.A.; et al. Core competencies for disaster medicine and public health. *Disaster Med. Public Health Prep.* **2012**, *6*, 44–52. [CrossRef] [PubMed]
28. Gulzar, S.A.; Faheem, Z.A.; Somani, R.K. Role of community health nurse in earthquake affected areas. *J. Pak. Med. Assoc.* **2012**, *62*, 1083–1086. [PubMed]
29. Rush, Z.; Depriest, K.; Mccauley, L. Climate Change-Related Hurricane Impact on Puerto Rico and the U.S. Virgin Islands, Environment Risk Reduction, and the Social Determinants of Health. *Nurs. Econ.* **2019**, *37*, 13–23.
30. Ahmadi, S.; Khankeh, H.; Sahaf, R.; da Lvandi, A.; Hosseini, S.A. Daily life challenges in an earthquake disaster situation in older adults: A qualitative study in Iran. *J. Clin. Diagn. Res.* **2018**, *12*, IC08–IC12. [CrossRef]

sustainability MDPI

Article

A Multi-Attribute Decision Support System for Allocation of Humanitarian Cluster Resources Based on Decision Makers' Perspective

Sara Rye [1,*] and Emel Aktas [2]

[1] School of Business, London South Bank University, London SE1 0AA, UK
[2] Cranfield School of Management, Cranfield University, Cranfield MK43 0AL, UK
* Correspondence: ryes@lsbu.ac.uk

Abstract: The rush of the humanitarian suppliers into the disaster area proved to be counter-productive. To reduce this proliferation problem, the present research is designed to provide a technique for supplier ranking/selection in disaster response using the principles of utility theory. A resource allocation problem is solved using optimisation based on decision maker's preferences. Due to the lack of real-time data in the first 72 h after the disaster strike, a Decision Support System (DSS) framework called EDIS is introduced to employ secondary historical data from disaster response in four humanitarian clusters (WASH: Water, Sanitation and Hygiene, Nutrition, Health, and Shelter) to estimate the demand of the affected population. A methodology based on multi-attribute decision-making (MADM), Analytical Hierarchy processing (AHP) and Multi-attribute utility theory (MAUT) provides the following results. First a need estimation technique is put forward to estimate minimum standard requirements for disaster response. Second, a method for optimization of the humanitarian partners selection is provided based on the resources they have available during the response phase. Third, an estimate of resource allocation is provided based on the preferences of the decision makers. This method does not require real-time data from the aftermath of the disasters and provides the need estimation, partner selection and resource allocation based on historical data before the MIRA report is released.

Keywords: disaster response; need estimation; resource based; MADM; AHP; MAUT; utility theory; humanitarian clusters; humanitarian supply

Citation: Rye, S.; Aktas, E. A Multi-Attribute Decision Support System for Allocation of Humanitarian Cluster Resources Based on Decision Makers' Perspective. *Sustainability* **2022**, *14*, 13423. https://doi.org/10.3390/su142013423

Academic Editors: Amir Khorram-Manesh and Krzysztof Goniewicz

Received: 14 September 2022
Accepted: 11 October 2022
Published: 18 October 2022

1. Introduction

The overall aim of the disaster relief operation is to ensure the survival and health of the maximum possible number of victims [1,2]. This operation is required to benefit the affected community's development and reduce the vulnerability of the population to future hazards. In the days and weeks immediately following a disaster, the basic relief supplies and services are provided free of charge to save and preserve human lives. This enables families to meet their basic needs for medical and health care, shelter, clothing, water, and food. However, the problem is in the early hours after the disaster strike, there is no official estimate of these needs. The first official UN report of preliminary Multi-Cluster/Sector Initial Rapid Assessment (MIRA) is released three days after the disaster strikes. This present problems as some quick decisions and actions need to be taken in the absence of detailed assessments and lack of appropriate Decision Support Systems (DSS) which may lead to loss of lives amongst others. For example, during the UK flood in 2014, even though good warning systems were in place [3], the lack of decision-making tools, led to the death of seven people and the destruction of 1700 homes. It is critical to understand that these negative effects happened in the presence of the exact knowledge of where and when the storm/flood would strike, in a developed country with a sufficient budget for prevention. Therefore, the lack of DSS in developing countries would be far more devastating. Like other decision-making problems with human elements, the preferences of decision makers also play a role in this resource allocation under uncertainty. The objective of this research is to provide a DSS for partner selection/ranking using only the data available before the release of MIRA report to reduce the partners' proliferation problem. So, this research addresses two questions: First to what extent is possible to estimate the resources required for humanitarian response operation in the absence of MIRA report within the first three days. Second to what extent is possible to optimise the resource allocation decisions within humanitarian response operation considering the preferences of the decision makers.

The preferences become important when you note that decision makers in disaster affected area, operate based on their background, beliefs, experience, and political views. For example, in some areas where the conflicts are an issue, some decision makers are reluctant towards the use of military relief supplies. Some decision makers due to experience might prefer government or NGO, International or local suppliers, UN or voluntary resources, and so on. To answer the above questions, this research aims to develop a DSS which could optimise the allocation of resources prior to the release of MIRA report and based on the decision makers' preferences. The DSS includes a framework for need assessment of the affected population to enhance the need-based resource allocation through decision makers' preferences. In this process, various humanitarian guidelines and official reports were used to argue that it is possible to outline minimum standard requirements for each disaster type and based on the affected countries' socio-economic characteristics. This estimates a list of requirements in disaster situation for affected population with priorities. This list can be the basis for need-based resource estimates. The estimates then are used to optimize the allocation of the resources available by humanitarian suppliers based on the principles of utility theory and resource-dependency theory. The agent-based optimisation technique which is where all DSS methods above overlap, are in general based on the principles of decision theory Neumann-Morgenstern in the 40s. This allows agents to select decision criteria, evaluate, and compare the options and act upon them. This can be viewed as combination of Utility theory and Probability theory [4]. Decision-making in a disaster situation, in particular fits well within both utility and probability as it is a decision scenario under uncertainty. The literature in this ilk are mainly divided in two branches; Rational choice and Expected utility (EU) and Behavioural and Prospect theory [5]. The former has arisen from mathematical literature, and provides clear formulations, whereas the latter is more practice-based and tries to show the controversies in the Expected utility theory [6]. This research is not an attempt to focus on the challenges facing Utility theory or study how and why decision makers decide the way, they do. The research focused on Utility theory to maximise the preferences of the decision makers who decide based on the reasons out of scope of this research. In fact, the investigation into the reasoning behind their preferences can be the subject of further studies on Prospect theory by other scholars.

This research provides a technique for supplier ranking/selection in disaster response by analysing the archival data, and decision support tools. Using Linear programming optimisation, Analytical Hierarchy processing (AHP) and Multi-attribute utility theory (MAUT) a DSS is developed based on secondary data. The DSS includes Phase1-ESTIMATION of the need in four humanitarian clusters (WASH, Nutrition, Health and Shelter). This will be the basis for estimating the demand of the affected population. Phase 2-OPTIMISATION selects the set of suppliers (and their resources) based on the decision maker' preferences. Using the AHP technique, a matrix of hypothetical decision makers' preferences is built and used to find the value of each supplier in the eye of the decision maker. The Significance of EDIS is that despite using numerical data, it does not require data gathering at the time of the disaster and uses historic data. EDIS can be complementary to existing methods for task allocation and scheduling techniques in disaster management, as a quicker data feed. This research also provides an insight into decision-making to reduce the uncertainty based on the principles of resource- dependency theory and through collaboration, as the most suitable group of suppliers are selected to share their resources based on the optimisation technique using the principles of the utility theory. Methodological contribution is a design to simulate the decision-making under uncertainty by taking into account the opinion of human agents (decision maker). It also uses mathematical optimisation in addition to the opinion of human agents, which integrates the heuristic and mathematical approaches of decision-making. It also bridge the gap in needs prioritisation by providing numerical priorities. Practical contribution is that by providing a range of it enables the decision maker to decide based on their budget limitations and personal preferences. It also gives different humanitarian organisations the chance to customise the model using their own database if required.

The structure of the paper is organised as follows. We present a literature review followed by an elaboration of data sources. The method is then outlined where input and output are provided. The results section expands on input/output and provides details of the optimization through AHP. The process of collecting the preferences of the decision makers through a questionnaire is outlined and then the ranking of the suppliers through MAUT is provided. The discussion outlines the answers to the research questions, elaborates the contribution and then presents the limitations and the future research directions.

2. Literature Review

The present research addresses the partner proliferation problem in disaster response networks as one of the most recurring problems in humanitarian operations. The existing experiences of failure in disaster management operations in large-scale disasters, signals the necessity to investigate an effective disaster relief management, which is successful in minimising the negative effects of the disasters [7] specifically with the focus on reducing the problem of partner proliferation. Due to counterproductive effects of this phenomenon on the whole disaster relief operation, the quality of response is damaged [8]. The proliferation of actors is induced due to the extreme requirements of the disaster which forces to mobilise and recover all the available sources [9] and therefore all available partners are encouraged to participate.

The negative effect of this reactionary response [10] is twofold. First, the mandatory growth in the relief budget in the public sector (UN, Red Cross and governments) as well as the fund raising by the private sector (such as NGOs) exceeds the absorption capacity of an overstretched humanitarian industry. This pushes the inexperienced actors including the public image seeking companies into activities outside their area of expertise [11,12]. This situation leads to the oversupply of uncoordinated and inexperienced partners [13]. This rush of all available partners creates a range of partners from competent and incompetent, reputable and disreputable, opportunistic and committed, well-established and just-formed in addition to individuals, tourists and also companies which aim to generate a favourable public image, to increase their long-term profit. They enter the disaster-effected area in a chaotic pattern and cause the proliferation problem Figure 1. This as mentioned before, results in the budget stretch leading to the oversupply of a range of heterogeneous uncoordinated and inexperienced partners [13].

Figure 1 shows the chaotic pattern of partners' rushing into the affected area of Hurricane Katrina. This increases the load on the affected populations, local authorities, and coordination structures for information or services. It also increases the costs due to replicated offices and overheads, produces a counterproductive duplication and confusion of efforts, and leads to competition between agencies for donations, facilities, and publicity.

The second negative effect of proliferation is the increase in the risks of inappropriate aid, due to the time pressure of competition and the rush for publicity. This increases the risk to the quality of the response and reputation of the humanitarian community through the actions of inexperienced or irresponsible agencies and damages the quality of the responses [8]. The damage is enhanced by the fact that this wasted effort could be used instead to take advantage of the capabilities of the partners within the network and creates competition between the agencies over funding [11,14]. The study suggests that one of the reasons for failure in disaster relief network lies in the incompatibility of the disaster relief situation with the existing collaborative structures used for managing the response operation.

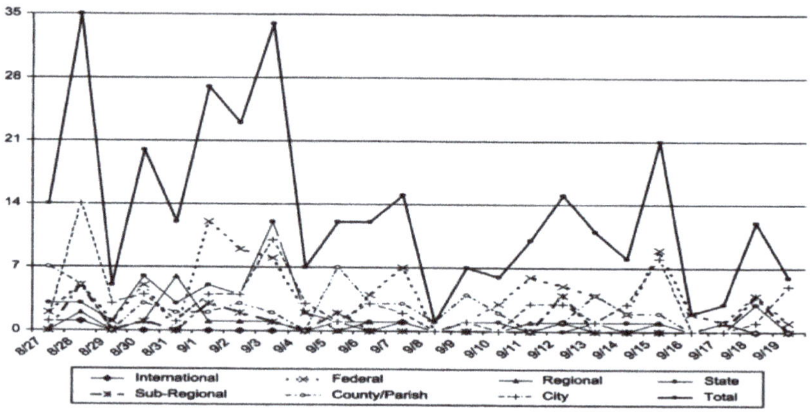

Figure 1. Partner's entry pattern into the affected area of Hurricane Katrina. Source: Comfort (2007).

The uncertainty and the lack of information [15] together with damaged infrastructure [16] unequal and ineffective distribution of demand and supply and their respective fluctuations [9,17], unsteady flow of the financial resources obtained by fund-raising from occasional donors [18] all make the planning and long-term outlook almost impossible. Additionally, long-term approaches in practice are usually profit-based whilst in disaster situations the non-financial factors such as the time value of commodities are much greater than the costs associated [18,19], which make the conventional profit-based values less accurate. Therefore, due to the lack of control and information in disaster situations, the existing structures such as supply chains or project-based collaborations might fall short in practice because these structures require a certain amount of knowledge about the supply, demand, timing, costs, etc. which are generally unknown in disaster situations.

This research proposes restructuring the relief network to accommodate the characteristics of the disaster situation to work with the minimum data available and without much pre-planning. The negative impacts of proliferation can be reduced if the partners are carefully selected according to the requirements of each particular disaster to make sure the interaction between heterogeneous partners does not have a counterproductive effect. An efficient operation needs to be supported with a suitable selection of partners who work together efficiently and guarantee the success of collaboration. The current study builds upon empirical research carried out in the field of decision making in disaster response operations as a response to calls [20] stating that an optimal network structure to assist in resolution of disasters is yet to be developed.

Dealing with the proliferation problem in a disaster situation falls under the heading of Decision Support Systems (DSS) in disaster situation [10,21]. The current literature mostly utilises DSS borrowed from logistics or production management studies into the disaster decision. The resource allocations generally include criteria-based optimisations. This criteria could include tangible characteristics of the resources including their location [22,23], Facilities [24], price [25], time [26–29], due date [30–33]. These are based on a fully informed decision environment and are time consuming to calculate or use complicated software and database which might not be available at the time of the disaster.

For example, task and resource allocation based on request from the aid centres assuming the data are available and reliable with no mention of the gap between the disaster strike and the data release [34]. They also are mostly based on the established distribution centres and fail to consider the ad hoc centres. The similar research considers community-based DSSs which tests all variations of the aid team to find the best [35] this trial and error is time consuming and there is no guarantee that the teams keep their members, performance and dynamic.

Others investigate distribution of resources [36,37], scheduling of supply chain for the delivery of resources [38], using genetic algorithms [39] integer linear programming in [40] to minimize the transportation cost, reinforcement learning [41] or MCDM to enhance the operational effectiveness of humanitarian activities [42]. The relief urgency index [43] using time-varying demand, population density, vulnerable population, damage, and last delivery to improve the relief distribution, fails to include the weight and the scalability of above factors. Other tools include stochastic optimization techniques knowing the exact number of national resources [44], using Nash equilibrium [45,46].

Other DSS rely on characteristics of the suppliers instead of resources. This could include measurable characteristics of the suppliers such as their attributes [26,47–49], partners' goal achievement probabilities [50] and performance indicators [51]. We argue that these criteria, although useful for planning and mitigation phases of disaster, are unsuitable for a disaster response due to the scarcity of data and time pressure associated with the disaster situation.

Additionally, regardless of the characteristics of the resources and/or suppliers, the decisions made by humans during disaster response, are highly affected by their preference. This has been addressed in few papers including risk preferences of decision makers [52], deep learning in resource prioritisation [53], mathematical models for resource optimisation based on community values in mitigation phase of disaster in few African countries [54], policy based resource optimisation for response [55]. The above criteria are often combined with mathematical optimisation techniques including AHP [56–59], Multi-attribute decision making under uncertain conditions [60–65], linear programming [10,66–68] and rule-based techniques [22], case-based reasoning [69] and spatial modelling of the resources [70]. It is noteworthy to mention this is a review of static models and dynamic models such as relief delivery models and route optimisations [71] or workflow modeling are not the focus of this research.

Based on the argument above, the research focuses on the partner selection in disaster situations as a solution to the partner proliferation problem. However, although a huge body of literature exist on the "how to restructure the selected partners", these approaches face a serious problem of duplication of efforts and the counterproductive effect of the operations during the disaster response operation. The existing research on this area mainly focuses on preparation, mitigation, and recovery phases by suggesting various long-term collaborative structures such as supply chains [72–75]. The problem arises from the high state of uncertainty in the response phase due to the temporary and urgent nature of the aid required, and the chaotic nature of disaster strike. This uncertainty affects the available data required for planning [15], the stream of financial resources [18] and unknown and fluctuating, supply and demand [9,15,17]. Due to the scarcity of the date before the release of MIRA report, this article develop a decision making framework (EDIS) for selecting suitable partners by reviewing the records of natural onset disasters, which have happened worldwide since 1980, and their data are available in various humanitarian databases (Emdat.be, 2014; Munichre.com, 2014;ReliefWeb, 2014; Gdacs.org, 2014). EDIS ultimately deals with the proliferation problem by ranking and selecting the most suitable partners based on the principals of the Decision theory and Resource-based theory.

The significance of this research is that in addition to dealing with the primary problem of the research (proliferation problem), it provides a framework for estimation of the needs, and resource optimisation through the allocation of the resources to the needs during the disaster response operation. This framework is noteworthy because currently the first official report of the disaster effects is released 72 h after the disaster strikes leading to a three-day gap between the decisions about the distribution of aid, and obtaining information about the actual needs amongst the affected population. The EDIS framework in this sense is an attempt to cover this gap by using the data available at the time of the disaster striking. This characteristic is also helpful because when a disaster strikes in many areas the people who decide about the allocation of the resources, are not trained in the field of decision making or logistics. Instead, they happen to be in the disaster-affected area before experts arrive, and this framework could help them to make decisions using historic data and without the use of any complicated software, only excel sheets.

3. Data

Various scholars and humanitarian organisations categorise the criteria or requirements in the response operations. The preliminary review identified myriads of criteria [2,20,76–79]. The list of these criteria of requirements is presented in Figure 2.

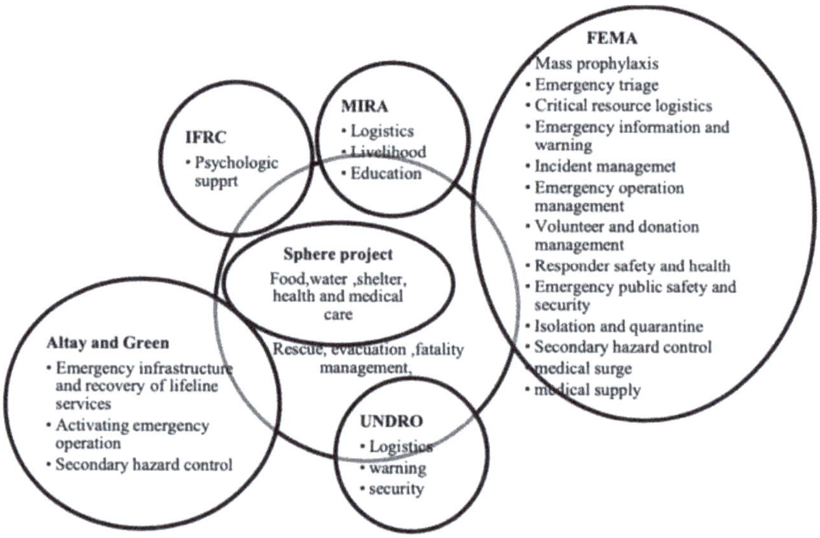

Figure 2. The requirements of the disaster affected area.

Figure 2 shows where these requirements overlap. The majority of the organisations emphasise on the importance of the key life-saving activities including food security and nutrition, shelter and settlement (including non-food items), water and sanitation and health actions. Additionally, except for one organisation [76] which focuses solely on saving the lives of the survivors, the rest of the sources agree that rescue, evacuation and fatality management, education and logistics are also important. Some criteria emphasise on the importance of secondary hazard control [20,79] whilst some criteria are only mentioned by one source only such as psychological support [78,80], warning and security [2], livelihood [81], emergency infrastructure and recovery of lifeline services and activating emergency operation [20], mass prophylaxis, emergency triage, critical resource logistics, emergency information and warning, incident management, emergency operation management, volunteer and donation management, responder safety and health, emergency public safety and security, isolation and quarantine, secondary hazard control, medical surge and medical supply [79]. To summarise, the key life-saving activities or mass care activities are shared by all above organisations and therefore are the focus of this study.

The minimum standards of needs for key life-saving activities is drawn from the previous practice in similar disasters, published by humanitarian organisations [2,20,76–79]. The significance of this method is that by knowing the number of affected population, and based on the minimum standard, the required units of aid for each disaster scenario can be calculated. This process in this article is called "need estimation".

The data required for the estimation phase is collected from standard minimum requirements published in the following. This includes the internal reports and working papers from variety of government archives including Census Bureau, Department of Laboure, military, European Central Bank [82], Federal Emergency Management Agency [79], various bodies of UN [1,2,83,84], World Health Organisation [85,86], Global Health Council [80,87,88], Office for the Coordination of Humanitarian Affairs [81,89–95] and various foundations and associations including OXFAM [96], The Association for Healthcare Resource & Materials Management, Health Industry Group Purchasing Association, Health Industry Distribution Association [97], Sphere project [76], National Voluntary Organisations Active in Disaster [98] in addition to other reports [99–101]. Table 1 shows the literature used in developing the need assessment technique.

Table 1. Data sources for needs-assessment.

Title of the Report	Publisher
A Case Study: Joint Needs Assessment after the West Sumatra Earthquake	ECB (2009)
Global Health Cluster Partners' survey	GHC. (2012),
Winter floods 2013/14	Hartwell-naguib and Roberts (2014)
Disaster emergency needs assessment	IFRC (2000)
IFRC shelter kit	IFRC (2009a)
World disaster report	IFRC (2009b)
Mass fatality management following the South Asian tsunami disaster: case studies in Thailand, Indonesia, and Sri Lanka	Morgan et al. (2006)
Multi/cluster-sector initial and rapid assessment (MIRA) Community level assessment	OCHA (n.d)
MIRA report—Pakistan Floods	OCHA (2012a)
MIRA report -In preparedness for disasters and emergencies A joint initiative between Government and the humanitarian community	OCHA (2012b)
MIRA Report Pakistan Floods	OCHA (2012c)
The Philippines second-phase MIRA report for tropical storm WASHI (Sending)	OCHA (2012d)
Inter-agency initial rapid needs assessment preliminary report, (October).	OCHA (2013a)
Joint Rapid Damage and Needs Assessment Report,	OCHA (2013b)
MIRA report Philippines typhoon Haiyan.	OCHA (2013c)
Central African republic multi-cluster/sector initial rapid assessment	OCHA (2014)
Sylhet phase 1 rapid emergency assessment	OXFAM (2012)
Emergency Relief Logistics: Evaluation of Disaster Response Models Based on Asian Tsunami Logistics Response.	Patrice (2008)
Target capabilities list	U.S department of homeland security (2007)
Medical-surgical supply formulary by disaster scenario.	AHRMM and HIDA and HIGPA (n.d.)
The sphere project	Sphere project (2011)
Shelter after disaster	UNDRO (1982)
An Overview of Disaster Management.	UNDRO (1992)
Shelter project	UNHCR (2010)
Emergency handbook	UNICEF (2005)
National voluntary organisations active in disaster	VOAD (2011)
Management of dead bodies after disasters	WHO (2011)
Classification and minimum standards for foreign medical teams in sudden onset	WHO (2013)

The resources in Table 1 were used to consolidate a need-based list of life-saving activities. This list was then categorized based on the humanitarian cluster system offered by Inter-Agency Standing Committee [77] to address the right of the affected population to receive the assistance required to live with dignity. This minimum standard requirement will be used in the first step of the methodology as described below.

The Effect of Type of Disaster on Need Estimation

The demand also may vary based on the type of the disaster because the type of disaster influences the extent of the effects. For example, earthquake causes the highest rate of death within different type of disasters. Additionally, some linguistic measures [76] shows that in an earthquake or high wind, food scarcity is not an issue, whilst it is quite probable in tsunami. For example, based on these data, it is unlikely that the affected population suffers from the food scarcity in the aftermath of earthquakes or winds, whilst it Is quite probable in after a tsunami. By adding to the effects of the different types of disasters, Table 2 is created. The following ranks are applied to the situation If Small = 1, Rare = 2, Few = 3, Moderate = 4, Many = 5, Common = 6, High = 7. It is noteworthy that the ranks need to be considered as priorities and not the actual numbers. Therefore, we started the priorities from 1 for simplification. It is possible to start it from any other number such as 0.57, 0.58, 0.59, or even start from 1000; 1100; 1200 as long as it makes it possible to show higher priorities. The result of this accumulation is summarised in Table 2 as ranked from 1–7, (1) being the lowest weight to (7) to the highest weight effect. The numbers are only representatives of weights and is not to be treated as actual numbers.

Table 2. Weights of the effects in various types of disasters.

Effect	Cluster	Complex Emergency	Earthquake	High Wind	Flood	Tsunami	Eruption
Deaths	Fatality management	5	5	3	3	5	Varies *
Severe injuries	Health Cluster	Varies *	5	4	3	3	4
Increased risk of communicable diseases	WASH cluster	7	Varies *	1	Varies *	Varies *	5
Food scarcity	Food cluster	6	2	2	Varies *	6	5
Major population displacements	Shelter cluster	6	2	2	6	Varies *	6

* The word "varies" is transferred from its original [76] and implies that the different records and scholars never agreed on a number on the specific disasters.

Table 2 shows that when earthquakes strike, fatality management, and medical mass care require the highest level of resources followed by food and shelter. Another conclusion is that after floods, the most required resources are shelter whilst after a flash flood and tsunami the highest priority is food cluster. Because the data set was void of information about the eruptions, the definition from [102] was used for this disaster type. It suggests that in eruptions the population displacement is often a consequence. Therefore, in general the eruption response prioritises are temporary shelter materials; safe water and basic sanitation; food supplies; and the short-term provision of basic health services and supplies. Using this data, decision makers could know roughly that when an earthquake strikes fatality management needs more participants than food supplying Suppliers. However, this rule does not indicate prioritising the population, and in applying this rule, it should always be taken into consideration that the live population has a higher priority. As a result, the mass care needs of the live population should be dealt with first before fatality management is put into place. This data is further used in combination to minimum standard requirement to estimate the needs as described as follows in the method.

4. Method

Decision-making methods suitable for a disaster network allocation, can be viewed as a multi-criteria decision-making problem [103]. Some scholars emphasize on the importance of DSS techniques in addressing specific disaster response problems [22,70]. The DSS designed for this research for allocation of the resources to the affected population is called EDIS (Estimating for DISaster response) Framework. EDIS follows two consecutive phases combining the existing decision techniques and determinants, suitable for the characteristics of the disaster response. The first step is "estimation" of the minimum resources required for the affected population and the second step is "optimisation" of these requirements by the decision makers as illustrated in Figure 3.

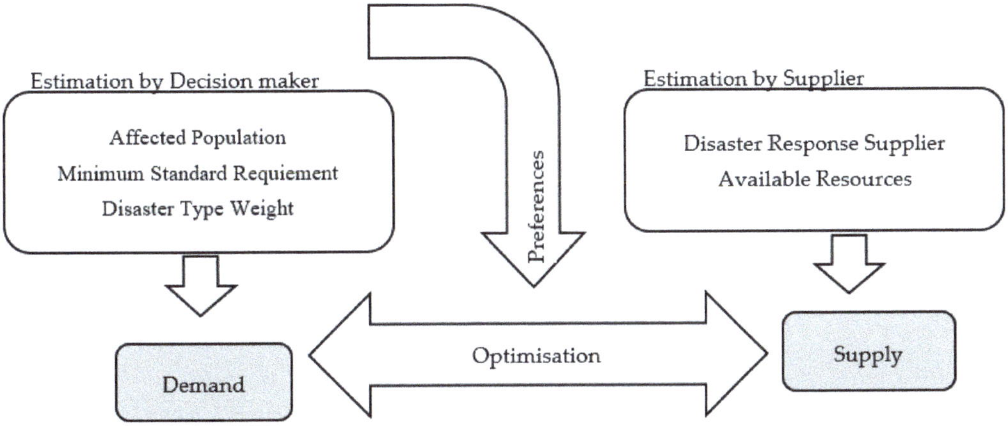

Figure 3. Inputs and outputs of the paper.

The principles of the resource-based view outlines that if the collaboration is to be successful it needs to focus on the resources, also based on the principles of the resource-dependency theory the companies collaborate in order to acquire critical resources and reduce uncertainty [104] which is the case in the disaster situation. The idea is to use the historic data about how many units of resources are required in similar situations in order to estimate the approximate needs. The rest would be an optimisation problem using the mathematical programming based on the principles of the utility theory. This insight outlines the design of the research to investigate two propositions.

This research addresses two questions: First to what extent is possible to estimate the resources required for humanitarian response operation in the absence of MIRA report within the first three days. Second to what extent is possible to optimise the resource allocation decisions within humanitarian response operation considering the preferences of the decision makers. This question is answered by a scenario-based decision making process to optimise the balance of available resources in possession of suppliers (supply) to the needs of the affected area (demand) as illustrated in Figure 3. The focus on this research are natural onset disasters or disasters with no-notice [22] such as eruption or earthquake.

This system categorises the minimum standard needs of affected population as Shelter, Nutrition, WASH (water and sanitation), and Health in 43 main needs. For simplicity and illustration purpose an example of the result of this accumulation is articulated in Table 3.

Table 3 accumulates data from different resources leads to an average number. For example, IFRC (Cited by WHO, pp. 48–49) states: "200 people/day 10–20 beds for overnight observation, Supplies to treat 30,000 people. For a month, per 12–14 h shift: 1 Doctor, 1 Pharmacist/Nurse, 1Curative/Community Health Nurse, 1 Midwife/Nurse, 2 General Technicians" from this statement, we can conclude that for 200 people/day we require a maximum of 20 beds, 1 doctor, 3 nurses and 2 other medical personnel and 1000 units of treatment supplies (30,000 for 30 days).

There are two points to keep in mind when looking at the above numbers. Minimum requirements for each cluster are expressed based on the person or household needs. A household is defined as a group of people who eat from a common pot, and share a common stake, interpreting and improving their socio-economic status from one generation to the next [105]. There are many options available for food as long as it provides the 2100 kcal required for each person [76] and complies with the cultural norms of the affected society. Additionally, the demand also may vary based on the type of the disaster.

Table 3. The examples of minimum requirements for life saving activities.

Humanitarian Cluster	Specification	Per Person	Per Household
WASH	Transportation containers (10–20 L)	N/a	1
	Storage containers (10–20 L)	N/a	1
	Blankets	1	
	Total basic water needs	7.5–15 L/day	
	Patients	60 L/day	
	Open wells	1/400	
	Toilets	1/50 people	
Nutrition	Salt, iodised edible	1	1
	Fish, canned, sardines, vegetable oil, 150 g	2	1
	Pasta, durum wheat meal	1	1
	Rice, white, long grain, irri6/2	1	1
	Oil, rapeseed	1	1
	Beans, white, small	1	1
Shelter and settlement	Tarpaulins (4 m × 6 m)		1
	Ropes (30 m)		1
	Saws		1
	Roding, small and largo nail (1/2 kg each)		1
	Shovels		1
	Hoe		1
	Machete		1
Health cluster	Doctors	4.57	100
	Nurses	5.9	100
	Others	6	100

Optimisation

For the optimisation of partner selection, a DSS is required that embeds the partner selection criteria for partner configuration. For the particular case of this research the decision methods used in literature were compared to identify the most suitable technique to be used in the research. A review shows a variety of hard methods (with quantitative and numerical values) and heuristic methods (with linguistic and quantitative values) in the decision-making field. As mentioned before the process of optimization in this research includes balancing the available suppliers' resources (supply) to the needs of the affected area (demand). Therefore, a multi-criteria [53,106–109] resource based [55] DSS which accommodates the characteristics of the disaster response is required [103]. These characteristics may include the time pressure [24], big database [110] and multiple perspective of decision makers [111].Variety of hard methods (with quantitative and numerical values) and heuristic methods (with linguistic and quantitative values) in the decision-making field can be used. The suitability of them is assessed in Table 4.

Table 4. Criteria suitable for disaster response DSS.

Method	Accommodating Preference Subjective Values	Rank Reversal Problem	Accommodate the Interaction of Subjective Expert Advise	Only Offers Local Optimal	Difficult for Average User	Require Strong Data Set
AHP	YES	YES				
ANP		YES	YES			
Heuristic algorithms				NO		
Evolutionary Algorithm					NO	
Fuzzy logic						NO
Neural network						NO
TOPSIS						
Mathematical programming					NO	

Table 4 indicates the strength and weaknesses of each method. There is one specific group of hard or mathematical methods capable of accommodating numbers and quantitative values (as opposed to fuzzy or qualitative values) such as goal programming and integer programming [112]. These methods for the purpose of this research seem to be unsuitable because they formulate the problem in objective terms and fail to accommodate subjective attributes, here subjective preferences of decision makers. In addition, due to the high load of computation, these methods are not suitable for this research, a big dataset.

Another set of methods, which are vastly used in this area are evolutionary algorithms [107], however they become very slow when the number of selections arises and they might offer only a local optimal solution [67]. Additionally, the main drawback of all above methods is that they require a high level of specialised knowledge that is likely to be well beyond what possessed by disaster response decision makers. Alternatively, neural network analysis is suitable in disaster response networks for large data sets for training [53,113], however the quality of estimation in disaster situation under certainty is not trustworthy for training. Expert systems such as fuzzy logic are suitable for linguistically expressed expert's experience for multi-criteria optimisation [114,115]. Because this method is based on drawing fuzzy based rules out of the series of data, and in the absence of data, the rules cannot be confidently drawn. Both fuzzy methods and neural networks are only as strong as their database, so in the absence of such a strong database the rule-based system may fail [116]. This is noteworthy to mention that there is no record of decision makers' choices of suppliers in the disaster response in the literature despite a good record of disaster impacts in the literature.

Another group of methods, such as Multi-Attributive Decision-Making (MADM) as part of Multi-Attributive Utility Theory (MAUT) used for disaster response [65,109] also seems more suitable for optimization in this research. The reason is their capability of accommodating the non- certain preferences of decision makers, and linguistic expert's opinion which are required for supplier selection. These may include Analytical Hierarchy Process (AHP), Analytical Network Process (ANP) and Technique for Order of Preference by Similarity to Ideal Solution (TOPSIS). MADM is a branch in the decision-making for choosing between a finite number of alternatives.

In the EDIS, we assume that the number of suppliers in disaster response is finite so it seems appropriate to use MADM. One of the weaknesses of MADM methods is the rank reversal problem [117], which means that result of the ranking (direction of maximising or minimising and the ranking method itself) differs with the quality of the information available and the set of criteria representing the reality. However, in the uncertain environment of the disaster response, the decision maker always has to settle for available or obtainable data. This is because of the time pressure [24] and the often destroyed infrastructure which makes it impossible to improve the quality of the data. Therefore, the low quality of the data is going to affect the result of their decision, no matter what decision-making method they choose. Thus, these methods still seem like good candidates. Within popular MADM methods ANP which is used for prioritization [118] is incapable of accommodating the subjective perspectives of decision makers [103], which is one of the elements of the optimisation model in EDIS.

Another option, Technique for Order Performance by Similarity to Ideal Solution (TOPSIS), is used for group decision-making under uncertainty of information in order to select suitable suppliers [58,119]. This method can rank alternatives regarding defined criteria by minimising their distance from a positive ideal solution and maximising their distance from the negative ideal solution. However, this method also is based on objective values and therefore it ignores the subjective decision maker preference required in our research.

The most suitable option within MADM is AHP, which is used extensively in supplier selection [59,120–122]. This method is a good method for our research because unlike the other MADM methods mentioned above, it accommodates the subjective values, including the decision maker's preferences. To summarise Table 4, due to time pressure inherent in disaster situation, a DSS methods with a high execution time such as evolutionary algorithms, which slows down towards the end, need to be avoided. They also require a high degree of technical mathematic understanding, which the average decision maker in disaster response network might not have.

Another characteristic of any DSS run by people is that their preferences may hugely influence the result. Thus, the methods in which the subjective preferences of decision maker are not accommodated should be excluded such as ANP or TOPSIS. For those reasons the final candidate for optimization here are AHP to rank the utility of disaster response suppliers based on the decision maker's preferences to allocate the resources in demand by affected population to the resources offered by supplier. This selection is based on the resources the supplier has in accordance to the estimated needs for the respected disaster impact.

5. Results

The present research suggests two steps; the first step estimates the needs required for a particular disaster, based on minimum standard requirement for disaster. The second step is to optimize the resource allocation using the principles of utility theory by ranking the decision maker's preferences and the disaster needs priorities into an AHP model. In summary the article provides an optimization technique between demand and supply of the disaster affected area. The results are classified based on the input and output demonstrated in Figure 2.

5.1. Input

The input is the demand estimated based on the affected population, minimum standard requirement, and the weight of the disaster type. The minimum requirements of life saving activities (Table 3) coupled with the weight of disaster type (Table 2) can provide an estimation for the required resources to address the humanitarian needs for that disaster type in that cluster. However, the socio-economic characteristics of the affected country can also influence the need estimation as discussed below.

5.1.1. Inputting the Effect of Socio-Economic Characteristics on Need Estimation

In addition, the economic characteristics of the affected regions could influence the priority of needs. Typically, the events that result in the highest numbers of fatalities are located in regions with increased risk and vulnerable populations. This is often compounded by limited infrastructure and poor integration of the health system into disaster preparedness, response, and recovery [86]. For example, more foreign medical care is required for a disaster, which strikes in Sub-Saharan Africa, than a disaster in the Middle East, due to the capabilities of medical infrastructure. Therefore, different levels of attention are required for various clusters in different types of disasters.

For example, after an earthquake, the food cluster in Japan and Philippines require different levels of attention, due to their different level of infrastructures. To address this issue the indicators of socioeconomic development have been included in the model. These indicators including lack of coping capability and susceptibility were drawn from the medical capabilities, and sanitation/nourishments of each country are annually calculated by the United Nation and published in the world risk report [123,124].

These indicators include the 'coping capability' indicators, which were calculated, based on (amongst other criteria) the number of physicians and hospital beds/per 10,000 inhabitants by UN. This indicator has been added to the model as weights, to signal the health cluster capability of the country. Furthermore, a 'susceptibility' indicator based on (amongst other criteria) access to the water sanitation and nourishment calculated by UN is also added to the model as a weight to signal the food and WASH cluster. These weights signal the criticality of the situation on a specific cluster in a particular country. It also provides an opportunity for comparison between different disasters as in Table 5.

Table 5. Comparing two different disasters with their weights.

Year	Origin	Cluster Weight	Lack of Coping Capability	Susceptibility	Cluster Weight for Earthquake	Cluster Priority
2005	Pakistan	FOOD		38.84	5	$=38.84 \times 5 = 194.2$
		WASH		38.84	5	$=38.84 \times 5 = 194.2$
		Health	87.39		Varies	87.39
		Shelter			2	$=100 \times 2 = 200$
		Other (Fatality)			2	$=100 \times 2 = 200$
2011	New Zealand	FOOD		16.19	5	$=16.19 \times 5 = 80.95$
		WASH		16.19	5	$=16.19 \times 5 = 80.95$
		Health	39.79		Varies	39.79
		Shelter			2	$=100 \times 2 = 200$
		Other (Fatality)			2	$=100 \times 2 = 200$

Table 5 shows that by comparing the 2005 disaster in Pakistan with the 2011 disaster in New Zealand, without knowing any other information, including the type of disaster, we can tentatively claim that the health cluster (in terms of hospital beds and physicians) in Pakistan is almost two times less likely to cope with the disaster effects than New Zealand. The reason is that Pakistan's lack of coping capability is 87.39% compared to New Zealand's, which is 39.79%. The same principle can be used to interpret the susceptibility based on access to food and nourishment. It shows that Pakistan (38.84% susceptibility) is three times more likely to suffer from mal-nourishment, lack of water, and sanitation than New Zealand (with 16.19% susceptibility).

These numbers should also be considered as probabilities or risk factors and not actual numbers. They are only to be used for signalling what areas of needs should be prioritised. Combining the criteria affecting the needs in a disaster situation (including evidence from previous experiences, the type of disaster, and economic aspects of the affected region), the priority for each task can be calculated. Assume we must choose between disaster response clusters in both Pakistan and New Zealand at the same time. Based on the data in Table 3 the priorities would be shelter and fatality management in both counties because their priorities are higher than other clusters and equal to 200. The next priority is food and WASH for Pakistan (both 194 points for priority), followed by the Health cluster for Pakistan (87.39 points for priority), then food and WASH for New Zealand (80.95 points for priority), followed by the Health cluster for New Zealand (30.79). This data is obtainable and calculated without knowing any other information about the disaster including its type.

5.1.2. Estimating the Required Resources: An Example

The affected number for Pakistan earthquake 2005 is used for an example. The total of 75,000 injured and 2,800,000 displaced population are the basis for this calculation. There are few assumptions associated with this example. First, assuming there is an overlap between the injured and displaced population, and for that reason we then assumed that the injured only use the health cluster and water for patient needs and the rest are being used by the displaced. There are four prominent categories of needs, one for each humanitarian cluster including health, nutrition, WASH and shelter. Multiplying the needs for one person in Table 1 and estimated number of people in need of that particular help, would provide the total number of needs required for that cluster. So the need for each cluster is calculated as: [Total unit required for a cluster = Minimum standard requirement * estimated impact]. A sample of 21 needs for the illustrative purposes are distributed between four humanitarian clusters is presented in Table 6 combining the result of Tables 2 and 5.

Table 6. Needs estimation for Pakistan earthquake 2005.

Humanitarian Cluster	Specification	Per Person	Number	Estimated Need	Cluster Priority
WASH	Transportation containers (10–20 L)	0.2	2,800,000	560,000	194
	Storage containers (10–20 L)	0.2	2,800,000	560,000	194
	Blankets	1	2,800,000	2,800,000	194
	Total basic water needs	7.5–15 L/day	2,800,000	42,000,000	194
	Patients	60 L/day	75,000	4,500,000	194
	Open wells	1/400	2,800,000	7000	194
	Toilets	1/50 people	75,000	1500	194
Nutrition	Salt, iodised edible	1	2,800,000	2,800,000	194
	Fish, canned, sardines, veg oil, 150 g	2	2,800,000	5,600,000	194
	Pasta, durum wheat meal	1	2,800,000	2,800,000	194
	Rice, white, long grain, irri6/2	1	2,800,000	2,800,000	194
	Oil, rapeseed	1	2,800,000	2,800,000	194
	Beans, white, small	1	2,800,000	2,800,000	194
Shelter and settlement	Tarpaulins (4 m × 6 m)	0.2	2,800,000	560,000	200
	Ropes (30 m)	0.2	2,800,000	560,000	200
	Saws	0.2	2,800,000	560,000	200
	Roding, small and largo nail (1/2 kg each)	0.2	2,800,000	560,000	200
	Shovels	0.2	2,800,000	560,000	200
	Hoe	0.2	2,800,000	560,000	200
	Machete	0.2	2,800,000	560,000	200
Health cluster	Doctors	0.0457	75,000	3428	87.39
	Nurses	0.059	75,000	4425	87.39
	Others	0.06	75,000	4500	87.39

Table 6 is calculated based on the minimum standard requirement in Table 2. For example, in the health cluster the need for a doctor in Pakistan earthquake 2005, is 75,000 doctors or 16,605 L water/day. Additionally, the cluster priority column shows that the community is less likely to cope with shelter shortage than the other needs, so in allocating the resources, the shelter (200 cluster priority) needs to be prioritised slightly over nutrition and water (194 cluster priority) and then health needs (87 cluster priority). This is also confirmed by the number of displaced who would require shelter, water and food (2,800,000 people) as opposed to the number injured (75,000 people).

5.2. *Output: The Optimized Set of Resources Available from Different Suppliers*

By entering the preferences of the decision makers, their subjective views which can affect the decisions are taken into account. The supply is the optimised in terms of the ranks of suppliers who have resources available for the required response phase.

5.2.1. Building AHP Model Based on Decision Makers' Preferences

Due to the subjective nature of decisions, different decision makers, provided with the same options and data, make different decisions, based on their preferences. In disaster situation when we have different suppliers, choosing between different suppliers and their resources is important to optimise the allocation of resources. A set of questionnaires are conducted from experts in disaster management field. The data collection process is described below.

Collecting Decision Maker's Preferences

This questionnaire was provided to the participants which overall took three weeks to complete for 42 participants. The information about the research and invitation for participation was distributed amongst various organisations (Environment agency, Crisis departments of five different embassies, Business continuity departments of Munich RE,

Barclays Bank and Lloyds bank, and individuals who had connections with humanitarian organisations including UN, UNISDR, UNICEF, World Vision, Caritas International, British Red Cross, American Red Cross, Save the children and various specialised forums and groups related to disaster management on LinkedIn (including Business Continuity and Disaster Recovery Professionals, Business Continuity Management & Risk, Business Continuity/Disaster Recovery Network, Disaster & Emergency Management, Disaster, Disaster, Disaster Management—Multi Hazard Risk Assessment, Disaster Researchers and Disaster Management Professionals, Disaster Risk Management Practitioners, Emergency Preparedness Consultants/Trainers Group, GWU Institute for Crisis, Disaster and Risk Management, Humanitarian & Disaster Response Technology Network, Innovations in Disaster Management and Emergency Response !,Natural disasters and natural hazards, Natural Hazards and Disaster Risk Management, Performance Management, Professionals in Emergency Management, World Conference on Disaster Management). 68 people initially expressed interest and were sent the questionnaire but at the end 42 filled questionnaires were returned.

The respondents are asked to identify in respect to each one, the criteria for partner selection which criterion is more important and how much more important on a scale of 1 to 9. This is the basis for questionnaire 1 (decision preference). These criteria include the type of partners (Government, NGO, Military, International organisations such as Red Cross and UN and volunteers), size, experience of the partners, their surge capacity (the ability to rapidly expand beyond normal capacity to meet the increased demand) and their cluster (WASH, nutrition, health, shelter). The first questionnaire is given to both groups of participants in order to identify their preferences. The goal, criteria, and sub-criteria considered in this questionnaire are articulated in Figure 4.

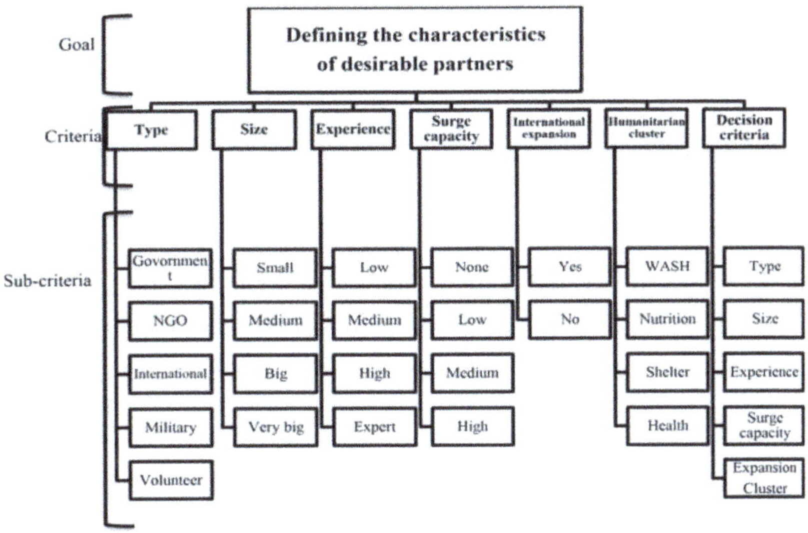

Figure 4. Components of the questionnaire about the selection decision.

The first row in Figure 4 shows that the goal of this questionnaire is to define the characteristics of the desirable partners in the view of each decision maker. The second row gathers the data about the characteristics of the desired partner in terms of the following criteria: *Type of the partner* in respect of being governmental, NGO, International, Military or Volunteer organisation as sub criteria. *Size of the partners* based on ANLAP's (2012) categories for humanitarian organisations, being Small (under 10 million USD expenditure), Medium (between 10–49 million USD expenditure), Big (between 50–99 million USD expenditure) and Very big (more than 100 million USD expenditure). *Experience of the partners* being Low (Under 5 disasters), Medium (Under 10 disasters), High (under 50 disasters) and Expert (more than 50 disasters). *Partner's surge capacity* (the ability to rapidly expand beyond normal capacity to meet the increased demand) being None (0% of the total capacity), Low (under 10% of the total capacity), Medium (under 30% of the total capacity) and High (over 30% of the total capacity). *Partner's international expansion* being Yes (expanded internationally such as UN), No (expanded only locally such as local charities). *Partner's ability* to address the needs for humanitarian cluster being WASH, Nutrition, Health, and Shelter. So the numerical preferences for the above decision criteria being type, size, experience, surge capacity, expansion and cluster is collected through the questionnaire in Table 7.

Table 7. Pairwise Comparison Questionnaire to elicit decision-maker's preferences.

	How Much More Important								Equal	How Much Less Important								
1									Type of the partners									
Government	9	8	7	6	5	4	3	2	1	2	3	4	5	6	7	8	9	NGO
Government	9	8	7	6	5	4	3	2	1	2	3	4	5	6	7	8	9	Military
Government	9	8	7	6	5	4	3	2	1	2	3	4	5	6	7	8	9	International
Government	9	8	7	6	5	4	3	2	1	2	3	4	5	6	7	8	9	Volunteers
NGO	9	8	7	6	5	4	3	2	1	2	3	4	5	6	7	8	9	Military
NGO	9	8	7	6	5	4	3	2	1	2	3	4	5	6	7	8	9	International
NGO	9	8	7	6	5	4	3	2	1	2	3	4	5	6	7	8	9	Volunteers
Military	9	8	7	6	5	4	3	2	1	2	3	4	5	6	7	8	9	International
Military	9	8	7	6	5	4	3	2	1	2	3	4	5	6	7	8	9	Volunteers
Volunteer	9	8	7	6	5	4	3	2	1	2	3	4	5	6	7	8	9	International
2									Size of the partner									
Small	9	8	7	6	5	4	3	2	1	2	3	4	5	6	7	8	9	Medium
Small	9	8	7	6	5	4	3	2	1	2	3	4	5	6	7	8	9	Big
Small	9	8	7	6	5	4	3	2	1	2	3	4	5	6	7	8	9	Very big
Medium	9	8	7	6	5	4	3	2	1	2	3	4	5	6	7	8	9	Big
Medium	9	8	7	6	5	4	3	2	1	2	3	4	5	6	7	8	9	Very big
Big	9	8	7	6	5	4	3	2	1	2	3	4	5	6	7	8	9	Very big
3									Experience of the partners									
Low	9	8	7	6	5	4	3	2	1	2	3	4	5	6	7	8	9	Medium
Low	9	8	7	6	5	4	3	2	1	2	3	4	5	6	7	8	9	High
Low	9	8	7	6	5	4	3	2	1	2	3	4	5	6	7	8	9	Expert
Medium	9	8	7	6	5	4	3	2	1	2	3	4	5	6	7	8	9	High
Medium	9	8	7	6	5	4	3	2	1	2	3	4	5	6	7	8	9	Expert
High	9	8	7	6	5	4	3	2	1	2	3	4	5	6	7	8	9	Expert

Table 7. *Cont.*

	How Much More Important								Equal	How Much Less Important								
4									Partner's surge capacity									
None	9	8	7	6	5	4	3	2	1	2	3	4	5	6	7	8	9	Low
None	9	8	7	6	5	4	3	2	1	2	3	4	5	6	7	8	9	Medium
None	9	8	7	6	5	4	3	2	1	2	3	4	5	6	7	8	9	High
Low	9	8	7	6	5	4	3	2	1	2	3	4	5	6	7	8	9	Medium
Low	9	8	7	6	5	4	3	2	1	2	3	4	5	6	7	8	9	High
Medium	9	8	7	6	5	4	3	2	1	2	3	4	5	6	7	8	9	High
5									International expansion									
Yes	9	8	7	6	5	4	3	2	1	2	3	4	5	6	7	8	9	No
6									Humanitarian cluster									
WASH cluster	9	8	7	6	5	4	3	2	1	2	3	4	5	6	7	8	9	Nutrition cluster
WASH cluster	9	8	7	6	5	4	3	2	1	2	3	4	5	6	7	8	9	Shelter cluster
WASH cluster	9	8	7	6	5	4	3	2	1	2	3	4	5	6	7	8	9	Health cluster
Nutrition cluster	9	8	7	6	5	4	3	2	1	2	3	4	5	6	7	8	9	Shelter cluster
Nutrition cluster	9	8	7	6	5	4	3	2	1	2	3	4	5	6	7	8	9	Health cluster
Shelter cluster	9	8	7	6	5	4	3	2	1	2	3	4	5	6	7	8	9	Health cluster
7									Decision criteria									
Type	9	8	7	6	5	4	3	2	1	2	3	4	5	6	7	8	9	Size
Type	9	8	7	6	5	4	3	2	1	2	3	4	5	6	7	8	9	Experience
Type	9	8	7	6	5	4	3	2	1	2	3	4	5	6	7	8	9	Surge capacity
Type	9	8	7	6	5	4	3	2	1	2	3	4	5	6	7	8	9	International Expansion
Type	9	8	7	6	5	4	3	2	1	2	3	4	5	6	7	8	9	Cluster
Size	9	8	7	6	5	4	3	2	1	2	3	4	5	6	7	8	9	Experience
Size	9	8	7	6	5	4	3	2	1	2	3	4	5	6	7	8	9	Surge capacity
Size	9	8	7	6	5	4	3	2	1	2	3	4	5	6	7	8	9	International Expansion
Size	9	8	7	6	5	4	3	2	1	2	3	4	5	6	7	8	9	Cluster
Experience	9	8	7	6	5	4	3	2	1	2	3	4	5	6	7	8	9	Surge capacity
Experience	9	8	7	6	5	4	3	2	1	2	3	4	5	6	7	8	9	International Expansion
Experience	9	8	7	6	5	4	3	2	1	2	3	4	5	6	7	8	9	Cluster
Surge capacity	9	8	7	6	5	4	3	2	1	2	3	4	5	6	7	8	9	International Expansion
Surge capacity	9	8	7	6	5	4	3	2	1	2	3	4	5	6	7	8	9	Cluster
International Expansion	9	8	7	6	5	4	3	2	1	2	3	4	5	6	7	8	9	Cluster

The data gathered in this questionnaire was then used to calculate the preference weights using AHP. The preferences of the decision maker can be quantified using AHP. This is calculated by a set of pairwise comparison matrices where the verbal preference (e.g., extremely less/more important) is translated into numerical values (e.g., 1/9 to 9). The AHP weight calculated for these values can get values from zero to 1.0 or from 0% to 100% as shown in Figure 5.

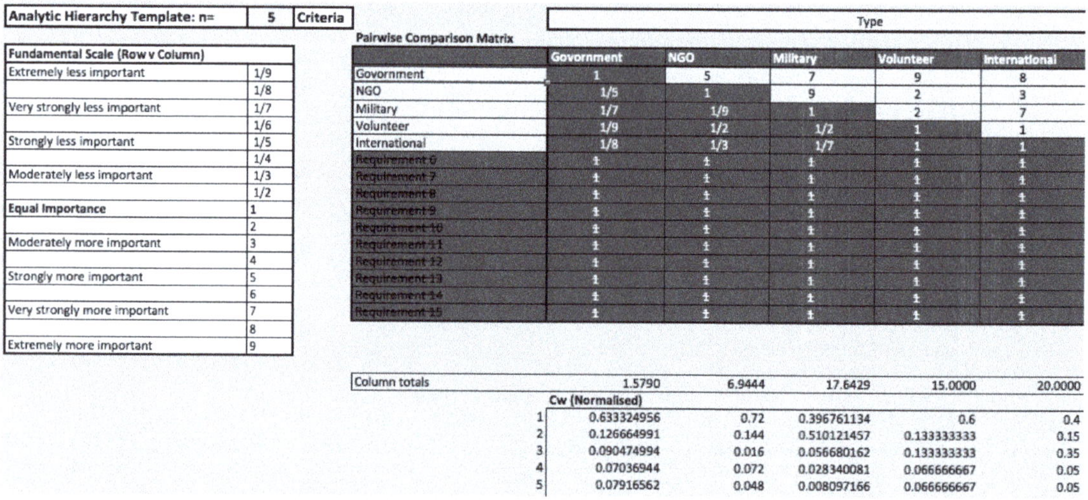

Figure 5. A snapshot of the process of calculating AHP preference.

Imagine we have a decision maker who prefers to be involved government organisation the most; in other words, if s/he wanted to decide based on the type of the organisation s/he would definitely choose the government over International organisations. A decision maker with the AHP values is calculated as the government had the highest value for this particular participant (60.8%) whilst the International organisations and volunteers had the lowest value (6.5%) as shown in Table 8.

Table 8. Example: The preferences of one of the participants towards the type of the partners.

	AHP	
1	0.608	60.80%
2	0.168	16.80%
3	0.094	9.40%
4	0.065	6.50%
5	0.065	6.50%

For example, in Figure 5 the government had the highest value for this participant (60.8%) whilst the international organisations and volunteers had the lowest value (6.5%). In other words, if s/he wanted to decide based on the type of the organisation s/he would definitely choose the government over international organisations. This process gives a full set of preference for each unit of resource per partner, presented in Table 9.

Table 9. Example of AHP for participant/unit of resource per partner.

Resources	AHP Weight	Partner 1	Partner 2	Partner 3	Partner 4	Partner 5
Total basic water needs	0.58407534	0.46365588	0.49915368	0.60237036	0.7427232	0.6225768
Rice	0.12190161	0.09676902	0.10417772	0.12571994	0.1550128	0.1299372
Tent	0.7279017	0.5778294	0.6220684	0.7507018	0.925616	0.775884
Doctors	0.09822288	0.07797216	0.08394176	0.10129952	0.1249024	0.1046976

Table 9 shows that the preference for doctors (a resource in the health cluster) for this participant is AHP = 0.98 or 9.8%; whilst s/he considered water (a resource in the WASH cluster) much more important (AHP = 0.58 or 58%). In addition, the AHP weight of each resource for each partner was calculated. For example, the water provided by Partner

4 had a higher preference (74%) than the water provided by partner 2 (49%) due to the preference this participant had towards the characteristics of these partners (including type, size, expansion and so on).

5.2.2. Calculating MAUT for Each Supplier

Based on the above priorities calculated by AHP, the MAUT produced for each supplier can be calculated as follows. $Ui(x)$ is a single utility function or preference function associated with candidate i, which represents the utility values the decision maker attaches to each candidate and is obtained by using the AHP process. To aggregate the scores of each attribute in the MAUT process, the linear additive utility form is the frequently simplified assessment procedure as given by Equation (1)—Utility function of the candidates based on the available resources:

$$V(yi) = \sum_{i=1}^{n} rij.ui(x).$$

where rij represents the resource j available to candidate i. The $V(yi)$ will be the value of the candidate i because of the resource j they have available. The AHP weights calculated before then were used to calculate the utility of each resource as well as the utility of that resource for that partner Table 10.

Table 10. An example of the utility for a participant.

Resource	Utility	Partner 1	Partner 2	Partner 3	Partner 4	Partner 5
Water	25.115	15.301	42.927	23.492	13.369	47.316
Rice	4.145	7.548	10.001	5.406	15.346	10.785
Tent	67.695	39.292	14.308	22.521	71.272	51.984
Doctors	6.778	4.834	3.442	6.078	7.744	8.899

For example, in Table 9 the utility of the water provided by Partner 1 is 15.30, whilst the utility of water for all the partners is 25.11. The total utility of all the resources that each partner holds can be calculated as the accumulated values of that partner's utilities. For example, for these particular participants, the utility of partners can be calculated and be used to rank the partners as exhibited in Table 11.

Table 11. Example of partners ranked/participant's preferences.

Rank	Partner	Total Utility	Type	Size	Expansion	Experience	Surge Capacity
1	Partner 5	1520.572	Government	Small	Yes	Low	Low
2	Partner 14	1371.679	Government	Small	No	Low	Low
3	Partner 18	1354.951	Government	Small	Yes	Low	Very high
4	Partner 12	1307.894	Government	Small	Yes	High	High
5	Partner 16	1164.387	Government	Medium	Yes	Low	Very high
6	Partner 6	1146.227	NGO	Small	No	Very high	Low
7	Partner 13	1052.240	Volunteer	Small	Yes	Medium	Low
8	Partner 3	1031.565	Volunteer	Medium	Yes	High	High
9	Partner 10	1030.562	Volunteer	Small	Yes	High	Very high
10	Partner 9	1016.646	Government	Medium	No	High	Very high

Table 11 shows an example of the rankings of the partners based on this participant's preferences. For example, Partner 5 is the most desirable partner with a utility of 1520. This also shows that the most desirable partners for these participants are small governmental entities. In addition, it seems that this participant does not value the experience or the surge capacity of the partners as critical requirements for a disaster response. Finally, the experts were asked to fill out the second questionnaire. An example of the accumulated data is exhibited in Table 12.

Table 12. An example of the result of the optimise resource-based decision-making.

Resource Name	Resource Code	Total Resources	Required Resources	Utility	Supplier 1	Supplier 2,	Supplier 300
Transportation container	N1	20.5065	221.4	0.0007	0.1324	0.1185	0.1087
Storage containers	N2	108.1904	221.4	0.0007	0.1467	0.0147	0.2348
Toilets	N4	21.0673	1107	0.0007	0.0411	0.0675	0.0675
Blankets	N6	22.3937	1107	0.0007	0.0235	0.0895	0.0205
basic water	N16	110.1125	16605	0.0007	0.3155	0.2421	0.6309
Patient water	N17	1.4999	66420	0.0007	0.0005	0.0062	0.0054
Open Well	N18	28.3749	4.428	0.0007	0.0661	0.0717	0.117
FISH150 g	N19	5573.1222	2.214	0.0007	23.1098	30.4462	12.8388
RICE,	N22	1074.4942	221.4	0.0017	3.0079	6.236	5.0621
SALT,	N23	107.6255	221.4	0.0017	0.044	0.6309	0.5722
PASTA	N27	54.8545	221.4	0.0017	0.1541	0.2788	0.0734
OIL, rapeseed	N29	114.2209	221.4	0.0017	0.2421	0.6016	0.4915
Tarpaulins	N31	109.3716	442.8	0.0099	0.6823	0.4989	0.1687
Ropes (30 m)	N32	55.6266	6642	0.0099	0.1264	0.3233	0.1003
Saws	N33	3.6562	1107	0.0099	0.0107	0.0193	0.0111
Roding	N34	21.323	110.7	0.0099	0.0862	0.1442	0.1011
Shovels	N35	232.2283	1107	0.0099	0.4906	0.8176	1.4122
Hoes	N36	22.5286	1107	0.0099	0.0535	0.0416	0.11
Machetes	N37	21.6605	1107	0.0099	0.0981	0.0937	0.0937
Doctors	N42	0.0372	0.5115	0.0103	0.0112	0.0133	0.0038
Nurses	N43	32.313	0.8775	0.0103	25.3685	30.1751	2.6237

Table 12 shows that for example, in this scenario the total available resources N42 = Doctors, are 0.0372 for each 100 people. However, the number of required doctors is more than 0.515 for 100 people. Although due to the scarcity of this resource, and the fact that the decision maker needs all the helps s/he could get, it is still possible to rank the Suppliers based on the decision maker's preference. As you see, the utility of the doctors that Supplier 2 can provide (0.133) is greater than the number doctors that Supplier 1 can provide (0.0112). In addition, as can be seen in this case the utility of the health cluster (0.103) is more than the other clusters. The utility of the shelter cluster is 0.099, whilst the utility of the nutrition is 0.017 and WASH is 0.0007. Therefore, if a decision maker must decide which need to prioritise, s/he should first consider choosing the Suppliers who can provide the doctors, nurses, etcetera, rather than the Suppliers who can provide, food, water, or shelter.

5.2.3. Ranking Suppliers Based on Their MAUT

To get a better understanding about how the Suppliers in different scenarios for different decision makers may differ, an example is presented in Table 13.

Table 13. An example of the Suppliers ranked based on MAUT.

Scenario1, Decision Maker 2		Scenario 2, Decision Maker 2		Scenario 1, Decision Maker 1		Scenario 2, Decision Maker 1	
Supplier Number	MAUT rank	Supplier Number	MAUT rank	Supplier Number	MAUT rank	Supplier Number	MAUT rank
153	1.132760	211	9.145249	41	0.633922	284	1.729715
41	1.093821	156	9.040183	2	0.627644	211	1.718803
103	1.091799	284	9.018674	34	0.626475	2	1.701977
49	1.087162	57	8.936134	147	0.624786	29	1.691246
34	1.074619	238	8.921111	188	0.624258	238	1.690334
89	1.059594	43	8.817729	89	0.619832	59	1.683765
147	1.045495	29	8.813828	128	0.618894	221	1.665627
47	1.042461	132	8.809210	49	0.618527	158	1.657653
258	1.041538	158	8.665270	103	0.614152	16	1.635905
2	1.038681	47	8.611685	64	0.605774	57	1.628362

Table 13 shows the ranking of the Suppliers based on the highest utility to the lowest for this example. Based on the preferences of decision maker 2 and the needs predicted in scenario 1, Supplier 153 with a total utility of 1.13 is the best option followed by Supplier 41 with 1.09 utility, etc.

6. Discussion

The present research is designed to provide a technique for Supplier ranking/selection in disaster response. The research employs various techniques including analysing the archival data, and decision support tools including Linear programming optimisation, Analytical Hierarchy processing (AHP), Multi-attribute utility theory (MAUT) to develop several decision techniques based on secondary data. This research provides an approach to Supplier configuration in disaster situation in two phases. The ESTIMATION process answers the first research questions is "how to estimate the needs of the affected population at the time of the disaster strike?". Using various resources, the minimum standard requirements for a disaster response in four humanitarian clusters (WASH, Nutrition, Health and Shelter) was defined. This estimation was used as the basis for estimating the demand of the affected population in disasters. This exceeds the use of minimum standard requirements provided by the Sphere project because it draws upon various sources to provide the data about the required units of medical help and nutrition.

This framework could also further be developed to provide data about fatality management, evacuation, and required well contamination teams. This also complements the existing literature on provide the priority of the disaster type, and tasks during each disaster type. Even though some linguistic priorities are practiced in the literature [76], the numerical priorities that can contribute to the quantification of the needs were missing. The priorities suggested in this research are required to be investigated further with the fuzzy logic analysis of the experts' opinions regarding the priorities of each, task/need for each disaster type/country. However, this is another extensive research in its own merit and is out of scope of this research. The OPTIMISATION process answers the second question "how to optimise the selected set of suppliers (and their resources) based on the decision maker' preferences. This is a framework for disaster response supplier selection using the principles of utility theory. In this step, the Suppliers are ranked based on their importance for hypothetical decision makers. Using the AHP technique, a matrix of hypothetical decision makers' preferences is built and used to find the value of each Supplier in the eye of the decision maker. This step can be defined as a resource allocation problem with the target of optimising the utility of the response Suppliers' set for each decision maker. The optimisation here is like a variety of supplier selections based on MCDM [125,126]. The variable which needs to be maximised is the utility of the suppliers in the eye of the agent (here the decision maker).

The EDIS can be complementary to the abundance of existing methods for task allocation and scheduling techniques [71,127,128] in disaster management, as a quicker data feed. Furthermore, the research shows that comparing to the existing decision models in humanitarian sector the EDIS could prevails the existing guideline based on highly specialised data in HAZUS [129] or highly subjective decision maker's preferences in HISS [130] from The European Interagency Security Forum (IESF). In a sense, EDIS gives numerical estimations, and clearly expressed choices of suppliers whilst it is using simple available data. Contribution to theory is that it provides a unique insight into the growing body of research a part of decision-making under uncertainty where it is attempted to reduce the uncertainty by "gaining accumulated access" to other firms' resources meaning that every member has access to the resources of all the other members. This is based on the principles of resource- dependency theory and through collaboration. Because the collaboration act in practice is no guarantee of a successful disaster response due to the interaction of contributors, the most suitable group of suppliers to accumulate and share their resources are selected based on the optimisation technique using the principles of the utility theory.

Methodological contribution is that this model provides a design to simulate the decision-making under uncertainty in the disaster situation by considering the opinion of human agents (decision maker). It also uses mathematical optimisation in addition to the opinion of human agents, which integrates the heuristic and mathematical approaches of decision-making. This also complements the existing literature by drawing upon various studies to provide the priority of the disaster type, and tasks during each disaster type. Even though some linguistic priorities are practiced in the literature (Sphere project, 2011), the numerical priorities that can contribute to the quantification of the needs were missing. Practical contribution is that by providing a range of it enables the decision maker to decide based on their budget limitations and personal preferences. It also gives different humanitarian organisations the chance to customise the model using their own database if required. The practical contribution of the article is the needs estimation tool. This framework uses various resources to articulate the minimum standard requirements for disaster response in four humanitarian charter clusters (WASH, Nutrition, Health, and Shelter).

The humanitarian organisations could use this tool to estimate the resources required to response to the needs of the affected population before the MIRA report is released. The significance is threefold. First, it is the first decision framework of its type that enables the decision maker to estimate the needs and select the partners using the data that are readily available for each country at the time of the disaster. Reliance on the available data at the time of the disaster, which are freely available to the public would reduce the cost of the data gathering, and the time required for collecting and analysing these data. Consequently, it speeds up the response time of the operation to the disaster by almost 72 h, which is vital at the time of the disaster. In addition, it is the only existing framework not limited to a certain type of disaster (although it just considers the five types of disasters) or geographical or chronological order. Another contribution is that the model has the capability of accommodating the socioeconomic characteristics of the affected population, which hugely influences the required aid in humanitarian response practices. The authors also believes that this model in long-term could facilitate establishing a centralised database for humanitarian response which is long overdue.

7. Limitations and Future Research Direction

The first limitation of this work is the lack of secondary data regarding the specific requirements of non-key-life-saving activities which led to the exclusion of them from the study. However, the principles of this research can be extrapolated to non-key life-saving activities when the data is available. However, data collection on this scale requires the co-operation of various humanitarian organisations including the UN, IFRC, and government related organisations, in addition to the private and public humanitarian organisations and charities (like the process in the sphere project) and is out with the scope of the current research. management, evacuation, and required well contamination teams.

Second, the priorities suggested in this research are required to be investigated further with the fuzzy logic analysis of the experts' opinions regarding the priorities of each, task/need for each disaster type/country. However, this is out of scope of this research. Nevertheless, this research provides the preliminary basis for the further development of such framework.

The third limitation is that the EDIS model is based on two major assumptions. The first assumption is that a data base for humanitarian suppliers already exists. However, creating and maintaining such a database requires the cooperation of the international humanitarian bodies. The model cannot be fully tested before the creation of a standardised accredited database containing data on humanitarian suppliers, their selection criteria, and regular updates of the database. This project can be further discussed with international humanitarian entities with regard to the applicability of launching a universal initiative for gathering data and building a universal humanitarian database. The model is built upon secondary data from various sources amongst others in which the data varies from case to case. Therefore, the model is only as accurate as its data feed.

The fourth limitation is that the optimisation constraints in this model are just the resources, the optimisation could be improved if other constraints such as time and cost could be considered. This could also be improved if the tasks can be separately defined in detail, and then the task allocation and resources related to the allocated task of each supplier could be optimised. Although the contribution of the current study is its model, further empirical research is required to develop an extensive database for the potential humanitarian suppliers at the industry level. The future research direction could follow different paths. For example, the EDIS model is based on the resources-based optimisation, it considers the decision makers' preference and characteristics in various other criteria such as experience, type, and size of the organisation, its surge capacity, and international expansion.

Further research is required to identify the actual non-resource based determinants of supplier selection in disaster response. Another suggestion is to provide a holistic research study involving all humanitarian actors to further identify and standardise the minimum requirements in a disaster response by considering the actual disaster type, and the geographical location and culture of each potential affected county. Another path could be the application of the EDIS model to various case studies and analyse the result and the areas of improvement. In addition, the EDIS model could be more accurately customised if it could analyse the data for each individual country, where it is possible to define exact scenarios for each disaster type, and the needs and suppliers required. This also may greatly improve the quality of estimations. The EDIS model is based on two major assumptions. The first assumption is that a pool of humanitarian partners already exists. However, creating and maintaining it requires the cooperation of the international humanitarian bodies.

The model cannot be fully tested before the creation of a standardised accredited database containing data on humanitarian partners, their selection criteria, and regular updates of the database. This project can be further discussed with international humanitarian entities with regard to the applicability of launching a universal initiative for gathering data and building a universal humanitarian database. Second, the model is built upon secondary data from various sources (Emdat.be, 2014, Munichre.com, 2014; ReliefWeb, 2013a; Gdacs.org, 2014), amongst others in which the data varies from case to case. Therefore, the model is only as accurate as its data feed. Although the contribution of the current study is its model, further empirical research is required to develop an extensive database for the potential humanitarian partners at the industry level.

The future research direction could follow different paths. For example, the EDIS model is based on the resources-based optimisation, it takes into account the decision makers' preference and characteristics in various other criteria such as experience, type, and size of the organisation, its surge capacity, and international expansion. Further research is required to identify the actual non-resource-based determinants of partner selection in collaborative networks with the focus on disaster response. Another suggestion is to provide a holistic research study involving all humanitarian actors in order to further identify and standardise the minimum requirements in a disaster response by considering the actual disaster type, and the geographical location and culture of each potential affected county. Another path could be the application of the EDIS model to various case studies and analyse the result and the areas of improvement.

Author Contributions: Conceptualisation: S.R.; methodology: S.R.; validation: S.R.; formal analysis: S.R.; investigation: S.R.; resources: S.R.; writing—original draft preparation: S.R.; Writing—review and editing: E.A. and S.R.; visualitaion: S.R.; supervision: E.A.; project administration: S.R. All authors have read and agreed to the published version of the manuscript.

Funding: This research received no external funding.

Institutional Review Board Statement: The study was conducted in accordance with the Declaration of Helsinki, and approved by the Ethics Committee of Brunel University as part of a PhD dissertation approved in September 2014.

Informed Consent Statement: Informed consent was obtained from all subjects involved in the study.

Data Availability Statement: The data presented in this study are available on request from the corresponding author. The data are not publicly available due to privacy of the humanitarian participants.

Conflicts of Interest: The authors declare no conflict of interest.

References

1. UNDRO. *Shelter after Disaster*; UNDRO: Geneva, Switzerland, 1982.
2. UNDRO. *An Overview of Disaster Management*; UNDRO: Geneva, Switzerland, 1992.
3. Environment Agency—What's in Your Backyard? Available online: http://apps.environment-agency.gov.uk/wiyby/default.aspx (accessed on 15 February 2021).
4. Russell, S.; Norvig, P. Artificial Intelligence: A Modern Approach. 1995. Available online: https://www.pearson.com/us/higher-education/program/Russell-Artificial-Intelligence-A-Modern-Approach-4th-Edition/PGM1263338.html (accessed on 29 April 2021).
5. Tversky, A.; Kahneman, D. Judgment under Uncertainty: Heuristics and Biases. *Science* **1974**, *185*, 1124–1131. [CrossRef] [PubMed]
6. Keykhah, M. The Shape of Uncertainty: Insurance Underwriting in the Face of Catastrophe Risk. Ph.D. Thesis, Oxford University, Oxford, UK, 2000.
7. Moe, T.L.; Pathranarakul, P.; Kyne, D. An integrated approach to natural disaster management: Public project management and its critical success factors. *Disaster Prev. Manag. Int. J.* **2006**, *15*, 396–413. [CrossRef]
8. Reinecke, I. International Disaster Response Law and the Coordination of International Organisations. *ANU Undergrad. Res. J.* **2010**, *2*, 143–163. [CrossRef]
9. Tierney, K.; Trainor, J. *Center Disaster*; MCEER: Buffalo, NY, USA, 2004; pp. 157–172.
10. Rolland, E.; Patterson, R.A.; Ward, K.; Dodin, B. Decision support for disaster management. *Oper. Manag. Res.* **2010**, *3*, 68–79. [CrossRef]
11. Telford, J.; Cosgrave, H. *Joint Evaluation of the International Response to the Indian Ocean Tsunami: Synthesis Report*; Tsunami Evaluation Coalition (TEC): London, UK, 2006; ISBN 0 85003 807 3.
12. Careem, M.; Silva, C.D.; Silva, R.D.; Raschidt, L.; Weerawarana, S. Sahana: Overview of a disaster management system. In Proceedings of the 2006 International Conference on Information and Automation, Shandong, China, 15–17 December 2006; pp. 361–366. [CrossRef]
13. Inomata, T. Towards a United Nations Humanitarian Assistance Programme for Disaster Response and Reduction: Lessons Learned from the Indian Ocean Tsunami Disaster, Geneva. 2006. Available online: https://digitallibrary.un.org/record/601740 (accessed on 29 April 2021).
14. Balcik, B.; Beamon, B.M.; Krejci, C.C.; Muramatsu, K.M.; Ramirez, M. Coordination in humanitarian relief chains: Practices, challenges and opportunities. *Int. J. Prod. Econ.* **2010**, *126*, 22–34. [CrossRef]
15. Van Wassenhove, L.N. Humanitarian aid logistics: Supply chain management in high gear. *J. Oper. Res. Soc.* **2006**, *57*, 475–489. [CrossRef]
16. Zhang, J.-H.; Li, J.; Liu, Z.-P. Multiple-resource and multiple-depot emergency response problem considering secondary disasters. *Expert Syst. Appl.* **2012**, *39*, 11066–11071. [CrossRef]
17. Comfort, L.K. Crisis Management in Hindsight: Cognition, Communication, Coordination, and Control. *Public Adm. Rev.* **2007**, *67*, 189–197. [CrossRef]
18. Oloruntoba, R.; Gray, R. Humanitarian aid: An agile supply chain? *Supply Chain Manag. Int. J.* **2006**, *11*, 115–120. [CrossRef]
19. Pettit, S.; Beresford, A. Critical success factors in the context of humanitarian aid supply chains. *Int. J. Phys. Distrib. Logist. Manag.* **2009**, *39*, 450–468. [CrossRef]
20. Altay, N.; Green, W.G., III. Interfaces with Other Disciplines OR/MS research in disaster operations management. *Eur. J. Oper. Res.* **2006**, *175*, 475–493. [CrossRef]
21. Simpson, N.C.; Hancock, P.G. Fifty years of operational research and emergency response. *J. Oper. Res. Soc.* **2009**, *60*, S126–S139. [CrossRef]
22. Sahebjamnia, N.; Torabi, S.A.; Mansouri, A. A hybrid decision support system for managing humanitarian relief chains. *Decis. Support Syst.* **2017**, *95*, 12–26. [CrossRef]
23. Nappi, M.M.L.; Souza, J.C. Disaster management: Hierarchical structuring criteria for selection and location of temporary shelters. *Nat. Hazards* **2014**, *75*, 2421–2436. [CrossRef]
24. Cavdur, F.; Sebatli, A. A decision support tool for allocating temporary-disaster-response facilities. *Decis. Support Syst.* **2019**, *127*, 113145. [CrossRef]
25. Mikhailov, L. Fuzzy analytical approach to partnership selection in formation of virtual enterprises. *Omega* **2002**, *30*, 393–401. [CrossRef]

26. Sarkis, J.; Talluri, S.; Gunasekaran, A. A strategic model for agile virtual enterprise partner selection. *Int. J. Oper. Prod. Manag.* **2007**, *27*, 1213–1234. [CrossRef]
27. Huang, M.; Fan, C. Research on the Partner Selection of Virtual Enterprise Based on Self-adaptive Genetic Algorithm. In Proceedings of the Third International Conference on Intelligent Information Hiding and Multimedia Signal Processing (IIH-MSP 2007), Kaohsiung, Taiwan, 26–28 November 2007.
28. Xiang, D.; Li, Q. Study on Partner Selection Method for Construction Supply Chain Using Tabu? Search Algorithm. In Proceedings of the 2012 International Conference on Information Management, Innovation Management and Industrial Engineering, Sanya, China, 20–21 October 2012; pp. 122–125.
29. Mohamed, A.M.; Abdelsalam, H.M. Optimal Composition of Virtual Enterprises with Interval Cost Parameters. In Proceedings of the 2012 8th International Conference on Informatics and Systems (INFOS), Giza, Egypt, 14–16 May 2012.
30. Zeng, Z.; Li, Y.; Li, S.; Zhu, W. A New Algorithm for Partner Selection in Virtual Enterprise. In Proceedings of the Sixth International Conference on Parallel and Distributed Computing Applications and Technologies (PDCAT'05), Dalian, China, 5–8 December 2005; pp. 884–886. [CrossRef]
31. Zhan, J. A Novel Partner Selection Solution Based on the Clonal Selection Algorithm. In Proceedings of the 2008 International Conference on Information Management, Innovation Management and Industrial Engineering, Taipei, Taiwan, 19–21 December 2008; Volume 1, pp. 191–194. [CrossRef]
32. Zhan, J. A Binary Ant Algorithm for Partner Selection Problem in the Virtual Enterprise. In Proceedings of the 2009 International Conference on E-Business and Information System Security, Wuhan, China, 23–24 May 2009; pp. 1–4. [CrossRef]
33. Xiao, J.; Qi, F.; Li, Y. Gravitational chaotic search algorithm for partners selection with due date constraint in virtual enterprise. In Proceedings of the Fourth International Workshop on Advanced Computational Intelligence, Wuhan, China, 19–21 October 2011; pp. 138–142. [CrossRef]
34. Jana, S.; Majumder, R.; Menon, P.P.; Ghose, D. Decision Support System (DSS) for Hierarchical Allocation of Resources and Tasks for Disaster Management. *Oper. Res. Forum* **2022**, *3*, 1–30. [CrossRef]
35. Hashemipour, M.; Stuban, S.M.F.; Dever, J.R. A community-based disaster coordination framework for effective disaster preparedness and response. *Aust. J. Emerg. Manag.* **2017**, *32*, 41.
36. Li, X.; Pu, W.; Zhao, X. Agent action diagram: Toward a model for emergency management system. *Simul. Model. Pract. Theory* **2019**, *94*, 66–99. [CrossRef]
37. Wang, Z.; Zhang, J. Agent-based evaluation of humanitarian relief goods supply capability. *Int. J. Disaster Risk Reduct.* **2019**, *36*, 101105. [CrossRef]
38. Othman, S.B.; Zgaya, H.; Dotoli, M.; Hammadi, S. Supply Chains. *Control Eng. Pract.* **2017**, *59*, 27–43. [CrossRef]
39. Wang, F.; Pei, Z.; Dong, L.; Ma, J. Emergency Resource Allocation for Multi-Period Post-Disaster Using Multi-Objective Cellular Genetic Algorithm. *IEEE Access* **2020**, *8*, 82255–82265. [CrossRef]
40. Faiz, T.I.; Vogiatzis, C.; Noor-E-Alam, M. A Column Generation Algorithm for Vehicle Scheduling and Routing Problems. *Comput. Ind. Eng.* **2019**, *130*, 222–236. [CrossRef]
41. Sun, J.; Zhang, Z. A post-disaster resource allocation framework for improving resilience of interdependent infrastructure networks. *Transp. Res. Part D Transp. Environ.* **2020**, *85*, 102455. [CrossRef]
42. Joshi, S.; Sharma, M.; Das, R.P.; Muduli, K.; Raut, R.; Narkhede, B.E.; Shee, H.; Misra, A. Assessing Effectiveness of Humanitarian Activities against COVID-19 Disruption: The Role of Blockchain-Enabled Digital Humanitarian Network (BT-DHN). *Sustainability* **2022**, *14*, 1904. [CrossRef]
43. Das, R.; Hanaoka, S. An agent-based model for resource allocation during relief distribution. *J. Humanit. Logist. Supply Chain Manag.* **2014**, *4*, 265–285. [CrossRef]
44. Doan, X.V.; Shaw, D. Resource allocation when planning for simultaneous disasters. *Eur. J. Oper. Res.* **2019**, *274*, 687–709. [CrossRef]
45. Majumder, R.; Warier, R.R.; Ghose, D. Game-Theoretic Model Based Resource Allocation During Floods. *arXiv* **2021**, arXiv:2112.01439.
46. Nagurney, A.; Flores, E.A.; Soylu, C. A Generalized Nash Equilibrium Network Model for Post-Disaster Humanitarian Relief. *Anna. Rev. CENIC Cienc. Biol.* **2016**, *152*, 28. Available online: https://supernet.isenberg.umass.edu/articles/Generalized_Nash_Equilibrium_for_Disaster_Relief.pdf (accessed on 13 September 2022). [CrossRef]
47. Yu, C.X.; Wong, T.N.; Wang, G. An agent-based negotiation model to support partner selection in a virtual enterprise. In Proceedings of the 40th International Conference on Computers & Indutrial Engineering, Awaji, Japan, 25–28 July 2010; pp. 1–6. [CrossRef]
48. Zhang, Y.; Geng, Z. Simulation analysis based on Multi-Agent for partner selection of cooperative R&D in virtual enterprise. In Proceedings of the 2010 Sixth International Conference on Natural Computation, Yantai, China, 10–12 August 2010; pp. 2940–2943. [CrossRef]
49. Yang, F.; Lin, P.-G.; Xu, R.-Z. An Emergency-Driven Virtual Organization Model for Emergency Management Based on Ontology. In Proceedings of the 2008 4th International Conference on Wireless Communications, Networking and Mobile Computing, Dalian, China, 12–14 October 2008; pp. 1–4. [CrossRef]
50. Mun, J.; Shin, M.; Jung, M. A goal-oriented trust model for virtual organization creation. *J. Intell. Manuf.* **2009**, *22*, 345–354. [CrossRef]

51. Baldo, F.; Rabelo, R.J.; Vallejos, R. A framework for selecting performance indicators for virtual organisation partners' search and selection. *Int. J. Prod. Res.* **2009**, *47*, 4737–4755. [CrossRef]
52. Schätter, F.; Hansen, O.; Wiens, M.; Schultmann, F. A decision support methodology for a disaster-caused business continuity management. *Decis. Support Syst.* **2019**, *118*, 10–20. [CrossRef]
53. Chaudhuri, N.; Bose, I. Exploring the role of deep neural networks for post-disaster decision support. *Decis. Support Syst.* **2020**, *130*, 113234. [CrossRef]
54. Chacko, J.; Rees, L.P.; Zobel, C.W.; Rakes, T.R.; Russell, R.S.; Ragsdale, C.T. Decision support for long-range, community-based planning to mitigate against and recover from potential multiple disasters. *Decis. Support Syst.* **2016**, *87*, 13–25. [CrossRef]
55. Arora, H.; Raghu, T.; Vinze, A. Resource allocation for demand surge mitigation during disaster response. *Decis. Support Syst.* **2010**, *50*, 304–315. [CrossRef]
56. Lin, C.-W.R.; Chen, H.-Y.S. A fuzzy strategic alliance selection framework for supply chain partnering under limited evaluation resources. *Comput. Ind.* **2004**, *55*, 159–179. [CrossRef]
57. Li, X.; Wang, J.; Yu, Y. An Optimal Partner Selection Approach Based on Prospect Theory. In Proceedings of the 2008 IEEE Symposium on Advanced Management of Information for Globalized Enterprises (AMIGE), Tianjin, China, 28–29 September 2008; pp. 1–5. [CrossRef]
58. Erkayman, B.; Gundogar, E.; Yılmaz, A. An Integrated Fuzzy Approach for Strategic Alliance Partner Selection in Third-Party Logistics. *Sci. World J.* **2012**, *2012*, 486306. [CrossRef]
59. Kara, S.S.; Ayadi, O.; Cheikhrouhou, N. An Extensive Group Decision Methodology for Alliance Partner Selection Problem in Collaborative Networked Organisations. *Int. J. Appl. Logist.* **2012**, *3*, 1–19. [CrossRef]
60. Lavrac, N.; Ljubic, P.; Urbancic, T.; Papa, G.; Jermol, M.; Bollhalter, S. Trust Modeling for Networked Organizations Using Reputation and Collaboration Estimates. *IEEE Trans. Syst. Man Cybern. Part C Appl. Rev.* **2008**, *37*, 429–439. [CrossRef]
61. Chang, M.-S.; Tseng, Y.-L.; Chen, J.-W. A scenario planning approach for the flood emergency logistics preparation problem under uncertainty. *Transp. Res. Part E Logist. Transp. Rev.* **2007**, *43*, 737–754. [CrossRef]
62. Wu, C.; Barnes, D.; Rosenberg, D.; Luo, X. An analytic network process-mixed integer multi-objective programming model for partner selection in agile supply chains. *Prod. Plan. Control* **2009**, *20*, 254–275. [CrossRef]
63. Zhao, L.; Fu, J.L. Game Analysis on Reputation Signals Restricting the Adverse Selection from Alliance Partners. In Proceedings of the 2011 IEEE International Conference on Grey Systems and Intelligent Services, Nanjing, China, 15–18 September 2011; pp. 163–165.
64. Kannan, D.; Khodaverdi, R.; Olfat, L.; Jafarian, A.; Diabat, A. Integrated fuzzy multi criteria decision making method and multi-objective programming approach for supplier selection and order allocation in a green supply chain. *J. Clean. Prod.* **2013**, *47*, 355–367. [CrossRef]
65. Peng, Y.; Zhang, Y.; Tang, Y.; Li, S. An incident information management framework based on data integration, data mining, and multi-criteria decision making. *Decis. Support Syst.* **2011**, *51*, 316–327. [CrossRef]
66. Ustun, O.; Demirtas, E.A. An integrated multi-objective decision-making process for multi-period lot-sizing with supplier selection. *Omega* **2008**, *36*, 509–521. [CrossRef]
67. Jarimo, T.; Salo, A. Multicriteria Partner Selection in Virtual Organizations With Transportation Costs and Other Network Interdependencies. *IEEE Trans. Syst. Man Cybern. Part C Appl. Rev.* **2008**, *39*, 124–129. [CrossRef]
68. Mircea, I.; Şerban, R.; Todose, D. Linear programming models applied in selection of partners in a virtual organization. In Proceedings of the 4th International Conference of ASECU–Development: Cooperation and Competitiveness, Bucharest, Romania, 22–24 May 2008; pp. 22–24.
69. Amailef, K.; Lu, J. Ontology-supported case-based reasoning approach for intelligent m-Government emergency response services. *Decis. Support Syst.* **2013**, *55*, 79–97. [CrossRef]
70. Keenan, P.B.; Jankowski, P. Spatial Decision Support Systems: Three decades on. *Decis. Support Syst.* **2018**, *116*, 64–76. [CrossRef]
71. Özdamar, L.; Ekinci, E.; Küçükyazici, B. Emergency Logistics Planning in Natural Disasters. *Ann. Oper. Res.* **2004**, *129*, 217–245. [CrossRef]
72. Maon, F.; Lindgreen, A.; Vanhamme, J. Developing supply chains in disaster relief operations through cross-sector socially oriented collaborations: A theoretical model. *Supply Chain Manag. Int. J.* **2009**, *14*, 149–164. [CrossRef]
73. Eßig, M.; Tandler, S. Disaster Response Supply Chain Management (SCM): Integration of Humanitarian and Defence Logistics by Means of SCM. In *Economic Impacts of Crisis Response Operations—An Underestimated Factor in External Engagement*; Landesverteidigungsakademie (LVAk)/Institut für Friedenssicherung und Konfliktmanagement (IFK): Vienna, Austria, 2009; pp. 283–310.
74. Tatham, P.; Spens, K. Towards a humanitarian logistics knowledge management system. *Disaster Prev. Manag. Int. J.* **2011**, *20*, 6–26. [CrossRef]
75. Wu, C.; Barnes, D. A dynamic feedback model for partner selection in agile supply chains. *Int. J. Oper. Prod. Manag.* **2012**, *32*, 79–103. [CrossRef]
76. van Zutphen, T.; Damerell, J. Sphereproject, Humanitarian Charter and Minimum Standards in Humanitarian Response. 2011. Available online: www.practicalactionpublishing.org/sphere (accessed on 15 February 2016).
77. IASC. Cluster Approach (IASC)—UNHCR | Emergency Handbook. Available online: https://emergency.unhcr.org/entry/41813/cluster-approach-iasc (accessed on 15 February 2021).

78. van Andrew Collins, A.; Maunder, N.; McNabb, M. World Disaster Report, Geneva. 2009. Available online: https://reliefweb.int/report/world/world-disasters-report-2009-focus-early-warning-early-action (accessed on 15 February 2016).
79. U.S. Department of Homeland Security. *Target Capabilities List*; U.S. Department of Homeland Security: Washington, DC, USA, 2007.
80. IFRC. *IFRC Shelter Kit*; IFRC: Geneva, Switzerland, 2009.
81. OCHA. *Multi/Cluster-Sector Initial & Rapid Assessment (MIRA) Community Level Assessment*; OCHA: New York, NY, USA, 2013; pp. 1–26.
82. ECB. *A Case Study: Joint Needs Assessment after the West Sumatra Earthquake*; ECB: Frankfurt, Germany, 2009; pp. 1–7.
83. UNICEF. *Emergency Handbook*; UNICEF: New York, NY, USA, 2005.
84. IFRC; UN-HABITAT; UNHCR. Shelter Project 2010. Available online: https://reliefweb.int/report/world/shelter-projects-2010 (accessed on 15 February 2021).
85. World Health Organisation. *Classification and Minimum Standards for Foreign Medical Teams in Sudden Onset*; World Health Organisation: Geneva, Switzerland, 2013; Available online: https://www.who.int/publications/i/item/classification-and-minimum-standards-for-foreign-medical-teams-in-sudden-onset-of-disasters (accessed on 15 February 2021).
86. World Health Organization. *SpringerReference*; World Health Organisation: Geneva, Switzerland, 2012. [CrossRef]
87. GHC. *Global Health Cluster Partners' Survey*; GHC: Glasgow, UK, 2012; pp. 1–30.
88. IFRC. *Disaster Emergency Needs Assessment*; IFRC: Geneva, Switzerland, 2000.
89. OCHA. *Multi-Sect tor Initial Rapid Assessmment (MIIRA) Report Pakistan Floods*; OCHA: New York, NY, USA, 2012.
90. OCHA. *Central African Republic Multi-Cluster/Sector Initial Rapid Assessment*; OCHA: New York, NY, USA, 2014.
91. OCHA. *Joint Rapid Damage and Needs Assessment Report*; OCHA: New York, NY, USA, 2013.
92. OCHA. *Multi-Sector Initial Rapid Assessment for Pakistan (MIRA) In Preparedness for Disasters and Emergencies A Joint Initiative between Government & the Humanitarian Community*; OCHA: New York, NY, USA, 2012.
93. OCHA. *MIRA Multi-Cluster/Sector Initial Rapid Assessment Philippines Typhoon Haiyan*; OCHA: New York, NY, USA, 2013.
94. OCHA. *Inter-Agency Initial Rapid Needs Assessment Preliminary Report*; OCHA: New York, NY, USA, 2013.
95. OCHA. *The Philippines Second-Phase Multi Cluster Rapid Needs Assessment for Tropical Storm Washi (Sendong)*; OCHA: New York, NY, USA, 2012; pp. 17–19.
96. OXFAM. *SYLHET Phase 1 Rapid Emergency Assessment*; OXFAM: Oxford, UK, 2012.
97. Association for Healthcare Resource and Materials Management; The Health Industry Distributors Association; The Health Industry Group Purchasing Association. Medical-Surgical Supply Formulary by Disaster Scenario. Available online: https://www.kyha.com/assets/docs/PreparednessDocs/disasterformulary.pdf (accessed on 15 February 2021).
98. VOAD. National Voluntary Organizations Active in Disaster. 2011. Available online: https://www.nvoad.org/ (accessed on 15 February 2021).
99. Hartwell-Naguib, S.; Roberts, N. Winter Floods 2013/14. 2014. Available online: https://researchbriefings.files.parliament.uk/documents/SN06809/SN06809.pdf (accessed on 15 February 2021).
100. Morgan, O.W.; Sribanditmongkol, P.; Perera, C.; Sulasmi, Y.; Van Alphen, D.; Sondorp, E. Mass Fatality Management following the South Asian Tsunami Disaster: Case Studies in Thailand, Indonesia, and Sri Lanka. *PLoS Med.* **2006**, *3*, e195. [CrossRef]
101. Tabbara, L. Emergency Relief Logistics: Evaluation of Disaster Response Models Based on Asian Tsunami Logistics Response. In *Based on Asian Tsunami Logistics Response*. 2008. Available online: http://driverspack.org/download/agile-framework-rmcproject (accessed on 15 February 2021).
102. IFRC/ICRC Emergency Items Catalogue | Shelter Cluster, (n.d.). Available online: https://www.sheltercluster.org/working-group-nfi-practices/documents/ifrcicrc-emergency-items-catalogue (accessed on 15 February 2021).
103. Crispim, J.A.; De Sousa, J.P. Partner selection in virtual enterprises: A multi-criteria decision support approach. *Int. J. Prod. Res.* **2009**, *47*, 4791–4812. [CrossRef]
104. Barringer, B.R.; Harrison, J.S. Walking a Tightrope: Creating Value Through Interorganizational Relationships. *J. Manag.* **2000**, *26*, 367–403. [CrossRef]
105. Baas, S.R.; Battista, S.; Federica, J. Disaster Risk Management Systems Analysis, PreventionWeb, Rome. 2008. Available online: https://www.preventionweb.net/publication/disaster-risk-management-systems-analysis-guide-book (accessed on 15 February 2021).
106. Fuqing, Z.; Yi, H.; Dongmei, Y. A multi-objective optimization model of the partner selection problem in a virtual enterprise and its solution with genetic algorithms. *Int. J. Adv. Manuf. Technol.* **2005**, *28*, 1246–1253. [CrossRef]
107. Zhao, J.; Jiao, L.; Xia, S.; Fernandes, V.B.; Yevseyeva, I.; Zhou, Y.; Emmerich, M.T. Multiobjective sparse ensemble learning by means of evolutionary algorithms. *Decis. Support Syst.* **2018**, *111*, 86–100. [CrossRef]
108. Lee, J.; Bharosa, N.; Yang, J.; Janssen, M.; Rao, H. Group value and intention to use—A study of multi-agency disaster management information systems for public safety. *Decis. Support Syst.* **2011**, *50*, 404–414. [CrossRef]
109. Petkov, D.; Petkova, O.; Andrew, T.; Nepal, T. Mixing Multiple Criteria Decision Making with soft systems thinking techniques for decision support in complex situations. *Decis. Support Syst.* **2007**, *43*, 1615–1629. [CrossRef]
110. Fertier, A.; Barthe-Delanoë, A.-M.; Montarnal, A.; Truptil, S.; Bénaben, F. A new emergency decision support system: The automatic interpretation and contextualisation of events to model a crisis situation in real-time. *Decis. Support Syst.* **2020**, *133*, 113260. [CrossRef]
111. Hall, D.; Guo, Y.; Davis, R.A.; Cegielski, C. Extending Unbounded Systems Thinking with agent-oriented modeling: Conceptualizing a multiple perspective decision-making support system. *Decis. Support Syst.* **2005**, *41*, 279–295. [CrossRef]

112. Talluri, S.; Baker, C. A quantitative framework for designing efficient business process alliances. In Proceedings of the International Conference on Engineering and Technology Management, Managing Virtual Enterprises: A Convergence of Communications, Computing, and Energy Technologies (IEMC 96), Vancouver, BC, USA, 18–20 August 1996; pp. 656–661. [CrossRef]
113. Qiu, J.; Wang, Z.; Ye, X.; Liu, L.; Dong, L. Modeling method of cascading crisis events based on merging Bayesian Network. *Decis. Support Syst.* **2014**, *62*, 94–105. [CrossRef]
114. Gardašević-Filipović, M.Z.Š. Multicriteria Optimization in a Fuzzy Environment: The fuzzy analytic hierarchy, Yugosl. *J. Oper. Res.* **2010**, *20*, 71–85.
115. Hasani, S.; El-Haddadeh, R.; Aktas, E. A disaster severity assessment decision support tool for reducing the risk of failure in response operations. In *Risk Analysis IX*; Wessex Institute of Technology: Southampton, UK, 2014. [CrossRef]
116. Hans, C. Supporting partner identification for virtual organisations in manufacturing. *J. Manuf. Technol. Manag.* **2008**, *19*, 497–513. [CrossRef]
117. Hodgett, R.E. Multi-Criteria Decision-Making in Whole Process Design. Ph.D. Thesis, Newcastle University, Newcastle upon Tyne, UK, 2013.
118. Verdecho, M.-J.; Alfaro-Saiz, J.-J.; Rodriguez-Rodriguez, R. Prioritization and management of inter-enterprise collaborative performance. *Decis. Support Syst.* **2012**, *53*, 142–153. [CrossRef]
119. Liao, C.-N.; Kao, H.-P. An integrated fuzzy TOPSIS and MCGP approach to supplier selection in supply chain management. *Expert Syst. Appl.* **2011**, *38*, 10803–10811. [CrossRef]
120. Zolghadri, M.; Amrani, A.; Zouggar, S.; Girard, P. Power assessment as a high-level partner selection criterion for new product development projects. *Int. J. Comput. Integr. Manuf.* **2011**, *24*, 312–327. [CrossRef]
121. Badea, A.; Prostean, G.; Goncalves, G.; Allaoui, H. Assessing Risk Factors in Collaborative Supply Chain with the Analytic Hierarchy Process (AHP). *Procedia Soc. Behav. Sci.* **2014**, *124*, 114–123. [CrossRef]
122. Shuai, J.-J. A Fuzzy MCDM Partnership Selection Model—Case of the IC Design House. In Proceedings of the 2009 Fourth International Conference on Innovative Computing, Information and Control (ICICIC), Kaohsiung, Taiwan, 7–9 December 2009; pp. 1452–1455. [CrossRef]
123. Unu-ehs, WorldRisk Report. 2011. Available online: https://reliefweb.int/report/world/worldriskreport-2011-can-disaster-be-prevented (accessed on 27 January 2021).
124. OCHA. WorldRiskReport 2012: Environmental Degradation Increases Disaster Risk Worldwide. 2012. Available online: https://reliefweb.int/report/world/world-risk-report-2012-environmental-degradation-increases-disaster-risk-worldwide (accessed on 27 January 2021).
125. Fiedrich, F.; Gehbauer, F.; Rickers, U. Optimized resource allocation for emergency response after earthquake disasters. *Saf. Sci.* **2000**, *35*, 41–57. [CrossRef]
126. Nourjou, R.; Hatayama, M.; Tatano, H. Introduction to spatially distributed intelligent assistant agents for coordination of human-agent teams' actions. In Proceedings of the 2011 IEEE International Symposium on Safety, Security, and Rescue Robotics, Kyoto, Japan, 1–5 November 2011; pp. 251–258. [CrossRef]
127. Kangas, M. Creative and playful learning: Learning through game co-creation and games in a playful learning environment. *Think. Ski. Creat.* **2010**, *5*, 1–15. [CrossRef]
128. Zografos, K.G.; Androutsopoulos, K.N. A decision support system for instegrated hazardous materials routing and emergency response decisions. *Transp. Res. Part C Emerg. Technol.* **2008**, *16*, 684–703. [CrossRef]
129. Schneider, P.J.; Schauer, B.A. HAZUS—Its Development and Its Future. *Nat. Hazards Rev.* **2006**, *7*, 40–44. [CrossRef]
130. Available online: https://gisf.ngo/wp-content/uploads/2014/09/0158-World-Vision-2008-HISS-CAM-flowchart.pdf (accessed on 17 February 2021).

sustainability

Article

A Fuzzy Linguistic Multi-Criteria Decision-Making Approach to Assess Emergency Suppliers

Huilin Li *, Jiaqi Yang and Ziquan Xiang

School of Transportation and Logistics Engineering, Wuhan University of Technology, Wuhan 430063, China
* Correspondence: huilin.li@whut.edu.cn

Abstract: Under the influence of COVID-19, various emergency supplies have repeatedly broken links, seriously affecting normal life and hindering the sustainable development of enterprises and society. Therefore, suitable emergency suppliers are crucial. To prioritize and select suitable emergency suppliers, key indicators were determined, and evaluation models were established based on the characteristics of epidemic situations and epidemic prevention materials. The application of the MCDM (multi-criteria decision-making) issue combining fuzzy SWARA (the stepwise weight assessment ratio analysis) and the actor analysis method to emergency supplier selection studies, called the fuzzy SWARA-based actor analysis method, is used to identify appropriate suppliers for optimizing pre-preparation. Results of evaluation system weight computations by the Fuzzy SWARA-based actor analysis method show that the overall prioritization of four non-economic factors in ranking orders are "Delivery Capacity", "Flexible Supply Capacity", "Quality", and "Social Evaluation and Reputation". For the inclusion of conflicting standards and the unquantifiable feature, economic and non-economic factors were discussed separately and evaluated by language variables. Additionally, the fuzzy actor analysis indicated that economic factors and non-economic factors need to be considered comprehensively for emergency supplier selection. This method has good operability and reference value, convenient for the final choice making according to actual situation.

Keywords: emergency supplies; multi-criteria decision making; fuzzy set; actor analysis method; linguistic variables

Citation: Li, H.; Yang, J.; Xiang, Z. A Fuzzy Linguistic Multi-Criteria Decision-Making Approach to Assess Emergency Suppliers. *Sustainability* **2022**, *14*, 13114. https://doi.org/10.3390/su142013114

Academic Editor: Krzysztof Goniewicz

Received: 7 September 2022
Accepted: 10 October 2022
Published: 13 October 2022

1. Introduction

In recent years, the frequent occurrence of various natural disasters and emergencies has caused varying degrees of casualties and property loss. Especially in the past two years under COVID-19 outbreak, the supply chain phenomenon seriously affected the normal life of the masses, hindered the development speed of enterprises and society, and deepened scholars' thinking of the emergency supply chain of logistics management research.

Emergency management operations generally consist of four parts: prevention, preparation, response, and recovery. The process of emergency supply chain system is shown in Figure 1. The main work in the prevention stage is the establishment of relevant emergency mechanisms, laws, and regulations by the main government departments in society, to reduce hidden dangers and strengthen the ability to deal with emergency events. The preparation stage is to advance deployment and arrangement to resist possible emergencies and ensure the effectiveness of rescue after the occurrence of the event to the greatest extent, such as the advance purchase of epidemic prevention materials, the location of emergency supplies reserve centers, the deployment of emergency facilities, and other issues. The response stage is the key element of emergency management. Various rescue methods are needed to reduce the losses and casualties caused by emergencies and reduce the negative impact on society as a whole after the incident, such as the distribution of emergency relief supplies, transportation, and scheduling of emergency relief supplies. The recovery stage involves the reconstruction of disaster areas and the recovery of people's lives after the response stage. Strictly, the prevention stage does not belong to the category of logistics management. In the field of emergency logistics management, the first step should be the preservation of emergency materials, that is, the preparation stage. In the preparation stage, to ensure the best rescue effect after an emergency, reliable suppliers should be selected from numerous emergency suppliers and a good supply system should be established. In disaster relief practices, a good cooperative relationship between relief agencies and suppliers can simplify the procurement process and improve the availability and rapid delivery of supplies. In addition, establishing a close relationship with suppliers can achieve discounts in bulk pricing. Regardless of the scale and importance of procurement in emergency logistics, only a few studies focus on the issue of emergency supply procurement decisions [1].

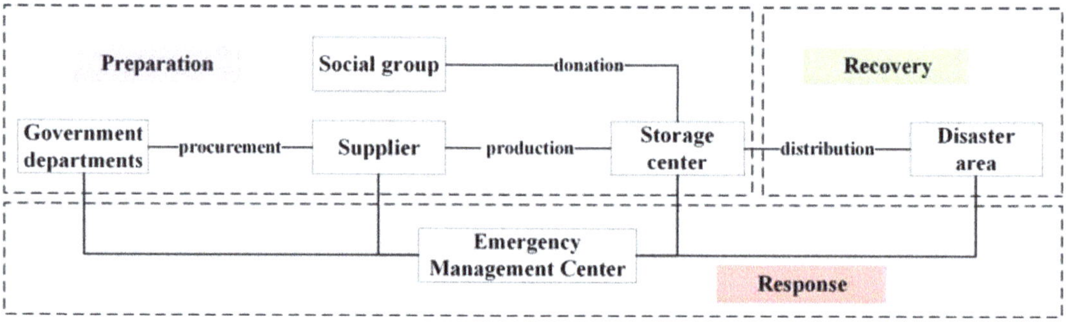

Figure 1. Emergency supply chain system flow chart.

Suppliers are the critical link to any supply chain as an important strategic decision, and supplier selection helps achieve a solid relationship between supply and demand [2,3]. Consequently, the selection of emergency suppliers is an important part of the emergency supply chain management, which is a typical problem. There is a large body of literature on supplier selection decision-making in the commercial supply chain, such as supplier selection criteria [4]. However, not much attention has been paid to these factors in emergency logistics management, because disaster management is more closely related to the relationship between economic and non-economic factors. Previous standards in the commercial supply chain can provide guidance for this study, and the emergency supply chain also uses some of the same indicators, including price, quality, delivery capacity, etc. The contributions of this paper are as follows:

Firstly, the evaluation index system of emergency suppliers for large emergencies was established, and 20 evaluation indicators for emergency suppliers were listed in a relatively comprehensive way, which has targeted and comprehensive coverage, and further improves the evaluation index system of emergency suppliers.

Secondly, different from other fuzzy multi-criteria decision-making methods, this paper focused on the decision preferences of economic factors and non-economic factors and adopted the decision weights of experts to evaluate and select emergency suppliers by the fuzzy SWARA-based actor analysis method. Through the corresponding relationship between triangular fuzzy and decision language variables, the scores of qualitative indicators of different experts were converted into objective values, and the weights of non-economic factors were obtained.

Finally, sensitivity analysis was used to verify the influence of economic and non-economic factors on the preference decision of emergency supplier selection, and the priority ranking under different decision preferences was obtained.

In this study, the scientific selection of emergency suppliers is emphasized. The evaluation indicators and evaluation method are two key research points in the evaluation and selection of emergency suppliers. Based on the characteristics of an emergency, by initiating the application of the MCDM issue combining fuzzy stepwise weight assessment ratio analysis (SWARA) and the actor analysis method to emergency supplier selection studies, this study bears significance for it illustratively identifies the evaluation system that is critical to prioritization and selection of alternative suppliers. In the process of supplier selection and evaluation, qualitative indicators need to be quantified because many qualitative indicators are involved. Therefore, linguistic variables are introduced in this method, and the corresponding relationship between linguistic variables and fuzzy sets is established to transform the evaluation of qualitative indicators by experts. Linguistic variables were used to determine standard ratings expressed as fuzzy numbers. The evaluation indicator weights of emergency suppliers were determined using the SWARA method. The ranking of each alternative supplier was determined by the actor analysis method on fuzzy sets, which considers non-economic factors.

The remainder of this paper is organized as follows. Section 2 presents the literature review and outlines the innovative points and contributions of this study. Section 3 puts forward the key evaluation indicators for emergency suppliers. Section 4 describes the methods and processes. Section 5 applies the method to numerical examples of emergency supplier prioritization. Section 6 presents the sensitivity analysis. Section 7 discusses managerial implications. Finally, Section 8 concludes the study and offers future research directions.

2. Literature Review

We focus our attention on the literature on supplier evaluation decision-making methods and evaluation indicators for the criteria.

In the field of emergency logistics management, the first step should be to reserve emergency materials. To ensure the best rescue effect after an emergency, reliable suppliers must be selected. In general, a reliable supplier should follow the principles of right price, right time, right place, right quality, and right quantity. At present, research on the evaluation or selection of commercial suppliers has produced rich results. Several evaluation indicators were proposed, including quantity discounts, transportation costs, carbon taxes, price discounts, delivery times, service levels, supplier capabilities, and delivery times [5–9]. Wang and Su [10] proposed a generic DSS framework based on activity-based costing to evaluate and select suppliers. According to the characteristics of logistics service outsourcing enterprises, Peng [11] established a logistics service outsourcing supplier evaluation and selection index system as measured by cost, operational efficiency, basic quality, and technical level, aiming for the evaluation and selection of logistics outsourcing service suppliers based on the hierarchical analysis method. However, for different industries, the selection basis of suppliers is different; in particular, the selection of emergency material suppliers is more special, and must be considered in terms of the material quality guarantee and timely supply capacity as the main factor. Hu and Dong [12] considered humanitarian assistance extremely important in supplier selection and incorporated it into the selection strategy. The supplier selection criteria include price discounts offered by suppliers based on order quantity, required delivery time, and physical inventory. Ruan et al. [13] built a balanced "helicopter and vehicle" intermodal network by selecting emergency distribution centers (EDCs) and allocating medical assistance points, considering helicopter travel time, transfer time, and vehicle delivery time.

Both quantifiable economic and qualitative non-economic factors are involved in supplier selection decisions; the conflict between the indicators is the existence, which is a typical multi-criteria decision-making problem. The multi-criteria decision-making (MCDM) approach, based on the evaluation of multiple conflict guidelines, provides an effective framework for supplier comparison. Evaluation methods, such as AHP, ANP, TOPSIS, DEA, TCO, and GRA, are widely used in the supplier selection problem [14]. TOPSIS is fully called Technique for Order Preference by Similarity to an Ideal Solution. The basic principle is to rank the distance between the evaluation object and the optimal solution and the worst solution [15–17]. In Boran's [18] study, the TOPSIS method combined with an intuitive fuzzy set is proposed, and it was used in a group decision-making environment to select appropriate suppliers. Based on a set of standards applicable to the Industry 4.0 environment, Kaur and Singh [19] used the fuzzy analytic hierarchy process and the ideal scheme similarity ranking technique (FAHP-TOPSIS) method to evaluate suppliers. Çalık [20] developed a new group decision-making approach based on Industry 4.0 components for selecting the best green supplier by integrating AHP and TOPSIS methods under the Pythagorean fuzzy environment. Chen [21] proposed a novel decision-making model of TOPSIS integrated entropy-AHP weights to select the appropriate supplier. Zhang et al. [22] solved the uncertain attribute values and weights in MCDM problems by combining the ER approach and stochastic multi-criteria acceptability analysis-2 (SMAA-2). Bai et al. [23] used the gray-BWM-TODIM method to evaluate and select socially sustainable suppliers. Social sustainability attribute weights were determined using the gray-BWM approach, and then the gray-TODIM method was used to rank suppliers. Nekooie et al. [24] proposed a fuzzy objective planning method with soft priority between the objectives. Wang and Cai [25] built a distance-based VIKOR multi-criteria group decision-making (MCGDM) model for processing heterogeneous information to appropriately and flexibly solve the problem of emergency supplier selection with a compromise solution, which is more acceptable and suitable in practice. Badi [26] used a hybrid grey theory-MARCOS method for decision-making regarding the selection of suppliers in the Libyan Iron and Steel Company (LISCO) to help it compete. Tavana [27] proposed an integrated approach for supplier selection by combining the fuzzy AHP method with the fuzzy multiplicative multi-objective optimization based on ratio analysis. Giannakis [28] developed a sustainability performance measurement framework for supplier evaluation and selection by the Analytic Network Process (ANP) method. Chou and Chang [29] used linguistic values to evaluate the ratings and weights of selection factors and proposed a strategy alignment fuzzy simple multiple attribute rating (SMART) technique to solve the supplier selection problem. Weng [30] presented the analytic hierarchy process (AHP) and grey relational analysis (GRA) as potential multi-criteria decision-making (MCDM) methods for spare parts planning (SPP) software selection. Bakeshlou et al. [31] established a multi-objective fuzzy linear planning model with 17 criteria and divided it into five clusters, solved by a mixed fuzzy multi-objective decision model (MODM). Fallahpour et al. [32] improved the existing DEA-AI model, introduced a new artificial intelligence method for supplier selection, and integrated the Kourosh and Arash methods into a robust DEA model obtained by genetic programming (GP).

This is a sophisticated problem because supplier selection is often a multi-standard group decision-making problem involving conflicting standards. Fuzzy set theory has been widely used in management decision making. The fuzzy set theory proposed by Zadeh [33] provides an effective method for addressing fuzzy problems. The judgment of decision makers is represented by fuzzy numbers, thereby quantifying the evaluation level. Muneeb [34] proposed a decentralized bi-level VSP where demand and supply are normal random variables and objectives are fuzzy in nature. Many others have solved evaluation and selection problems using fuzzy set theory [35–38]. Based on this, aiming at the fuzzy concepts that often appear in decision-making problems, a new multi-criteria decision-making method is proposed to solve the supplier selection problem.

In summary, most previous studies have focused on the evaluation or selection of suppliers, and the fields of application are mostly in commercial supply areas, using classic evaluation methods. A comparison of supplier selection methods is shown in Table 1. Additionally, many scholars have made innovations from the perspective of fuzzy theory, and a variety of fuzzy multi-criteria decision-making methods have been formed. Meanwhile, the emergency supplier selection decision issues as a multi-standard group decision-making problem involving conflicting standards and unquantifiable features. There are many non-economic factors to be considered, economic and non-economic factors should be discussed separately. In order to fully demonstrate the importance of non-economic factors and their mutual comparison, the fuzzy SWARA-based actor analysis method is used to evaluate emergency suppliers. Meanwhile, the lack of research on emergency supply evaluation fields thus makes it necessary to conduct an emergency suppliers' criteria system and method, and fuzzy set theory is suitable for this issue. Therefore, the actor analysis method combined with the fuzzy SWARA method is proposed to solve the multiple-criteria decision-making (MCDM) problem, which evaluates unquantifiable indicators using language variables.

Table 1. Comparison of supplier selection methods.

Method	Features	References
TOPSIS method	Simple calculation, full use of original data, and less information loss, but strong subjectivity.	[15–19]
Analytic hierarchy process (AHP)	Comprehensive consideration of qualitative and quantitative. However, when there are too many indicators, the data statistics are large. The weight of the indicators is difficult to determine.	[20,21,27]
Grey relation analysis (GRA)	The computation amount is small, low data requirements, less workload, but it must be a gray system, and the optimal value of some indicators is difficult to determine.	[23,26,30]
Analytic network process (ANP)	Reflects the dependence between the hierarchical structure but needs to study the relationship between the factors; the workload is relatively large.	[28]
Fuzzy comprehensive evaluation (FCE) method	According to the membership degree theory of fuzzy mathematics, the qualitative evaluation is transformed into a quantitative evaluation method. The result is clear and systematic, suitable for solving nondeterministic problems, but the calculation is complex and subjective.	[24,33,34]
DEA method	Not affected by the dimensional and subjective factors, the results obtained are the relative evaluation values.	[31,32]

3. Evaluation Indicators Analysis

Compared with ordinary materials, epidemic prevention materials are highly irreplaceable, with more uncertainties and high timeliness in the delivery process, that need more reliable channels [39–42]. If the quality of supplies is not guaranteed, insufficient quantity, or a low qualified rate, it may cause problems in the subsequent rescue response stage. As the supplier of emergency supplies, it should have a better supply capacity and a higher response capacity in both delivery time and quantity. In addition, a high response level in the supply chain ensures the effectiveness and supply of emergency supplies. The emergency suppliers' evaluation and selection criteria system established in this study is shown in Figure 2, which includes five main indicators: flexible supply capacity, delivery capacity, price, quality, social evaluation, and reputation. The following is an explanation of these indicators.

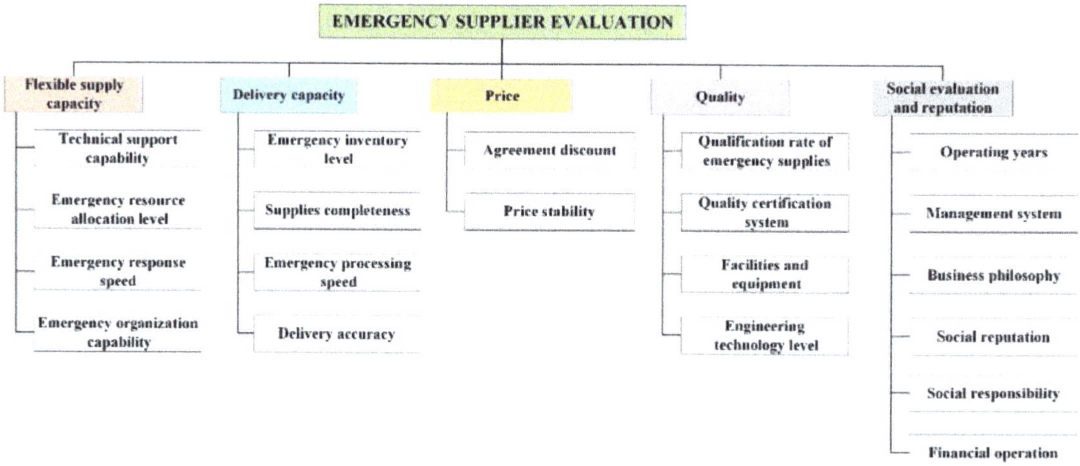

Figure 2. The emergency suppliers' evaluation and selection criteria.

1. Flexible supply capacity.

After the replenishment demand for emergency materials is issued, different enterprises have different emergency response speeds and resource allocation capabilities. In addition, when encountering material damage or other technical problems, the response capabilities of different companies also differ. Therefore, it is necessary to choose suppliers with more flexible supply capabilities.

2. Delivery capacity.

Priority is given to suppliers with strong delivery capacity due to differences in delivery quantity, timeliness, completion rate, and accuracy.

3. Price.

This indicator is used to measure the economic factors in the procurement cost of emergency material reserves. Even if the emergency work itself is weakly economical, the more efficient the rescue, the higher the economic cost, but the price and cost factors must be comprehensively considered. This includes price stability, bulk agreement preferential price, etc. Here, refers to the unit cost of the material allocated to the distribution center.

4. Quality.

The quality of emergency materials determines the quality of the rescue after emergencies. This includes the product qualification rate, quality certification system, engineering technology level, etc.

5. Social evaluation and reputation.

The evaluation and reputation of enterprises in society must be considered, including whether they have a good image in the hearts of the people and a high social reputation. The difference is that disaster relief has a strong public welfare nature. If the social evaluation degree of the suppliers is not high, it may cause unfair doubts in the public.

In general, the evaluation and selection indicators of the emergency materials suppliers should closely focus on the characteristics of the emergency rescue work, consider the connection between the indicators and the working process, and highlight the emergency ability of the supplier enterprises, so as to choose. At the same time, the above analysis shows that the indicators selected by emergency materials suppliers can be basically divided into two categories; one is economical indicators, where the smaller the evaluation value, the better. Price is an economic indicator. The other is the non-economical indicator; the greater the evaluation value, the better. Flexible supply capacity, delivery capacity, quality, social evaluation, and reputation are non-economical indicators.

4. Methodology

4.1. Fuzzy Set Theory

Definition 1. *R is a real number set, $F(R)$ represents all the fuzzy sets, and a fuzzy set $M \in F(R)$ on R is called a fuzzy number [43].*

① $x_0 \in R$, *such that* $\mu_M(x_0) = 1$.
② *For any* $\alpha \in [0,1]$, $A_\alpha = [x, \mu_{A_\alpha} \geq \alpha]$ *is the closed interval.*

Definition 2. *In fuzzy mathematics, the membership function of fuzzy sets can be represented by a triangular distribution:*

$$\mu_M(x) = \begin{cases} \frac{x}{m-l} - \frac{l}{m-l} & x \in [l, m] \\ \frac{x}{m-u} - \frac{u}{m-u} & x \in [m, u] \\ 0 & others \end{cases} \tag{1}$$

where, $l \leq m \leq u$, l and u represent the lower limit and upper limit of M, respectively, and m is the most likely value.

The triangular fuzzy number can be defined by $(l < x < u)$, and represents the non-fuzzy number when l, m, and u are equal. $M = \{x \in R | l \leq m \leq u\}$.

Its image is shown in Figure 3.

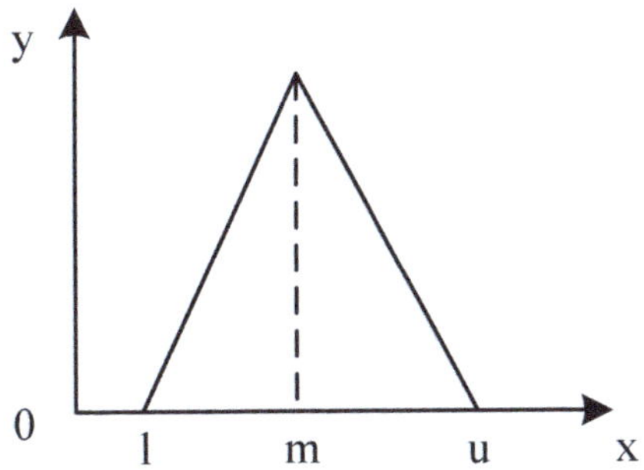

Figure 3. Triangular distribution function.

The fuzzy number of the triangular distribution is represented as $M = [l, m, u](l \leq m \leq u)$. If the size of the fuzzy number is compared, it needs to be de-fuzzy, and the average comprehensive representation method is selected to de-fuzzy. According to the Equation (2), the defuzzification value $P(M)$ is as follows.

$$P(M) = (l + m + u)/3 \tag{2}$$

Definition 3. *Set up triangular fuzzy numbers M_1 and M_2, $M_1 = (l_1, m_1, u_1)$, $M_2 = (l_2, m_2, u_2)$, $M_1 + M_2 = (l_1 + l_2, m_1 + m_2, u_1 + u_2)$, $M_1 - M_2 = (l_1 - l_2, m_1 - m_2, u_1 - u_2)$, $M_1 * M_2 = (l_1 l_2, m_1 m_2, u_1 u_2)$, $\gamma * M_1 = (\gamma l_1, \gamma m_1, \gamma u_1)$.*

4.2. Fuzzy SWARA Method

The stepwise weight assessment ratio analysis (SWARA) method is a new multi-criteria decision-making method proposed by Kersuliene et al. [44] to determine standard weights [45]. An important feature of SWARA is the ability to assess the accuracy of experts regarding the weighting criteria in the methodological process. Experts play a crucial role in the process of judging the criteria and weights. Each expert sets the priority of each criterion, and then considers the total results to rank all factors. In this method, the highest priority will be assigned to the most valuable indicator, and the lowest priority will be assigned to the lowest value evaluation indicator.

Considering that the knowledge, experience, and information of experts are different, their scores directly affect the accuracy of the final results in the evaluation process. In order to weaken the decisive role of subjective factors in the traditional SWARA method and reduce the influence of a single decision maker's preference, the fuzzy SWARA method is adopted in this paper. According to the level of knowledge and experience of experts, combined with the fuzzy set, different experts are given the weight and the indicators weight are obtained. Here, is a description of fuzzy SWARA.

Step 1. Relative importance of different indicators and the corresponding order of defuzzification values. Each decision expert expresses the relative importance of each indicator. The triangular fuzzy number for each indicator can be obtained according to the corresponding linguistic variable. The defuzzification value of each indicator is then obtained [46–49]. The defuzzification values of the different indicators are arranged in descending order [50,51].

Step 2. The correlation parameter s_j ($j \geq 2$) between two adjacent indicators before and after is determined. The correlation parameter s_j ($j \geq 2$) can be determined according to different rules. In this study, the difference between the defuzzification values of two adjacent indicators is used to calculate the correlation parameter.

Step 3. Calculate the comparison coefficient k_j according to Equation (3).

$$k_j = \begin{cases} 1, & j = 1 \\ s_j + 1, & j > 1 \end{cases} \tag{3}$$

Step 4. Calculate the relative weight q_j according to Equation (4).

$$q_j = \begin{cases} 1, & j = 1 \\ \frac{q_{j-1}}{k_j}, & j > 1 \end{cases} \tag{4}$$

Step 5. Calculate the final weight ω_j according to Equation (5).

$$\omega_j = \frac{q_j}{\sum_{k=1}^{n} q_k} \tag{5}$$

4.3. Actor Analysis Method

Actor analysis is a comprehensive factor evaluation method. The economic and non-economic factors are unified according to their relative importance, and the factors are comprehensively analyzed from different degrees [52]. In this study, the fuzzy SWARA method was combined with the actor analysis method to determine the priority of the alternatives.

Step 1: Calculation of the importance value of economic factors T_j.

$$T_j = \frac{\frac{1}{c_j}}{\sum_{j=1}^{n} \frac{1}{c_j}} \tag{6}$$

There are n alternatives, and c_j is the cost value reflected by the economic factors of the alternative, which is the economic cost. The higher the cost, the worse the economy; therefore, taking the reciprocal for comparison, the larger the result, the better is the economy.

Step 2: Calculation of the importance value of non-economic factors T_f.

(1) The pairs of alternatives are compared using a single factor. According to the importance evaluation value given by the experts, the proportion value of the better one is

1 point, and the worst one is 0. Therefore, the relative importance value T_{di} of every single non-economic factor for different alternatives is obtained. *Gi* is the specific gravity value of the alternatives for a single factor.

$$T_{di} = \frac{G_i}{\sum_{j=1}^{n} G_i} \tag{7}$$

(2) The relative importance value T_{di} of every single non-economic factor is multiplied by its weight value W_i and accumulated to obtain the importance factor T_f. The number of non-economic factors is m.

$$T_f = \sum_{i=1}^{m} W_i T_{di} \tag{8}$$

Step 3: Calculation of the importance values F_i.

The importance values of the alternatives are superimposed according to economic and non-economic factors to obtain the ranking of alternatives. M, N are the relative importance of economic factors (objective factors) and non-economic factors (subjective factors) respectively, $M + N = 1$.

$$F_i = MT_j + NT_f \tag{9}$$

5. Case Analysis

A schematic of the research methodology is shown in Figure 4. First, the weights of the experts were determined according to the triangular fuzzy set method. The SWARA method of triangular fuzzy sets was then used to determine the weights of the evaluation indicators. Finally, the actor analysis method was used to determine the priority of each alternative enterprise.

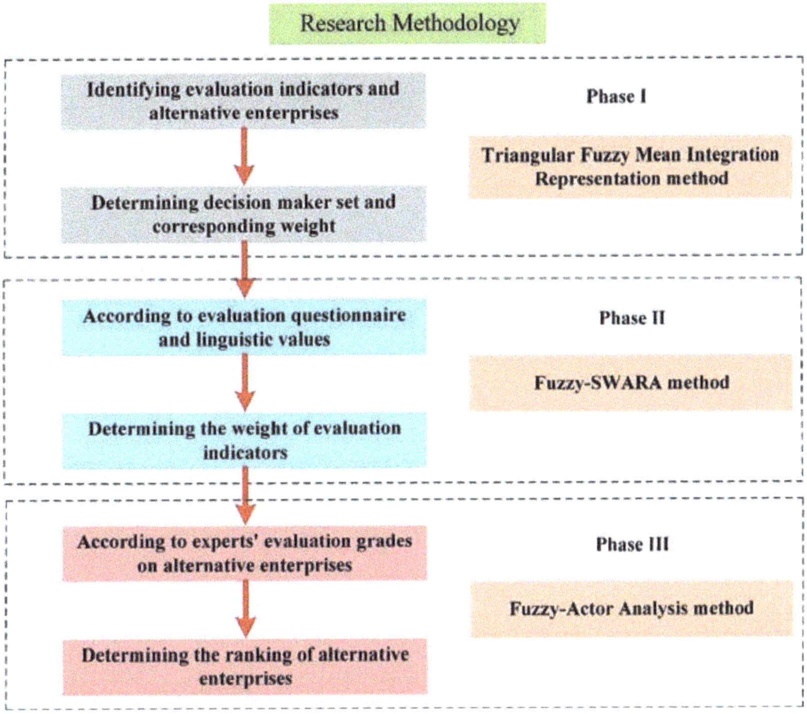

Figure 4. The schematic diagram of the research methodology.

It is assumed that city J needed to carry out reserve work of emergency relief materials, and the cooperative emergency suppliers needed to be determined. Originally, ten companies are selected. After a preliminary judgment and evaluation by three experienced experts in the emergency industry, the remaining five enterprises served as alternatives.

The indicator set was determined as $C = \{C_1, C_2, C_3, C_4, C_5\}$, C_1 corresponding to flexible supply capacity, C_2 to delivery capacity, C_3 to price, C_4 to quality, and C_5 to social evaluation and reputation, respectively. Here, C_3 is the economic indicator, C_1, C_2, C_4, and C_5 are non-economic indicators. The unit prices of the five alternatives are 18, 22, 30, 15, and 20. A questionnaire for the evaluation of indicators was established and sent to three experienced experts. The evaluation values in the questionnaire were designed according to the importance scale tables in Tables 2 and 3 [53].

Table 2. Importance scales for evaluating decision makers.

Linguistic Variable Value	Fuzzy Number	Linguistic Variable Value	Fuzzy Number
Extremely important (EI)	(0.8, 0.9, 1.0)	Middle (M)	(0.4, 0.5, 0.6)
Very important (VI)	(0.7, 0.8, 0.9)	Unimportant (U)	(0.3, 0.4, 0.5)
Important (I)	(0.6, 0.7, 0.8)	Very unimportant (VU)	(0.1, 0.2, 0.3)

Table 3. Correspondence of linguistic variable values.

Linguistic Variable Value	Triangular Fuzzy Number
Extremely Good (EG)/Extremely High (EH)	(0.8, 0.9, 1.0)
Very Very Good (VVG)/Very Very High (VVH)	(0.7, 0.8, 0.9)
Very Good (VG)/Very High (VH)	(0.6, 0.7, 0.8)
Good (G)/High (H)	(0.5, 0.6, 0.7)
Medium Good (MG)/Medium-High (MH)	(0.4, 0.5, 0.6)
Fair (F)/Medium (M)	(0.3, 0.4, 0.5)
Medium Bad (MB)/Medium Low (ML)	(0.2, 0.3, 0.4)
Bad (B)/Low (L)	(0.1, 0.2, 0.3)

Phase 1: Determining decision maker set and corresponding weight, alternative enterprise set, and evaluation indicators set.

The alternative enterprise set is $E = \{E_1, E_2, E_3, E_4, E_5\}$. The evaluation indicators set is $C = \{C_1, C_2, C_3, C_4, C_5\}$. The set of decision-makers is represented by $A = \{A_1, A_2, A_3\}$, and the relative importance value of decision-makers are calculated according to the importance scale of Table 2. The order $\varepsilon = (\varepsilon_1, \varepsilon_2, \varepsilon_3)^T$ as the importance weight of the expert group. The weight of the three decision makers can be obtained according to Table 2 and Equation (10). The results are presented in Table 4.

$$\varepsilon_k = \frac{P(M_k)}{\sum_{k=1}^{p} P(M_k)}, \ k = 1, 2, \ldots, p \tag{10}$$

$$\varepsilon = (\varepsilon_1, \varepsilon_2, \varepsilon_3)^T = (0.3750, 0.2917, 0.3333) \tag{11}$$

Table 4. Weight of decision makers.

Decision-Maker	A1	A2	A3
Linguistic variable	EI	I	VI
Triangular fuzzy number	(0.80, 0.90, 1.00)	(0.60, 0.70, 0.80)	(0.70, 0.80, 0.90)
Weight	0.3750	0.2917	0.3333

Phase 2: Determine the weight of non-economic factors.

Decision makers assigned the importance of the indicators based on the linguistic variable values in Table 3. The aggregation triangular fuzzy number was obtained using Equation (11). The defuzzification value was calculated using Equation (2). The obtained defuzzification value P(C_j) was sorted in descending order, according to Equations (3)–(5), as shown in Table 5. The weights of four non-economic indicators were obtained as follows:

$$W = (W_1, W_2, W_4, W_5) = (0.2604, 0.2767, 0.2583, 0.2046) \quad (12)$$

Table 5. Significance of the evaluation indicators.

Indicators	A1	A2	A3	Aggregated Fuzzy Number	Crisp Values *P* (C_j)	W_j
C1	EG	VVG	VVG	(0.7375, 0.8375, 0.9375)	0.8375	0.2604
C2	EG	EG	EG	(0.8000, 0.9000, 1.0000)	0.9000	0.2767
C4	VVG	VG	VVG	(0.7292, 0.8292, 0.9292)	0.8292	0.2583
C5	MG	MG	VG	(0.4667, 0.5667, 0.6667)	0.5667	0.2046

Phase 3: Calculate the importance values.

According to the Equations (6)–(8), Tables 6–8, and the price, the importance values of economic and non-economic factors were calculated.

$$T_{jE1}, T_{jE2}, T_{jE3}, T_{jE4}, T_{jE5} = (0.2214, 0.1812, 0.1326, 0.2656, 0.1991) \quad (13)$$

$$T_{fE1}, T_{fE2}, T_{fE3}, T_{fE4}, T_{fE5} = (0.2981, 0.0928, 0.2912, 0.1351, 0.1828) \quad (14)$$

Table 6. Decision makers' evaluation grades of alternative enterprises.

Enterprises	E1			E2			E3			E4			E5		
Decision-Maker	A1	A2	A3	A1	A2	A3	A1	A2	A3	A1	A2	A3	A1	A2	A3
C1	G	VG	G	MG	G	MG	VG	VVG	VG	MG	G	G	M	MG	MG
C2	VG	G	G	M	MG	M	G	MG	G	VG	VG	G	VVG	VG	G
C3	VH	H	VH	H	H	MH	VH	VH	H	VH	H	H	VH	H	MH
C4	G	MG	M	MB	M	MB	MG	M	M	B	MB	MB	M	MG	MG
C5	MG	G	MG	M	MG	G	VG	G	VG	MG	M	MG	MG	MG	M

Table 7. Comparison results on non-economic factors.

Comparison Results on C1								Comparison Results on C2							
Enterprises	E1	E2	E3	E4	E5	G_i	T_{dC1}	Enterprises	E1	E2	E3	E4	E5	G_i	T_{dC2}
E1	\	1	0	1	1	3	0.3	E1	\	1	1	0	0	2	0.2
E2	0	\	0	0	1	1	0.1	E2	0	\	0	0	0	0	0
E3	1	1	\	1	1	4	0.4	E3	0	1	\	0	0	1	0.1
E4	0	1	0	\	1	2	0.2	E4	1	1	1	\	0	3	0.3
E5	0	0	0	0	\	0	0	E5	1	1	1	1	\	4	0.4
Comparison Results on C4								**Comparison Results on C5**							
Enterprises	E1	E2	E3	E4	E5	G_i	T_{dC4}	Enterprises	E1	E2	E3	E4	E5	G_i	T_{dC5}
E1	\	1	1	1	1	4	0.4	E1	\	1	0	1	1	3	0.3
E2	0	\	0	1	0	1	0.1	E2	0	\	0	1	1	2	0.2
E3	0	1	\	1	1	3	0.3	E3	1	1	\	1	1	4	0.4
E4	0	0	0	\	0	0	0	E4	0	0	0	\	0	0	0
E5	0	1	0	1	\	2	0.2	E5	0	0	0	1	\	1	0.1

Table 8. Comparison results summary.

Enterprises	E1	E2	E3	E4	E5	W_i
C1	0.3	0.1	0.4	0.2	0	0.2604
C2	0.2	0	0.1	0.3	0.4	0.2767
C4	0.4	0.1	0.3	0	0.2	0.2583
C5	0.3	0.2	0.4	0	0.1	0.2046

Let $M = N = 0.5$. The importance values of the alternatives were obtained. and the order of importance was $E_1 > E_3 > E_4 > E_5 > E_2$. Therefore, E_1 is the best choice.

$$F_{E1}, F_{E2}, F_{E3}, F_{E4}, F_{E5} = (0.2598, 0.1370, 0.2119, 0.2003, 0.1910) \tag{15}$$

6. Sensitivity Analysis

To verify the effectiveness of the method, sensitivity analysis is carried out in this section. The relative importance of economic factors and non-economic factors are adjusted, and the remaining indicators are kept unchanged to test the stability of the fuzzy linguistic multi-criteria decision-making method. Make the scenario S1 = Tj:Tf = (0.1, 0.9), the relative importance weights of the economic factor indicators Tj and Tf are set to 0.1, 0.9, respectively. There are nine scenarios, S1 = Tj:Tf = (0.1, 0.9), S2 = Tj:Tf = (0.2, 0.8), S3 = Tj:Tf = (0.3, 0.7), S4 = Tj:Tf = (0.4, 0.6), S5 = Tj:Tf = (0.5, 0.5),S6 = Tj:Tf = (0.6, 0.4),S7 = Tj:Tf = (0.7, 0.3), S8 = Tj:Tf = (0.8, 0.2), S9 = Tj:Tf = (0.9, 0.1).

In each scenario, the importance values of alternative emergency suppliers were calculated respectively, which are shown in Table 9 and Figure 5. As can be seen from the results, the obtained enterprise priorities are not exactly the same in the nine different scenarios. When the important values of economic factors and non-economic factors are the same, $E_1 > E_3 > E_4 > E_5 > E_2$ can be obtained. When the importance value of economic factors is higher and decision-making preference is toward economic factors, 1 and 4 have higher priority. When the importance value of non-economic factors is higher and the decision preference is toward non-economic factors, the priority of 1 and 3 is high.

Table 9. Sensitivity analysis of rankings by F_{Ei}.

Scenarios	Tj	Tf	F_{E1}	F_{E2}	F_{E3}	F_{E4}	F_{E5}	Rankings
S1	0.1	0.9	0.2904	0.1016	0.2753	0.1482	0.1845	$E_1 > E_3 > E_5 > E_4 > E_2$
S2	0.2	0.8	0.2827	0.1105	0.2595	0.1612	0.1861	$E_1 > E_3 > E_5 > E_4 > E_2$
S3	0.3	0.7	0.2751	0.1193	0.2436	0.1743	0.1877	$E_1 > E_3 > E_5 > E_4 > E_2$
S4	0.4	0.6	0.2674	0.1282	0.2278	0.1873	0.1893	$E_1 > E_3 > E_5 > E_4 > E_2$
S5	0.5	0.5	0.2598	0.1370	0.2119	0.2003	0.1910	$E_1 > E_3 > E_4 > E_5 > E_2$
S6	0.6	0.4	0.2522	0.1458	0.1960	0.2134	0.1926	$E_1 > E_4 > E_3 > E_5 > E_2$
S7	0.7	0.3	0.2444	0.1547	0.1802	0.2265	0.1942	$E_1 > E_4 > E_5 > E_3 > E_2$
S8	0.8	0.2	0.2368	0.1636	0.1643	0.2395	0.1958	$E_4 > E_1 > E_5 > E_3 > E_2$
S9	0.9	0.1	0.2291	0.1724	0.1485	0.2525	0.1975	$E_4 > E_1 > E_5 > E_2 > E_3$

It can be concluded that the triangle fuzzy SWARA factor analysis method used in emergency supplies supplier selection is reliable, can not only reflect the importance weights of different experts themselves and the ratings of the target enterprise, more can adjust the economic factors and non-economic factors to reflect the decision-making preference in practical application. It is convenient for decision-making departments to make final decisions, which has good operability and reference value.

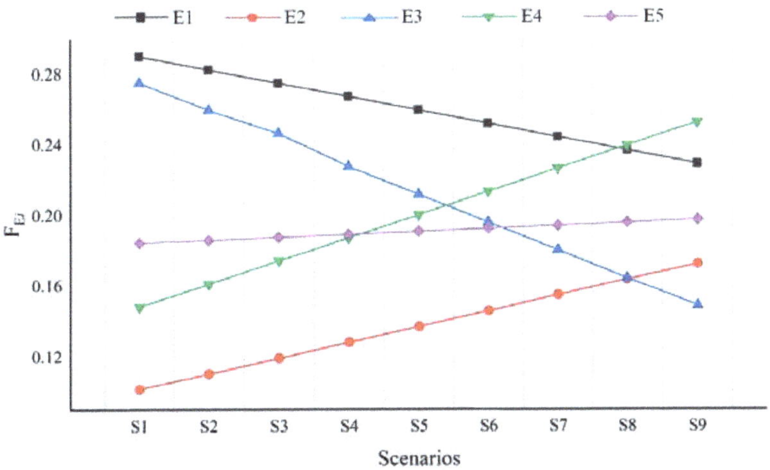

Figure 5. Sensitivity analysis of rankings by F_{Ei}.

7. Discussion

Various natural disasters and emergencies occurred frequently in recent years; after the disaster, to minimize adverse effects, we must attach importance to disaster relief work. Therefore, it is necessary to establish an effective emergency supply chain, among which a reasonable selection of emergency suppliers is an important link for all departments to cope with new challenges and build a modern emergency support mode. Based on the analysis of the evaluation indicators of emergency suppliers, the fuzzy SWARA method was used to give the indicators' weights, and the fuzzy SWARA-based actor analysis method was used to establish the evaluation model of emergency suppliers considering the final decision preference. Thus, the best choice under different decision-making preferences can be obtained, which provides a scientific theoretical basis for decision-making departments to make final decisions, and to ensure the smooth development of emergency rescue work. This study has the following management implications:

(1) The evaluation index system of emergency suppliers proposed in this paper is developed from five aspects of flexible supply capacity, delivery capacity, price, quality, social evaluation, and reputation. The quantifiable economic factors and non-quantifiable non-economic factors are fully considered, which can provide more comprehensive reference for management decision makers. Among them, the flexible supply capacity, emergency delivery capacity, and quality factors are closely related to the timeliness, stability, and reliability of supplies delivery. The acceptable price level is determined by the financial expenditure capacity of the management department, and the social evaluation and reputation will involve the public's view on the fairness and credibility of the management department. That means there are antinomic relationships among some indicators. In the decision-making process, it should be fully considered and relatively appropriate suppliers should be chosen to avoid some disadvantages of suppliers, which can not only guarantee the rescue work, but also maintain a good social image of the emergency management department.

(2) Since January 2020, novel coronavirus pneumonia has been spreading worldwide. Novel coronavirus pneumonia is a new type of public health emergency. It needs comprehensive emergency management and needs a coordinated response from different countries and regions. It is necessary to strengthen international macroeconomic policy coordination, maintain a stable and smooth supply chain of the global industrial chain, and jointly cope with the new crown pneumonia epidemic. At the same time, in the process of emergency management, reserve inventory, emergency demand, and supplier supply capacity should be deeply analyzed, and the uncertain impact of emergency inventory management should

be considered. In order to maximize the efficiency of emergency resource allocation, strong unified organization and implementation are needed in terms of material sources, material distribution, social security, and other measures. Emergency supplier evaluation and selection is an important link affecting the efficiency of emergency resource allocation, which has an important impact on the response and efficiency of the whole emergency supply chain.

(3) Under uncertain conditions, the total cost input of emergency rescue will increase with the improvement of the requirements on service level and reliability. Therefore, in the practical decision making of emergency supplier selection, the final decision maker should give certain decision-making preferences and fully consider the financial expenditure ability, so as to achieve the ideal decision-making goal within the reasonable total cost budget.

8. Conclusions

Due to the uncertainty and abruptness of natural disasters and emergencies, coupled with the complexity and changeability of the rescue process, the emergency rescue management has put forward high requirements. In order to respond quickly and effectively, emergency suppliers can be determined in advance, and the emergency material supply plan can be arranged to ensure emergency supply.

(1) This paper combined the fuzzy theory and the actor analysis method; fuzzy numbers are used to represent uncertainty and fuzziness, which improves the scientific and feasibility of decision making. Fuzzy numbers were used to convert the evaluation language of experts and establish a triangular fuzzy actor analysis method using the constraint nature of triangular fuzzy numbers. To get closer to the actual decision-making situation, the weight of each indicator was determined according to the situation of the experts. The weight of each indicator is determined using the fuzzy SWARA method. The triangle fuzzy actor analysis method determined the priority ranking of different emergency suppliers, which fully considered the decision preference for economic and non-economic factors.

Additionally, the specific application process of the method is given through a numerical example in this paper, and the optimal selection strategy of emergency supplies suppliers under different decision preferences is obtained by combining the sensitivity analysis of economic and non-economic factors. This method provides an evaluation method for emergency suppliers selection, which has reference value in practice. The results show that when the preferences of economic factors and non-economic factors are different, the optimal choice is different. When the important values of economic factors and non-economic factors are the same, we can obtain $E_1 > E_3 > E_4 > E_5 > E_2$. When the decision preference is toward economic factors, E_1 and E_4 have higher priority. When the decision preference is toward non-economic factors, E_1 and E_3 have higher priority. This also indicates that in practical decision-making, disaster needs and financial situation need to be closely linked to achieve the best supply of materials within the range of reasonable economic expenditure.

Different from other qualitative or quantitative evaluation methods, the results of AHP, COPRAS, SWARA, and TOPSIS are mainly determined by the subjective evaluation of external experts, but they cannot directly reflect the antinomic relationship between economic and non-economic factors, which is not conducive to the reference and choice of the final decision-making departments. The method proposed in this paper can not only reflect the importance weights of different experts themselves and the ratings of the target enterprise, but it can also adjust the important value of the economic factors and economy factors to reflect the actual application of the decision preference. This method has good operability and reference value, which is convenient for the decision-making departments to make the final choice according to their own actual situation.

(2) The evaluation scope of emergency supplies suppliers has a wide range, especially for different types of suppliers involved in different indicators. This paper mainly puts forward a single supplier selection scheme from the perspective of epidemic prevention

supplies, and there is still a lot of research space. In future research, the following aspects should be studied. First, it can be considered to increase the evaluation and analysis of specific materials, to solve the problem of supplier selection of emergency materials in a more targeted manner. Second, considering the impact scope of large emergencies, a single supplier may not be able to meet the actual demand, so the selection and configuration of emergency suppliers can be carried out from the perspective of multi-supplier collaborative supply. Third, it can study the emergency supply chain of multi-product, multi-level, and multi-inventory, considering the existing inventory and the supply guarantee ability of suppliers. The dynamic demand can be expressed by appropriate random function, which fully reflects the behavior of multi-level supply chain and completes the allocation of emergency materials. Finally, in the future, it can be considered to further extend the research from trapezoidal fuzzy sets, intuitionistic fuzzy sets, interval intuitionistic fuzzy sets, Z-number theory, and other fuzzy sets, so as to express uncertainty and fuzziness more precisely [54–56].

Author Contributions: Conceptualization, Z.X. and H.L.; formal analysis, H.L.; funding acquisition, J.Y.; methodology, Z.X. and H.L.; project administration, J.Y.; software, H.L. and Z.X.; supervision, J.Y.; writing—original draft, Z.X. and H.L.; writing—review and editing, H.L. and Z.X. All authors have read and agreed to the published version of the manuscript.

Funding: This research was supported by the National Natural Science Foundation of China (51279153) and supported by the Fundamental Research Funds for the Central Universities (2021-zy-010).

Institutional Review Board Statement: Not applicable.

Informed Consent Statement: Not applicable.

Data Availability Statement: Not applicable.

Conflicts of Interest: The authors declare no conflict of interest.

References

1. Balcik, B.; Ak, D. Supplier selection for framework agreements in humanitarian relief. *Prod. Oper. Manag.* **2014**, *23*, 1028–1041. [CrossRef]
2. Aktas, E.; Ulengin, F. Penalty and reward contracts between a manufacturer and its logistics service provider. *Logist. Res.* **2016**, *9*, 8. [CrossRef]
3. Zhou, R.J.; Li, L.J. Joint capacity planning and distribution network optimization of coal supply chains under uncertainty. *AIChE J.* **2018**, *64*, 1246–1261. [CrossRef]
4. Alkhatib, S.F.; Darlington, R.; Yang, Z.; Nguyen, T.T. A novel technique for evaluating and selecting logistics service providers based on the logistics resource view. *Expert Syst. Appl.* **2015**, *42*, 6976–6989. [CrossRef]
5. Schramm, V.B.; Cabral, L.P.B.; Schramm, F. Approaches for supporting sustainable supplier selection-A literature review. *J. Clean. Prod.* **2020**, *273*, 123089. [CrossRef]
6. Rashidi, K.; Noorizadeh, A.; Kannan, D.; Cullinane, K. Applying the triple bottom line in sustainable supplier selection: A meta-review of the state-of-the-art. *J. Clean. Prod.* **2020**, *269*, 122001. [CrossRef]
7. Taherdoost, H.; Brard, A. Analyzing the process of supplier selection criteria and methods. *Procedia Manuf.* **2019**, *32*, 1024–1034. [CrossRef]
8. Chen, Z.; Ming, X.; Zhou, T.; Chang, Y. Sustainable supplier selection for smart supply chain considering internal and external uncertainty: An integrated rough-fuzzy approach. *Appl. Soft Comput.* **2020**, *87*, 106004. [CrossRef]
9. Xu, J.; Zhai, J. Research on the Evaluation of Green Innovation Capability of Manufacturing Enterprises in Innovation Network. *Sustainability* **2020**, *12*, 807. [CrossRef]
10. Wang, K.L.; Su, Q. Suppliers selection and evaluation using activity-based costing. *Comput. Integr. Manuf. Syst. Beijing* **2001**, *7*, 53–57. [CrossRef]
11. Peng, J. Selection of logistics outsourcing service suppliers based on AHP. *Energy Procedia* **2012**, *17*, 595–601. [CrossRef]
12. Hu, S.; Dong, Z.S. Supplier selection and pre-positioning strategy in humanitarian relief. *Omega* **2019**, *83*, 287–298. [CrossRef]
13. Ruan, J.H.; Wang, X.P.; Chan, F.T.S.; Shi, Y. Optimizing the intermodal transportation of emergency medical supplies using balanced fuzzy clustering. *Int. J. Prod. Res.* **2016**, *54*, 4368–4386. [CrossRef]
14. Chai, J.; Ngai, E.W.T. Decision-making techniques in supplier selection: Recent accomplishments and what lies ahead. *Expert Syst. Appl.* **2020**, *140*, 112903. [CrossRef]

15. Dos Santos, B.M.; Godoy, L.P.; Campos, L.M.S. Performance Evaluation of Green Suppliers using Entropy-TOPSIS-F. *J. Clean. Prod.* **2018**, *207*, 498–509. [CrossRef]
16. You, S.Y.; Zhang, L.J.; Xu, X.G.; Liu, H.C. A New Integrated Multi-Criteria Decision Making and Multi-Objective Programming Model for Sustainable Supplier Selection and Order Allocation. *Symmetry* **2020**, *12*, 302. [CrossRef]
17. Tang, H.; Shi, Y.; Dong, P. Public blockchain evaluation using entropy and TOPSIS. *Expert Syst. Appl.* **2018**, *117*, 204–210. [CrossRef]
18. Boran, F.E.; Genç, S.; Kurt, M.; Akay, D. A multi-criteria intuitionistic fuzzy group decision making for supplier selection with TOPSIS method. *Expert Syst. Appl.* **2009**, *36*, 11363–11368. [CrossRef]
19. Kaur, H.; Singh, S.P. Multi-stage hybrid model for supplier selection and order allocation considering disruption risks and disruptive technologies. *Int. J. Prod. Econ.* **2021**, *231*, 107830. [CrossRef]
20. Çalık, A. A novel Pythagorean fuzzy AHP and fuzzy TOPSIS methodology for green supplier selection in the Industry 4.0 era. *Soft Comput.* **2021**, *25*, 2253–2265. [CrossRef]
21. Chen, C.H. A novel multi-criteria decision-making model for building material supplier selection based on entropy-AHP weighted TOPSIS. *Entropy* **2020**, *22*, 259. [CrossRef] [PubMed]
22. Zhang, X.; Gong, B.; Yang, F.; Ang, S. A stochastic multicriteria acceptability analysis–evidential reasoning method for uncertain multiattribute decision-making problems. *Expert Syst.* **2019**, *36*, e12426. [CrossRef]
23. Bai, C.; Kusi-Sarpong, S.; Badri Ahmadi, H.; Sarkis, J. Social sustainable supplier evaluation and selection: A group decision-support approach. *Int. J. Prod. Res.* **2019**, *57*, 7046–7067. [CrossRef]
24. Nekooie, M.A.; Sheikhalishahi, M.; Hosnavi, R. Supplier selection considering strategic and operational risks: A combined qualitative and quantitative approach. *Prod. Eng.* **2015**, *9*, 665–673. [CrossRef]
25. Wang, X.; Cai, J. A group decision-making model based on distance-based VIKOR with incomplete heterogeneous information and its application to emergency supplier selection. *Kybernetes* **2017**, *46*, 501–529. [CrossRef]
26. Badi, I.; Pamucar, D. Supplier selection for steelmaking company by using combined Grey-MARCOS methods. *Decis. Mak. Appl. Manag. Eng.* **2020**, *3*, 37–48. [CrossRef]
27. Tavana, M.; Shaabani, A.; Mansouri Mohammadabadi, S.; Varzgani, N. An integrated fuzzy AHP-fuzzy multimoora model for supply chain risk-benefit assessment and supplier selection. *Int. J. Syst. Sci. Oper. Logist.* **2021**, *8*, 238–261. [CrossRef]
28. Giannakis, M.; Dubey, R.; Vlachos, I.; Ju, Y. Supplier sustainability performance evaluation using the analytic network process. *J. Clean. Prod.* **2020**, *247*, 119439. [CrossRef]
29. Chou, S.Y.; Chang, Y.H. A decision support system for supplier selection based on a strategy-aligned fuzzy SMART approach. *Expert Syst. Appl.* **2008**, *34*, 2241–2253. [CrossRef]
30. Weng, S.S.; Chen, K.Y.; Li, C.Y. Application of the analytic hierarchy process and grey relational analysis for vendor selection of spare parts planning software. *Symmetry* **2019**, *11*, 1182. [CrossRef]
31. Bakeshlou, E.A.; Khamseh, A.A.; Asl, M.A.G.; Sadeghi, J.; Abbaszadeh, M. Evaluating a green supplier selection problem using a hybrid MODM algorithm. *J. Intell. Manuf.* **2017**, *28*, 913–927. [CrossRef]
32. Fallahpour, A.; Olugu, E.U.; Musa, S.N.; Khezrimotlagh, D.; Wong, K.Y. An integrated model for green supplier selection under fuzzy environment: Application of data envelopment analysis and genetic programming approach. *Neural Comput. Appl.* **2016**, *27*, 707–725. [CrossRef]
33. Zadeh, L.A. Fuzzy Sets. *Inf. Control* **1965**, *8*, 338–353. [CrossRef]
34. Muneeb, S.M.; Nomani, M.A.; Masmoudi, M.; Adhami, A.Y. A bi-level decision-making approach for the vendor selection problem with random supply and demand. *Manag. Decis.* **2019**, *6*, 1164–1180. [CrossRef]
35. Rabbani, M.; Foroozesh, N.; Mousavi, S.M.; Farrokhi-Asl, H. Sustainable supplier selection by a new decision model based on interval-valued fuzzy sets and possibilistic statistical reference point systems under uncertainty. *Int. J. Syst. Sci. Oper. Logist.* **2019**, *6*, 162–178. [CrossRef]
36. Sharaf, I.M. Global supplier selection with spherical fuzzy analytic hierarchy process. In *Decision Making with Spherical Fuzzy Sets*; Springer: Cham, Switzerland, 2021; pp. 323–348. [CrossRef]
37. Zhou, Z.; Dou, Y.; Liao, T.; Tan, Y. A preference model for supplier selection based on hesitant fuzzy sets. *Sustainability* **2018**, *10*, 659. [CrossRef]
38. Qu, G.; Zhang, Z.; Qu, W.; Xu, Z. Green supplier selection based on green practices evaluated using fuzzy approaches of TOPSIS and ELECTRE with a case study in a Chinese Internet company. *Int. J. Environ. Res. Public Health* **2020**, *17*, 3268. [CrossRef]
39. Liu, C. Supplier selection evaluation of shipbuilding enterprises based on entropy weight and multi-attribute decision making. In *Proceedings of the Fifth International Forum on Decision Sciences*; Springer: Singapore, 2018; pp. 255–268. [CrossRef]
40. Qin, J.; Liu, X.; Pedrycz, W. An extended TODIM multi-criteria group decision making method for green supplier selection in interval type-2 fuzzy environment. *Eur. J. Oper. Res.* **2017**, *258*, 626–638. [CrossRef]
41. Wang, L.E.; Liu, H.C.; Quan, M.Y. Evaluating the risk of failure modes with a hybrid MCDM model under interval-valued intuitionistic fuzzy environments. *Comput. Ind. Eng.* **2016**, *102*, 175–185. [CrossRef]
42. Yazdani, M.; Torkayesh, A.E.; Chatterjee, P. An integrated decision-making model for supplier evaluation in public healthcare system: The case study of a Spanish hospital. *J. Enterp. Inf. Manag.* **2020**, *33*, 965–989. [CrossRef]
43. Zarbakhshnia, N.; Soleimani, H.; Ghaderi, H. Sustainable third-party reverse logistics provider evaluation and selection using fuzzy SWARA and developed fuzzy COPRAS in the presence of risk criteria. *Appl. Soft Comput.* **2018**, *65*, 307–319. [CrossRef]

44. Keršuliene, V.; Zavadskas, E.K.; Turskis, Z. Selection of rational dispute resolution method by applying new step-wise weight assessment ratio analysis (SWARA). *J. Bus. Econ. Manag.* **2010**, *11*, 243–258. [CrossRef]
45. Sremac, S.; Stević, Ž.; Pamučar, D.; Arsić, M.; Matić, B. Evaluation of a Third-Party Logistics (3PL) Provider Using a Rough SWARA–WASPAS Model Based on a New Rough Dombi Agregator. *Symmetry* **2018**, *10*, 305. [CrossRef]
46. Rani, P.; Mishra, A.R.; Mardani, A.; Cavallaro, F.; Štreimikienė, D.; Khan, S.A.R. Pythagorean fuzzy SWARA–VIKOR framework for performance evaluation of solar panel selection. *Sustainability* **2020**, *12*, 4278. [CrossRef]
47. Rani, P.; Mishra, A.R.; Krishankumar, R.; Mardani, A.; Cavallaro, F.; Soundarapandian Ravichandran, K.; Balasubramanian, K. Hesitant fuzzy SWARA-complex proportional assessment approach for sustainable supplier selection (HF-SWARA-COPRAS). *Symmetry* **2020**, *12*, 1152. [CrossRef]
48. Agarwal, S.; Kant, R.; Shankar, R. Evaluating solutions to overcome humanitarian supply chain management barriers: A hybrid fuzzy SWARA—Fuzzy WASPAS approach. *Int. J. Disaster Risk Reduct.* **2020**, *51*, 101838. [CrossRef]
49. Mavi, R.K.; Goh, M.; Zarbakhshnia, N. Sustainable third-party reverse logistic provider selection with fuzzy SWARA and fuzzy MOORA in plastic industry. *Int. J. Adv. Manuf. Technol.* **2017**, *91*, 2401–2418. [CrossRef]
50. Garg, H.; Vimala, J.; Rajareega, S.; Preethi, D.; Perez-Dominguez, L. Complex intuitionistic fuzzy soft SWARA-COPRAS approach: An application of ERP software selection. *AIMS Math.* **2022**, *7*, 5895–5909. [CrossRef]
51. Ziquan, X.; Jiaqi, Y.; Naseem, M.H.; Zuquan, X.; Xueheng, L. Supplier Selection of Shipbuilding Enterprises Based on Intuitionistic Fuzzy Multicriteria Decision. *Math. Probl. Eng.* **2021**, *2*, 1775053. [CrossRef]
52. Macharis, C.; Turcksin, L.; Lebeau, K. Multi actor multi criteria analysis (MAMCA) as a tool to support sustainable decisions: State of use. *Decis. Support Syst.* **2012**, *54*, 610–620. [CrossRef]
53. Govindan, K.; Kadziński, M.; Ehling, R.; Miebs, G. Selection of a sustainable third-party reverse logistics provider based on the robustness analysis of an outranking graph kernel conducted with ELECTRE I and SMAA. *Omega* **2018**, *85*, 1–15. [CrossRef]
54. Chutia, R.; Saikia, S. Ranking intuitionistic fuzzy numbers at levels of decision-making and its application. *Expert Syst.* **2018**, *35*, e12292. [CrossRef]
55. Fu, Q.; Song, Y.; Fan, C.; Lei, L.; Wang, X. Evidential model for intuitionistic fuzzy multi-attribute group decision making. *Soft Comput.* **2019**, *24*, 7615–7635. [CrossRef]
56. Xie, D.; Xiao, F.; Pedrycz, W. Information quality for intuitionistic fuzzy values with its application in decision making. *Eng. Appl. Artif. Intell.* **2022**, *109*, 104568. [CrossRef]

healthcare

MDPI

Article

The Effect of Competency-Based Triage Education Application on Emergency Nurses' Triage Competency and Performance

Sun-Hee Moon and In-Young Cho *

College of Nursing, Chonnam National University, 160 Baekseo-ro, Dong-gu, Gwang-ju 61469, Korea; sunnymon@jnu.ac.kr
* Correspondence: kikiin1024@jnu.ac.kr

Abstract: The Korean Triage and Acuity Scale (KTAS) is used to determine emergency patient priority. The purpose of this study was to develop the Competency-Based Triage Education Application (CTEA) using KTAS and evaluate its effectiveness on emergency nurses' triage competency and performance. The developed CTEA mobile application comprised 4 lectures, 12 text-based cases, and 8 video-based triage scenarios. A quasi-experimental pre-post design with a comparison group (CG) was used to evaluate the effectiveness of the CTEA. Thirty-one participants were assigned to an intervention group (IG) and used the application for at least 100 min over one week. Thirty-five participants were assigned to a CG and underwent book-based learning, which covered the same content as the CTEA. Triage competency ($t = 2.55$, $p = 0.013$) and performance ($t = 2.11$, $p = 0.039$) were significantly improved in the IG. The IG's undertriage error was significantly reduced compared to that of the CG ($t = 2.08$, $p = 0.041$). These results indicated that the CTEA was effective in improving the emergency nurses' triage competency and performance. This application will be useful as a program for providing repeated and continuous triage education.

Keywords: triage; mobile applications; education; distance; competency-based education; KTAS

Citation: Moon, S.-H.; Cho, I.-Y. The Effect of Competency-Based Triage Education Application on Emergency Nurses' Triage Competency and Performance. *Healthcare* **2022**, *10*, 596. https://doi.org/10.3390/healthcare10040596

Academic Editors: Amir Khorram-Manesh, Krzysztof Goniewicz and Holger Muehlan

Received: 23 January 2022
Accepted: 21 March 2022
Published: 22 March 2022

1. Introduction

In modern emergency departments (EDs), the triage process is applied to quickly identify patients' acuity and classify their priority based on the severity of their conditions [1,2]. In EDs, emergency treatment is provided based on urgency rather than on a first-come, first-served basis; therefore, triage, which guides the allocation of limited medical resources—including health care providers and available medical equipment—according to patient's conditions, is an essential system for patient safety [1,2]. Typically, nurses are the main practitioners of triage in EDs, acting as gatekeepers at ED entrances [2,3]. Hence, educational support to ensure sufficient triage competency among emergency nurses is imperative.

Due to its proliferation, triage scales have been developed; in particular, a five-tier triage scale that divides patient urgency into five levels is mainly applied in modern EDs [4]. The triage scales used worldwide include the Canadian Triage and Acuity Scale (CTAS), the U.S. Emergency Severity Index (ESI), the Australasian Triage Scale (ATS), and the U.K. Manchester Triage System (MTS) [4]. In addition to these, a triage scale suitable for each country's emergency medical system has recently been developed. In 2016, the Korean Triage and Acuity Scale (KTAS) was established based on CTAS and used in EDs nationwide [5]. To ensure that nurses can use the KTAS to make accurate and rapid decisions, appropriate educational support is required.

Various training methods have been applied to assist triage nurses in making accurate and rapid decisions. According to existing review studies on triage education, the methods used primarily include brief lectures with case studies, simulations, live actors, computerized scenarios, and game-based learning [6–8]. Since the goal of triage education is to improve emergency nurses' competence in making accurate and rapid decisions through various educational methods [2,7,9], there is a need for more efficient and learner-friendly methods to be developed. Countries that have created a representative triage scale offer efficient triage education online [6]; recently, various techniques, such as virtual reality and augmented reality, have been introduced [10,11].

A few KTAS-based education programs have been developed, including the official hospital-KTAS provider course, an offline training program consisting of lectures and text-based case studies [12]. However, one-time education programs offered offline suffer from certain limitations. Specifically, to improve their triage competencies, emergency nurses need to experience triage repeatedly and continuously [3], which one-time courses do not offer. According to extant review studies, smartphone-based education significantly improved nursing and medical science practitioners' clinical competency, knowledge, attitude, performance, and confidence [13,14]. Since online education via mobile devices can be accessed freely and repeatedly without spatial and temporal constraints, a positive effect can be expected for app-based triage education centered on the KTAS.

Therefore, the purpose of this study was to develop a mobile-app-based online education program to improve emergency nurses' triage competency and verify the effectiveness of the education program. This study hypothesized that participants using the Competency-Based Triage Education Application (CTEA) would have greater (1) triage competency and (2) triage performance, compared to those learning triage using a book.

2. Materials and Methods

2.1. Design

This was a pre- and post-test quasi-experimental study with a comparison group, designed to evaluate the effect of the CTEA on emergency nurses' triage competency and performance.

2.2. The CTEA Development

The basic framework of the CTEA was designed based on a literature review and a qualitative study conducted by the research team to explore the educational needs of emergency nurses. The development of the preliminary educational contents was led by the first author, who has 12 years of experience working in EDs and more than 6 years of triage experience. The lecture content was developed with reference to four triage books from the Emergency Nurses Association and KTAS committees and one emergency medicine book [15–19]. The educational content included four lectures, 12 text-based case studies (covering abdominal pain, dyspnea, fever, vomiting, epistaxis, simple treatment, cough, behavior, dizziness, vaginal bleeding, and traffic accidents), and eight conversational scenarios (covering acute myocardial infarction, acute stroke, major trauma, congestive heart failure, acute hemorrhage, urticarial rash, appendicitis, and hyperventilation) (Figure 1). The case study was designed to equip the learners to solve the competency targeted KTAS quizzes. The CTEA was structured such that learners could ask the operator questions about triage cases and communicate freely with each other (learner to learner).

An expert group consisting of two emergency medicine professors and four emergency nursing professors who evaluated the validity of the educational content using content validity indices (CVIs). The overall CVI score of the educational contents was 0.92. In accordance with the experts' opinions, the vital signs of the triage cases and the dialogue of the scenario were modified.

The educational content was then converted to video form. Specifically, the first author created a 50 min video containing four lectures. The actors filmed the conversational scenarios in 8 videos, each 2–3 min long. The developed educational content was loaded into an Android-based hybrid mobile app (Figure 2). Learners were able to score "energy" points when viewing triage lectures, taking quizzes, and reviewing cases using the app, and they were able to check their ranking against other learners.

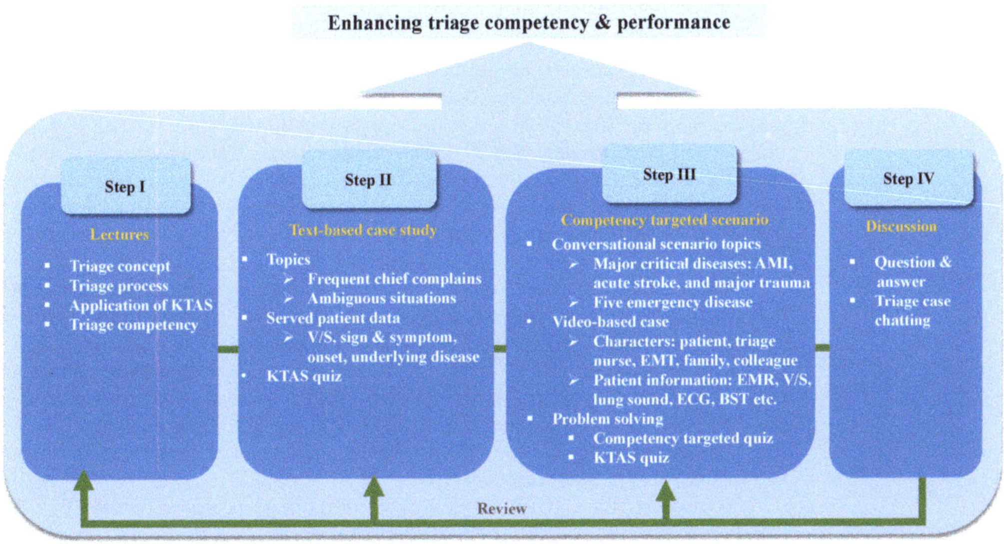

Figure 1. Triage education program. KTAS = Korean Triage and Acuity Scale, V/S = vital sign, AMI = acute myocardial infarction, EMT = emergency medical technician, EMR = electronic medical records, ECG = electrocardiogram, BST = blood sugar test.

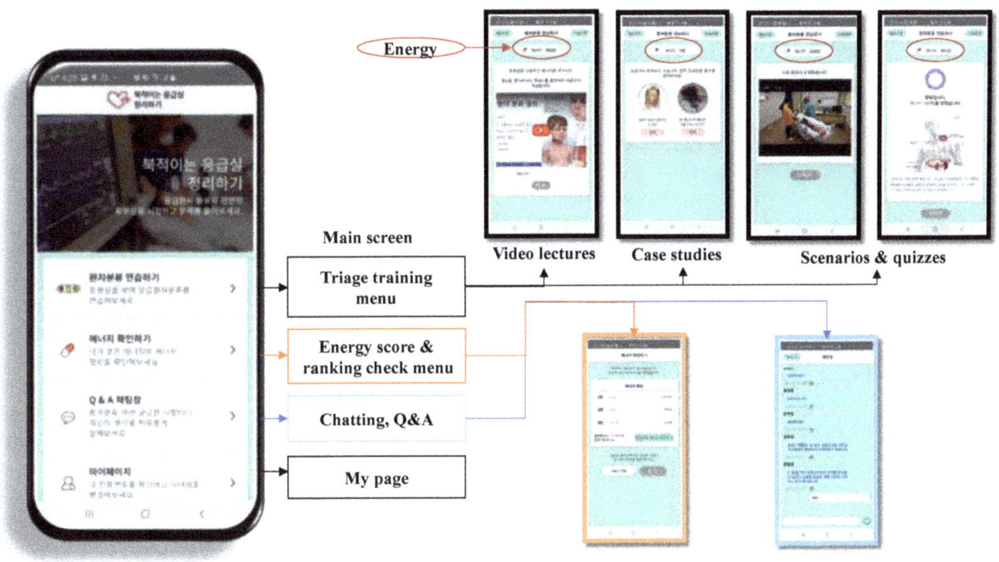

Figure 2. The Competency-Based Triage Education Application.

2.3. Outcome Measurements

To determine the nurses' KTAS competency, we measured four outcomes—critical thinking disposition, triage competency, triage knowledge, and triage performance.

Critical thinking disposition was the propensity to think critically to lead decision-making and problem-solving tasks [20]. In this study, critical thinking disposition was measured using a 5-point Likert scale developed by Kwon et al. in 2006 [20]. The scale consists of 35 items with potential total scores ranging from 35 to 175 points, with higher scores indicating higher critical thinking disposition. At the time of development, the scale received a Cronbach's α of 0.89 [20]. In this study, it received a Cronbach's α of 0.83.

Triage competency is the ability to allocate medical resources efficiently by determining care priority according to patients' health statuses [1]. In this study, triage competency was measured using a 5-point Likert scale developed by Moon et al. in 2018 [21]. The triage competency measure comprises 30 items with five sub-factors, including clinical judgment, expert assessment, management of medical resources, timely decisions, and communication [21]. The potential scores of the scale range from zero to 150, with higher scores indicating higher triage competency. The Cronbach's α of the scale in Moon et al.'s study was 0.91 [21], while in this study it was 0.96.

To measure triage knowledge, we developed a scale consisting of 32 preliminary items based on the four triage books mentioned previously. The content validity verification of the developed items was conducted by a panel of experts who participated in the CTEA's content validity verification. Among the 32 preliminary items, one item with a CVI score of 0.67 was deleted, resulting in 31 final items; the CVI of the final triage knowledge scale was 0.96. The items were answered by selecting one true/false answer for each of the 31 questions, and triage knowledge was calculated by totaling up the correct answers. The KR-20 of the triage knowledge scale was 0.56.

To measure triage performance we created 10 triage scenarios, drafted based on the experience of the first author and revised through research meetings. An expert panel verified the content validity of the scenarios written in conversational format. The CVI of the triage scenarios was 0.93. Videos, which were approximately 2 min in length, were created for the 10 triage scenarios, to which participants had to respond by assigning the videos a KTAS-based score from level 1 to level 5. The number of correct answers would then be summed up, overtriage error totaled up, and undertriage error totaled up. The KR-20 of the triage performance scale was 0.71.

2.4. Participants and Data Collection

Six EDs in four cities participated in this study from July 2020 to January 2021. The emergency medical system in Korea consists of the regional emergency center (REC), which is in charge of treating critical emergency patients, and the local emergency center (LEC), which is in charge of treating emergency patients in their local area. Of the EDs participating in this study, two were RECs and four were LECs. All EDs have been performing triage using KTAS since 2016. Three EDs each were assigned to the intervention and the comparison group (Figure 3). Thirty-eight emergency nurses were assigned to the intervention group and 37 to the comparison group. In total, 75 emergency nurses in the EDs responded to our online survey comprising six measures—critical thinking, triage competency, triage knowledge, triage performance, demographic factor (age, gender, educational level), and clinical experience (total nursing, emergency nursing, triage) before intervention.

The participants in the intervention group were provided with instructions on installing the CTEA. The participants read the guide and then downloaded and installed the CTEA from Play Store. Android smartphones were rented for Apple smartphone users. The participants in the intervention group underwent triage training using the CTEA for over 100 min in one week. The lengths of time the intervention group participants spent learning via the CTEA were saved in the program so that the administrator could monitor them. Five of the learners who studied for less than 100 min over the week were excluded from the intervention group. After one week of using the CTEA, the intervention was deemed complete and a post-survey in the same format as the pre-survey was conducted online. Of the 33 participants who completed learning in the intervention group, two participants did not respond to the post-survey and were excluded. The remaining 31 participants' data were analyzed.

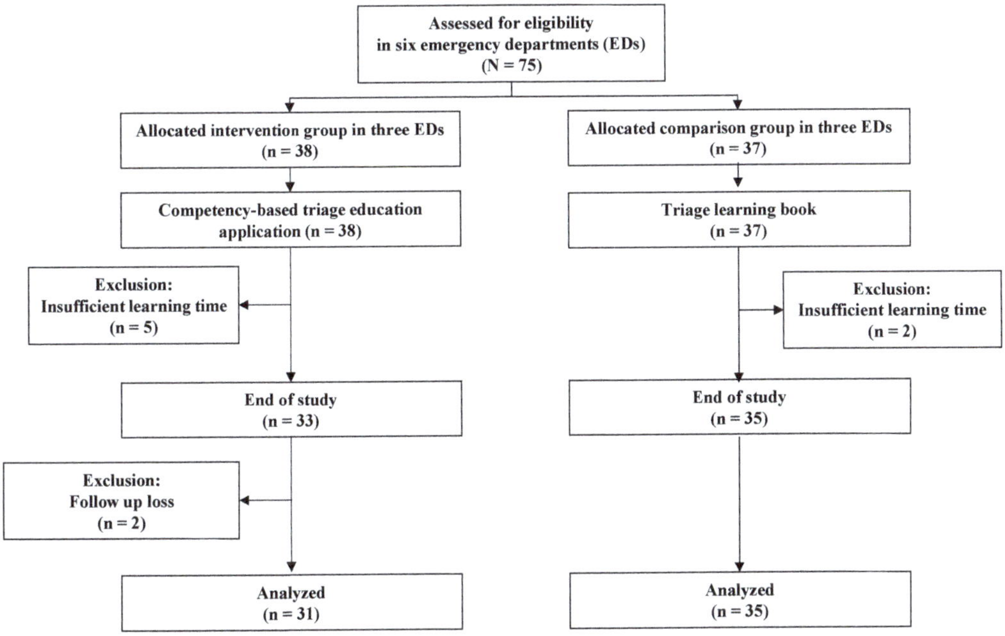

Figure 3. Participant's flow chart.

For the 37 participants in the comparison group, the 4 lecture materials and 12 text-based case studies (containing the same content as the CTEA material) were provided as a book. The comparison group participants completed 100 min of self-learning over one week using the triage book. The participants measured and reported their learning time to the researchers. After completing the learning, a post-survey in the same format as the pre-survey was conducted. Two of the comparison group participants were excluded due to insufficient self-learning time. The remaining 35 participants' data were analyzed.

The sample size calculation yielded G*Power 3.1.9.4. According to a meta-analysis on virtual patient education for health professionals, the effect size *d* was 0.8 [22]. In a two-tailed significance test with a power of 80% and an alpha level of 0.05, the sample size of each group was calculated to be 26. Therefore, the data used in this study's analysis met this criterion.

2.5. Data Analysis

The data were analyzed using IBM SPSS software, version 25.0(Armonk, NY: IBM Corp). The variables were analyzed based on frequencies, percentages, or means. We compared the baseline data of the two groups using chi tests for the categorical variables and *t*-tests for the continuous variables. To test the differences in critical thinking disposition, triage competency, triage knowledge, and triage performance, we calculated the difference between the pre-post means within each group and then compared the differences between the two groups using the independent *t*-test. As the pre-test result presented a difference in baseline triage knowledge, ANCOVA was applied to verify the difference in post-knowledge between the two groups using pre-knowledge as a covariate.

2.6. Ethical Approval

This study received approval from the University Institutional Review Board (No. 7001066-202002-HR-006). All participants willingly engaged in the data collection and intervention process and signed online informed consent forms. As a token of appreciation, all participants were awarded a $50 gift card at the end of the study.

3. Results

3.1. Baseline Characteristics

The average age of the participants was 32.15 ± 7.47 years, and most of them (56) were women (Table 1). The average total nursing experience was 8.85 ± 7.54 years. In accordance with the Career Development Model of Nurses, a clinical career was defined in four-stages: novice (under 1 year of nursing experience), advanced beginner (1~3 years of nursing experience), competent (3~7 years of nursing experience), and proficient nurses (7 or more years of nursing experience) [23]. The participants' average emergency experience was 4.04 ± 3.54 years, with 24 (36.4%) of them falling within the competent level. The participants' triage experience was 1.25 ± 1.46 years. Except for the triage knowledge score, the baseline variables of the two groups before intervention did not differ (t = 2.56, p = 0.013) (Table 2).

Table 1. Baseline characteristics of participants.

Characteristics	Classification	IG (n = 31) n (%) or Mean ± SD	CG (n = 35) n (%) or Mean ± SD	Total (N = 66) n (%) or Mean ± SD	χ2 or t (p)
Age	Total (years)	34.09 ± 8.19	30.42 ± 6.41	32.15 ± 7.47	2.00 (0.050)
	20~29	11 (16.7)	20 (30.3)	31 (47.0)	4.66 (0.097)
	30~39	12 (18.2)	12 (18.2)	24 (36.4)	
	≥40	8 (12.1)	3 (4.5)	11 (16.7)	
Gender	Female	26 (39.4)	30 (45.5)	56 (84.8)	0.04 (0.834)
	Male	5 (7.6)	5 (7.6)	10 (15.2)	
Education level	Associate degree	11 (16.7)	5 (7.6)	16 (24.2)	4.93 (0.085)
	Bachelor's degree	18 (27.3)	29 (43.9)	47 (71.2)	
	Over master's degree	2 (3.0)	1 (1.5)	3 (4.5)	
Experience in nursing	Total (year)	10.46 ± 8.19	7.42 ± 6.72	8.85 ± 7.54	1.65 (0.104)
	Novice (<1)	2 (3.0)	2 (3.0)	4 (6.1)	2.53 (0.471)
	Advanced beginner (1≤~<3)	4 (6.1)	7 (10.6)	11 (16.7)	
	Competent (3≤~<7)	6 (9.1)	11 (16.7)	17 (25.8)	
	Proficient (≥7)	19 (28.8)	15 (22.7)	34 (51.5)	
Experience in the ED	Total (year)	4.06 ± 3.12	4.02 ± 3.93	4.04 ± 3.54	0.05 (0.960)
	Novice (<1)	5 (7.6)	5 (7.6)	10 (15.2)	0.13 (0.989)
	Advanced beginner (1≤~<3)	9 (13.6)	11 (16.7)	20 (30.3)	
	Competent (3≤~<7)	11 (16.7)	13 (19.7)	24 (36.4)	
	Proficient (≥7)	6 (9.1)	6 (9.1)	12 (18.2)	
Experience of triage (year)		1.27 ± 1.77	1.23 ± 1.14	1.25 ± 1.46	0.10 (0.920)

IG = intervention group, CG = comparison group, SD = standard deviation, ED = emergency department.

3.2. Comparison of Outcomes

The first hypothesis in this study posited that the intervention group participants (those using the CTEA) would show higher triage competency than those in the comparison group. The intervention group's pre-post triage competency levels showed significant improvement compared with that of the comparison group (t = 2.55, p = 0.013) (Table 3). Specifically, after examining the sub-factors of the pre-post triage competency, the intervention group participants' clinical judgment (t = 2.39, p = 0.021) and timely decisions (t = 2.89, p = 0.005) showed significant improvement.

Table 2. Baseline outcome variables of participants.

Variables	IG (n = 31) Mean ± SD	CG (n = 35) Mean ± SD	Total (N = 66) Mean ± SD	t (p)
Critical thinking disposition	113.70 ± 9.62	112.34 ± 10.28	112.34 ± 10.28	−0.55 (0.581)
Triage competency	79.51 ± 16.68	82.88 ± 12.63	82.88 ± 12.63	0.93 (0.355)
Triage knowledge	20.35 ± 3.15	22.22 ± 2.77	22.22 ± 2.77	2.56 (0.013 *)
Triage accuracy	3.90 ± 1.86	4.02 ± 1.85	4.02 ± 1.85	0.27 (0.786)

IG = intervention group, CG = comparison group, SD = standard deviation, ED = emergency department, * $p < 0.05$.

Table 3. Comparison between pre- and post-outcomes of the two groups.

Variables	Groups	Pre (a) Mean ± SD	Post (b) Mean ± SD	Difference (b − a) Mean ± SD	t (p)
Critical thinking disposition	IG	113.70 ± 9.62	115.45 ± 10.31	1.74 ± 8.89	−0.47 (0.633)
	CG	112.34 ± 10.28	115.14 ± 10.93	2.80 ± 8.98	
Triage competency	IG	79.51 ± 16.68	86.25 ± 15.79	6.74 ± 14.42	2.55 (0.013 *)
	CG	82.88 ± 12.63	82.54 ± 12.65	-0.34 ± 7.40	
Clinical judgment	IG	34.12 ± 6.65	37.00 ± 6.37	2.87 ± 6.41	2.39 (0.021 *)
	CG	35.62 ± 5.33	35.45 ± 5.26	−0.17 ± 3.13	
Expert assessment	IG	10.00 ± 3.01	11.09 ± 2.59	1.09 ± 2.97	1.22 (0.225)
	CG	9.85 ± 2.46	10.20 ± 2.13	0.34 ± 1.79	
Management of medical resources	IG	11.29 ± 2.84	11.87 ± 2.26	0.58 ± 2.87	1.99 (0.051)
	CG	12.22 ± 2.27	11.62 ± 2.34	−0.60 ± 1.89	
Timely decisions	IG	10.51 ± 2.95	11.41 ± 2.93	0.90 ± 1.90	2.89 (0.005 *)
	CG	10.71 ± 2.29	10.31 ± 2.45	−0.40 ± 1.75	
Communication	IG	13.58 ± 3.26	14.87 ± 3.09	1.29 ± 3.01	1.30 (0.197)
	CG	14.45 ± 2.44	14.94 ± 2.02	0.48 ± 1.72	
Triage knowledge	IG	20.35 ± 3.15	22.41 ± 2.72	2.06 ± 2.95	3.11 (0.003 *)
	CG	22.22 ± 2.77	22.28 ± 2.39	0.05 ± 2.27	
Triage accuracy	IG	3.90 ± 1.86	4.77 ± 1.68	0.87 ± 2.34	2.11 (0.039 *)
	CG	4.03 ± 1.85	3.80 ± 1.71	−0.22 ± 1.88	

IG = intervention group, CG = comparison group, SD = standard deviation, * $p < 0.05$.

The second hypothesis of this study was that the intervention group participants would show higher triage accuracy than those in the comparison group. When the pre-post triage accuracy of the two groups was verified, the intervention group showed significant improvement (t = 2.11, $p = 0.039$). To evaluate the cause of triage error, the averages of the two groups' undertriage and overtriage were investigated and compared (Figure 4). The results revealed a significant reduction in the intervention group's undertriage error, compared to the comparison group (t = 2.08, $p = 0.041$). However, both groups showed a decrease in the average of overtriage error.

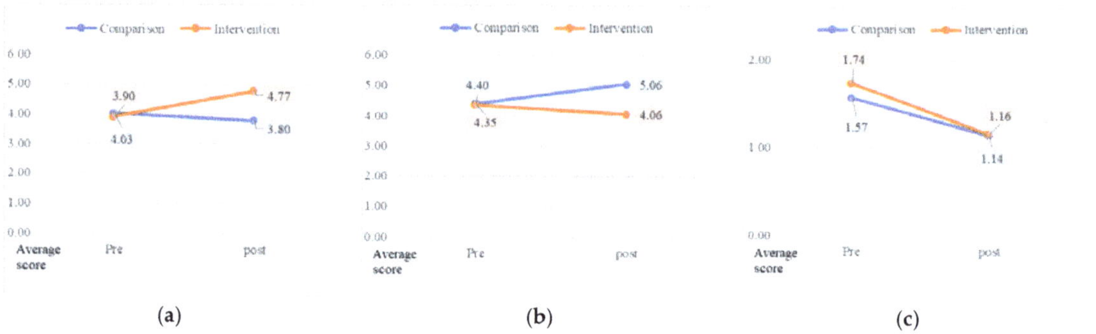

Figure 4. Triage accuracy and causes of triage error. (**a**) Triage accuracy. (**b**) Undertriage. (**c**) Overtriage.

There was no significant difference between the two groups regarding critical thinking disposition when the pre- and post-test values were compared (t = −0.47, p = 0.633). For triage knowledge, after controlling the baseline values, that is, the covariate, no difference was found (F = 3.52, p = 0.065).

4. Discussion

Due to the spread of COVID-19, various non face-to-face education methods have recently been developed and utilized. Smartphone-based learning is one of the representative non face-to-face education methods that emphasizes learner accessibility. Recent research has reported that smartphone-based education improves clinical competency, knowledge, performance, attitude, and confidence in nursing and medical science practice [13,14]. Since a smartphone-based triage education program was developed, distance training and repeat clinical decision-making practice was rendered possible [24,25]. The significance of this study was the development of a mobile education app for strengthening the triage competency of emergency nurses based on the KTAS and the verification of its effectiveness. This KTAS-based educational mobile app development and effectiveness verification was the first attempt in Korea. Furthermore, since the importance of repetitive education is emphasized for the advancement of triage [3], the CTEA can be a complementary method to official triage education that allows iterative and convenient learning.

The Emergency Nurses Association (ENA) establishes practice guidelines for triage qualifications; thus, it is necessary to strengthen triage competency by improving knowledge and skills through appropriate triage education courses [26]. Extant research also reported competency and knowledge improvement as the main effect of triage education. Previous research reported that nursing students' competency and knowledge significantly improved after they were provided with education, including role plays and lectures based on the Simple Triage and Rapid Treatment (START) triage [27]. In a disaster nursing education program comprising lectures and practical tasks, nursing students' disaster nursing knowledge, disaster triage performance, and disaster readiness increased [28]. In this study, after undergoing CTEA-based training, the participants' triage competency improved. However, although the mean difference in triage knowledge between the two groups in this study was significant, there was no significant difference when the baseline score was adjusted using ANCOVA. Compared to the previous face-to-face research, the CTEA was conducted in a non face-to-face manner, which, except for observing learning time, translated to the limited monitoring of learners. Thus, triage knowledge may not have improved. Additionally, the intervention group's triage knowledge pre-test score and the comparison group's triage knowledge pre- and post-test score were almost similar. This may be due to the ceiling effect.

Triage competency comprises five attributes: clinical judgment, expert assessment, management of medical resources, timely decisions, and communication [1]. Among the sub-factors of triage competency, clinical judgment and timely decisions showed significant improvement in this study. When emergency nurses perform triage, rapid and accurate decision-making is important, making it a crucial objective that must be achieved through triage education [1,7,18,26]. Therefore, improvements in clinical judgment and the ability to make timely decisions through the CTEA could be referred to as educational goals. However, sub-factors such as communication and expert assessment did not significantly improve in this study. As physical examination requires direct practice, it may have been difficult to achieve the same in mobile-based non face-to-face research. Other than the chat function, the CTEA did not have a feature that allowed participants to communicate with patients or medical staff. Due to these development limitations, communication ability may not have been improved. In cases where artificial intelligence plays the role of an emergency patient or where learners perform triage simulations with standard patients in a virtual space, improvements in learners' communication in non face-to-face education could be expected.

According to a review study, triage accuracy was reported to be 56.2~82.9% when analyzed based on written case scenarios or medical record review results [29]. Based on electronic medical records in the EDs using KTAS, the weighted kappa value was 0.69~0.83 for triage accuracy, which increased to 0.84 after problem-based learning [30,31]. In this study, triage accuracy significantly increased after using the CTEA; however, compared to a previous study [29], this was not high. Although the mobile-based education in this study had a limited effect on triage accuracy compared to face-to-face education, such education may be a good alternative; as triage education must be accessible and administered continuously and repeatedly to maintain triage accuracy [3] and mobile devices allow for such conveniences. Thus, if various mobile-based triage education programs are developed, triage quality can eventually be achieved and maintained.

There are two types of triage errors: undertriage and overtriage [32,33]. Undertriage is when treatment time for emergency patients is delayed due to underestimating the severity of the patients' condition at triage, potentially jeopardizing patients' safety [33]. Overtriage is when patients' conditions are overestimated, which can cause overcrowding in the ED and jeopardize patients' safety by endangering urgent patients [32]. Mistriage in the Korean EDs using KTAS resulted in an undertriage of 70.4% and overtriage of 29.6%, which was reported to have a higher underestimation error [31]. In this study, the incidence of undertriage was higher than that of overtriage when assessed using the video-based triage scenarios. The nurses' triage errors were reported to decrease when the web-based video education program developed using the KTAS was applied [34]. Similarly, in this study, when the mobile-based video scenario was applied, undertriage decreased significantly, and overtriage showed a decreasing pattern, although it was not statistically significant. Therefore, it could be said that the use of video-based scenarios for triage learning was effective and that it is necessary to develop various triage cases to ensure that learners can repeatedly access education more conveniently. In addition, since the incidence of undertriage in Korea's EDs using the KTAS was high, it may be necessary to develop an education program focused on reducing underestimation.

Gamification is the application of a game design in non-game contexts and has been widely used in education programs to motivate users, enhance psychological outcomes, and encourage behavioral change [35–37]. As in many other educational programs, gamification has also been introduced to triage education. A study on trauma triage education using serious game technology reported improvement in emergency physicians' decision heuristics [38]. According to review studies, game features commonly used in healthcare gamification include points, social interactions, leaderboards, progress statuses, levels, and immediate feedback [36]. The gamification strategies used in this study were "energy points," social interaction through chatting, levels, and immediate feedback. In a meta-analysis study verifying the effect of gamification in medical education, knowledge improvement and long-term knowledge retention were reported [39]. Although it was not possible to directly verify the educational effect of the gamification in this study design, if the same gamification strategy is used in future triage education, we expect continuity in the training effect.

This study had a few limitations. First, it measured the effectiveness of the CTEA program immediately after its use. Therefore, it was not possible to estimate the continuation of the educational effect on the participants and the interval requiring repeated education. If the effect of continuous education through the CTEA is confirmed, the application can be used more effectively as a complementary program for the official KTAS education. Second, this was a quasi-experimental study and participants were not randomly assigned. Randomization and blinding can assert strong causality and are suitable in research settings such as laboratories [40]. Many randomized studies examining the effectiveness of medical education have raised validity and reliability concerns; therefore, it has been suggested that they be categorized as quasi-experimental studies [40]. In this study, in accordance with the suggestions of a review [40], a randomized controlled trial, which was considered difficult in the educational field, was not unreasonably followed. Although random assignment could not be performed in this study, we attempted to maintain validity by assigning groups based on hospitals to avoid influence between participants and conducted a homogeneity test. Third, the book provided to the CG included 4 lectures and 12 text-based cases, except for the 8 videos provided to the IG. Although video-based contents could not be included in a paper-based book, differences in the amount of content provided may have affected the results. Fourth, this study was conducted only in six EDs in Korea; therefore, there was a limit to the generalizability of the results.

5. Conclusions

The development of the CTEA and its application to emergency nurses in this study improved triage competency and performance in the intervention group. Moreover, the CTEA was effective in reducing triage error. Therefore, the CTEA can be used as an educational program for continuous triage education because it is mobile-based and enables repetitive and convenient learning.

Author Contributions: Conceptualization, S.-H.M.; data curation, S.-H.M. and I.-Y.C.; investigation, S.-H.M.; methodology, S.-H.M.; project administration, S.-H.M.; software, S.-H.M. and I.-Y.C.; supervision, S.-H.M.; validation, S.-H.M.; visualization, I.-Y.C.; writing—review & editing, S.-H.M. and I.-Y.C.; funding acquisition, S.-H.M. All authors have read and agreed to the published version of the manuscript.

Funding: This work was supported by the National Research Foundation of Korea (NRF) grant funded by the Korea government (MSIT) (No. NRF-2017R1C1B5074027).

Institutional Review Board Statement: The study was conducted in accordance with the Declaration of Helsinki and approved by the Institutional Review Board (IRB) of Changwon National University IRB (No. 7001066-202002-HR-006).

Informed Consent Statement: Informed consent was obtained from all subjects involved in the study.

Data Availability Statement: Not applicable.

Conflicts of Interest: The authors declare no conflict of interest. The funders had no role in the design of the study; in the collection, analyses, or interpretation of data; in the writing of the manuscript; or in the decision to publish the results.

References

1. Moon, S.H.; Park, Y.H. Concept analysis of triage competency in emergency nursing. *J. Korean Crit. Care Nurs.* **2017**, *10*, 41–52.
2. Fry, M.; Burr, G. Review of the triage literature: Past, present, future? *Aust. Emerg. Nurs. J.* **2002**, *5*, 33–38. [CrossRef]
3. Moon, S.-H.; Jeon, M.-K.; Ju, D. Facilitators and Barriers of the Triage Process based on Emergency Nurses' Experience with the Korean Triage and Acuity Scale: A Qualitative Content Analysis. *Asian Nurs. Res.* **2021**, *15*, 255–264. [CrossRef] [PubMed]
4. Christ, M.; Grossmann, F.; Winter, D.; Bingisser, R.; Platz, E. Modern triage in the emergency department. *Dtsch. Ärzteblatt Int.* **2010**, *107*, 892. [CrossRef]
5. Park, J.; Lim, T. Korean triage and acuity scale (KTAS). *J. Korean Soc. Emerg. Med.* **2017**, *28*, 547–551.
6. Recznik, C.T.; Simko, L.M. Pediatric triage education: An integrative literature review. *J. Emerg. Nurs.* **2018**, *44*, 605–613.e609. [CrossRef]

7. Hardy, A.; Calleja, P. Triage education in rural remote settings: A scoping review. *Int. Emerg. Nurs.* **2019**, *43*, 119–125. [CrossRef]
8. Ricciardi, F.; De Paolis, L.T. A comprehensive review of serious games in health professions. *Int. J. Comput. Games Technol.* **2014**, *2014*, 9. [CrossRef]
9. Austin, E.E.; Blakely, B.; Tufanaru, C.; Selwood, A.; Braithwaite, J.; Clay-Williams, R. Strategies to measure and improve emergency department performance: A scoping review. *Scand. J. Trauma Resusc. Emerg. Med.* **2020**, *28*, 55. [CrossRef]
10. Foronda, C.L.; Shubeck, K.; Swoboda, S.M.; Hudson, K.W.; Budhathoki, C.; Sullivan, N.; Hu, X. Impact of virtual simulation to teach concepts of disaster triage. *Clin. Simul. Nurs.* **2016**, *12*, 137–144. [CrossRef]
11. Anderson, M.; Guido-Sanz, F.; Díaz, D.A.; Lok, B.; Stuart, J.; Akinnola, I.; Welch, G. Augmented Reality in Nurse Practitioner Education: Using a Triage Scenario to Pilot Technology Usability and Effectiveness. *Clin. Simul. Nurs.* **2021**, *54*, 105–112. [CrossRef]
12. Korean Triage and Acuity Scale Committee. KTAS Training Course. Available online: http://www.ktas.org/education/info.php (accessed on 5 June 2021).
13. Kim, J.H.; Park, H. Effects of smartphone-based mobile learning in nursing education: A systematic review and meta-analysis. *Asian Nurs. Res.* **2019**, *13*, 20–29. [CrossRef] [PubMed]
14. Koohestani, H.R.; Arabshahi, S.K.S.; Fata, L.; Ahmadi, F. The educational effects of mobile learning on students of medical sciences: A systematic review in experimental studies. *J. Adv. Med. Educ. Prof.* **2018**, *6*, 58.
15. Visser, L.S.; Montejano, A.S. An Orientation and Care Guide. In *Fast Facts for the Triage Nurse*, 2nd ed.; Springer: Berlin/Heidelberg, Germany, 2018.
16. Visser, L.S.; Montejano, A.S. *Rapid Access Guide for Triage and Emergency Nurses: Chief Complaints with High Risk Presentations*; Springer: Berlin/Heidelberg, Germany, 2018.
17. Manchester Triage Group. *Emergency Triage*; Wiley: Hoboken, NJ, USA, 2008.
18. Korean Triage and Acuity Scale Committee. *KTAS Provider Manual 2nd*; Koonja: Paju, Korea, 2021.
19. Tintinalli, J.E.; Stapczynski, J.S.; Ma, O.J.; Cline, D.M.; Meckler, G.D. *Tintinalli's Emergency Medicine: A Comprehensive Study Guide*, 8th ed.; McGraw-Hill Education: New York, NY, USA, 2016.
20. Kwon, I.S.; Lee, G.E.; Kim, G.D.; Kim, Y.H.; Park, K.M.; Park, H.S.; Sohn, S.K.; Lee, W.S.; Jang, K.S.; Chung, B.Y. Development of a critical thinking disposition scale for nursing students. *J. Korean Acad. Nurs.* **2006**, *36*, 950–958. [CrossRef]
21. Moon, S.H.; Park, Y.H. Development of a triage competency scale for emergency nurses. *J. Korean Acad. Nurs.* **2018**, *48*, 362–374. [CrossRef]
22. Cook, D.A.; Erwin, P.J.; Triola, M.M. Computerized virtual patients in health professions education: A systematic review and meta-analysis. *Acad. Med.* **2010**, *85*, 1589–1602. [CrossRef] [PubMed]
23. Jang, K.-S. A Study on Establishment of Clinical Career Development Model of Nurses. Ph.D. Thesis, Yonsei University, Seoul, Korea, 2000. Unpublished.
24. McCoy, L.; Lewis, J.H.; Dalton, D. Gamification and multimedia for medical education: A landscape review. *J. Osteopath. Med.* **2016**, *116*, 22–34. [CrossRef]
25. Montano, I.H.; de la Torre Díez, I.; López-Izquierdo, R.; Villamor, M.A.C.; Martín-Rodríguez, F. Mobile triage applications: A systematic review in literature and play store. *J. Med. Syst.* **2021**, *45*, 86. [CrossRef]
26. Emergency Nurses Association. Triage Qualifications and Competency. *J. Emerg. Nurs.* **2017**, *43*, 571–574. [CrossRef]
27. Aysha, Z.M.S.; Allam, Z.A. Efficacy of START Triage Algorithm Scenario-Based Education on Nursing Students' Knowledge, Attitude, Competencies, and Clinical Judgment. *IOSR J. Nurs. Health Sci. IOSR-JNHS* **2020**, *9*, 39–56.
28. Huh, S.S.; Kang, H.Y. Effects of an educational program on disaster nursing competency. *Public Health Nurs.* **2019**, *36*, 28–35. [CrossRef]
29. Tam, H.L.; Chung, S.F.; Lou, C.K. A review of triage accuracy and future direction. *BMC Emerg. Med.* **2018**, *18*, 58. [CrossRef] [PubMed]
30. Jang, K.; Jo, E.; Song, K.J. Effect of problem-based learning on severity classification agreement by triage nurses. *BMC Nurs.* **2021**, *20*, 256. [CrossRef] [PubMed]
31. Moon, S.-H.; Shim, J.L.; Park, K.-S.; Park, C.-S. Triage accuracy and causes of mistriage using the Korean Triage and Acuity Scale. *PLoS ONE* **2019**, *14*, e0216972. [CrossRef] [PubMed]
32. Lee, J.H.; Park, Y.S.; Park, I.C.; Lee, H.S.; Kim, J.H.; Park, J.M.; Chung, S.P.; Kim, M.J. Over-triage occurs when considering the patient's pain in Korean Triage and Acuity Scale (KTAS). *PLoS ONE* **2019**, *14*, e0216519. [CrossRef] [PubMed]
33. Grossmann, F.F.; Zumbrunn, T.; Frauchiger, A.; Delport, K.; Bingisser, R.; Nickel, C.H. At risk of undertriage? Testing the performance and accuracy of the emergency severity index in older emergency department patients. *Ann. Emerg. Med.* **2012**, *60*, 317–325.e313. [CrossRef]
34. Kim, H.-J.; Kang, H.-Y. Effects of a Web-Based Korean Triage and Acuity Scale Learning Program on Triage Self-Efficacy and Triage Performance Ability for Nurses in Emergency Department. *J. Korean Acad. Nurs.* **2019**, *49*, 171–180. [CrossRef]
35. Nah, F.F.-H.; Zeng, Q.; Telaprolu, V.R.; Ayyappa, A.P.; Eschenbrenner, B. Gamification of education: A review of literature. In Proceedings of the International Conference on HCI in Business, Crete, Greece, 22–24 June 2014; pp. 401–409.
36. Deterding, S.; Khaled, R.; Nacke, L.E.; Dixon, D. Gamification: Toward a definition. In Proceedings of the CHI 2011 Gamification Workshop Proceedings, Vancouver, BC, Canada, 7 May 2011; pp. 12–15.
37. Hamari, J.; Koivisto, J.; Sarsa, H. Does gamification work?—A literature review of empirical studies on gamification. In Proceedings of the 2014 47th Hawaii International Conference on System Sciences, Waikoloa, HI, USA, 6–9 January 2014; pp. 3025–3034.

38. Mohan, D.; Angus, D.C.; Ricketts, D.; Farris, C.; Fischhoff, B.; Rosengart, M.R.; Yealy, D.M.; Barnato, A.E. Assessing the validity of using serious game technology to analyze physician decision making. *PLoS ONE* **2014**, *9*, e105445. [CrossRef]
39. Zhao, J.; Zhou, K.; Ding, Y. Digital Games-Based Learning Pedagogy Enhances the Quality of Medical Education: A Systematic Review and Meta-Analysis. *Asia-Pac. Educ. Res.* **2021**, 1–12. [CrossRef]
40. Colliver, J.A.; Kucera, K.; Verhulst, S.J. Meta-analysis of quasi-experimental research: Are systematic narrative reviews indicated? *Med. Educ.* **2008**, *42*, 858–865. [CrossRef]

safety

Article

Addressing Uncertainty by Designing an Intelligent Fuzzy System to Help Decision Support Systems for Winter Road Maintenance

Mahshid Hatamzad [1,*], Geanette Polanco Pinerez [1] and Johan Casselgren [2]

[1] Department of Industrial Engineering, UiT/The Arctic University of Norway, 8514 Narvik, Nordland, Norway; geanette.polanco@uit.no
[2] Department of Engineering Sciences and Mathematics, Luleå University of Technology, 971 87 Luleå, Sweden; johan.casselgren@ltu.se
* Correspondence: mahshid.hatamzad@uit.no

Abstract: One of the main challenges in developing efficient and effective winter road maintenance is to design an accurate prediction model for the road surface friction coefficient. A reliable and accurate prediction model of road surface friction coefficient can help decision support systems to significantly increase traffic safety, while saving time and cost. High dynamicity in weather and road surface conditions can lead to the presence of uncertainties in historical data extracted by sensors. To overcome this issue, this study uses an adaptive neuro-fuzzy inference system that can appropriately address uncertainty using fuzzy logic neural networks. To investigate the ability of the proposed model to predict the road surface friction coefficient, real data were measured at equal time intervals using optical sensors and road-mounted sensors. Then, the most critical features were selected based on the Pearson correlation coefficient, and the dataset was split into two independent training and test datasets. Next, the input variables were fuzzified by generating a fuzzy inference system using the fuzzy c-means clustering method. After training the model, a testing set was used to validate the trained model. The model was evaluated by means of graphical and numerical metrics. The results show that the constructed adaptive neuro-fuzzy model has an excellent ability to learn and accurately predict the road surface friction coefficient.

Keywords: adaptive neuro-fuzzy inference system (ANFIS); prediction methods; road surface friction; road transportation safety; winter road maintenance

Citation: Hatamzad, M.; Polanco Pinerez, G.; Casselgren, J. Addressing Uncertainty by Designing an Intelligent Fuzzy System to Help Decision Support Systems for Winter Road Maintenance. *Safety* **2022**, *8*, 14. https://doi.org/10.3390/safety8010014

Academic Editors: Amir Khorram Manesh and Tom Brijs

Received: 1 November 2021
Accepted: 15 February 2022
Published: 17 February 2022

1. Introduction

1.1. Motivation

Low temperatures and heavy snowfall can be problematic for road users, especially in countries with long and harsh cold-weather conditions. Road safety can be significantly reduced due to slippery surface conditions and poor visibility [1]. Adverse weather can decrease the reliability and productivity of the surface transportation system. In addition, it increases traffic delays and the likelihood of vehicle accidents that may lead to severe injuries and fatalities [2]. To minimize these negative impacts, roads must be kept clear of ice and snow through chemical (salting) and mechanical (plowing) operations, referred to as winter road maintenance (WRM) techniques. WRM helps to increase the friction between tires and the road surface to prepare the road for normal traffic flow, meaning that the road users can drive as fast as in summer (effective WRM); however, this can result in high expenses (inefficient WRM).

Prediction of the road surface friction coefficient (RSFC) can help decision makers to plan in advance for the type and timing of WRM to improve decision support systems (DSS). The prediction of RSFC is a comprehensive calculation from different performance aspects using multiple physical dynamic variables (e.g., weather temperature, ice layer, snow height, etc.), which often shows a nonlinear relationship between road surface friction and the considered variables. In fact, sensors are not always able to measure road surface conditions (RSC) precisely, due to various reasons such as signal noise. Therefore, uncertainties need to be considered to enhance the accuracy of prediction models and improve the WRM performance.

1.2. Significance of the Topic

An accurate RSFC prediction model helps decision makers to effectively prepare for and respond to severe road conditions in winter (such as snowstorms and sharp reductions in RSFC), in order to maximize road safety for road users. Addressing uncertainty in a prediction model allows decision makers to systematically prevent hazards (such as fatal vehicle accidents) and strategically organize WRM resources to mitigate the detrimental impacts that a disaster can cause. In addition, avoiding the use of extra salt (chemicals) on the road surface minimizes cost and environmental impacts. In fact, high WRM quality and using an optimal salt quantity minimizes damage to vehicles, road infrastructure, vegetation, lakes, rivers, etc.

1.3. State-of-the-Art Method

There are several studies that present various methods to reach effective and efficient WRM. Shao and Lister [3], the authors used air temperature, wind speed, surface temperature, and dew-point as input variables to develop an automated road ice prediction model. Mohseni [4] applied a regression model to select the strongest features (pavement temperature, latitude, air temperature, elevation, and depth into the asphalt concrete layer) to develop a prediction model for low pavement temperature based on laboratory tests. Kangas et al. [5] developed a simulation model named RoadSurf using numerical weather forecasts as input to predict road surface temperature and condition. Moreover, developing sensor technologies has had a significant impact on monitoring road surface conditions in winter. Ye et al. [6] presented a review about developing and implementing advanced technologies to achieve safe and efficient WRM. Ewan et al. [7] investigated the reliability of an optical sensor to measure snow depth, water depth, and surface state (dry, wet, icy, etc.). Feng and Fu [8] investigated the performance of pavement sensors, and their results show that a sensor cannot always detect friction precisely. However, WRM effectiveness and efficiency can be improved by developing data-driven approaches using historical data collected by sensors. Ahabchane et al. [9] proposed a data-driven regression model using geometry, weather, and telemetry data to predict the amount of salt and abrasives in street segments. Pan et al. [10] applied deep neural networks to classify RSC according to images. Liu et al. [11] utilized machine learning algorithms (gradient-boosting) to develop road surface temperature forecasting. Roychowdhury et al. [12] applied neural networks to design a methodology to estimate RFSC. Panahandeh et al. [13] employed machine learning (ML) classification algorithms to predict RFCS for connected vehicles. Pu et al. [14] developed a daily RSFC prediction model using a long–short-term memory neural network based on the following three scenarios: (i) considering only daily friction data, (ii) selecting water thickness as an input variable, and (iii) selecting road surface temperature and water thickness as predictors. Their results showed that the second scenario had the highest accuracy. ML algorithms are powerful techniques to predict different nonlinear problems. Optical and road-mounted sensors are mostly used to measure data-related road surface conditions. Sometimes, numerical data derived from sensors can be associated with uncertainty due to imprecision, vagueness, or ambiguity. Song et al. [15] estimated maximum RSFC under uncertainty using deep learning. Matusko et al. [16] presented a new approach by adding neural networks to the friction estimator model, to enhance the estimation quality by compensating for the impacts of uncertainties. Kim et al. [17] designed a system for composite friction control, which included friction uncertainty using recurrent fuzzy neural networks. While previous research studies have contributed significantly to developing different dimensions of WRM, there has, thus far, been no study to predict RSFC by designing an adaptive neuro-fuzzy inference system (ANFIS), which is able to handle the uncertainty hidden in historical data extracted by sensors. An adaptive fuzzy RSFC prediction model with high accuracy plays an important role in making WRM plans in advance, in order to achieve effective and efficient WRM.

1.4. Contributions

Reviewing previous studies on WRM reveals that it is not easy to establish an accurate data-driven RSFC prediction model, due to dynamic weather conditions that can lead to variation in road surface conditions. In addition, historical data collected by sensors can be associated with uncertainty, which must be modeled. To model this complex problem, the main contribution of this study is the design of an ANFIS model to predict RSFC using real data measured by optical and road-mounted sensors. The ANFIS model fuzzifies the crisp data for simulating this complex problem, associated with uncertainty.

1.5. Outline of the Paper

The remainder of this paper is organized as follows. Section 2 explains the summary of ANFIS. The data and methods are defined in Section 3. In Section 4, we present results. Finally, in Section 5, a conclusion is drawn.

2. Adaptive Neuro-Fuzzy Inference System (ANFIS)

Crisp numerical data points can be fuzzified and represented by membership functions (MFs) [18]. In recent years, artificial intelligence methods, including fuzzy intelligent techniques, have been extensively used in different fields such as economics, medicine, and engineering. The ANFIS model was proposed by Jang in the 1990s [19] and can be considered as a universal estimator for predicting long- and short-term effects [20]. ANFIS is a five-layer adaptive network that illustrates the relationship between inputs and outputs to simulate complex problems associated with uncertainties by creating fuzzy variables [21]. The ANFIS network utilizes the learning ability of neural network concepts and the reasoning mechanisms of the Takagi–Sugeno fuzzy interference system (FIS) [22]. Due to using both fuzzy logic and neural networks, ANFIS can benefit from both models' principles in a single model. The inference system employs fuzzy "if-then" rules, which have a learning ability to estimate nonlinear functions [23].

3. Data and Methods

Figure 1 shows the framework of this study and its different steps, which are explained in this section.

3.1. Data Collection

Although there is an obvious relationship between road surface conditions and weather conditions, the proposed model's input variables are defined as conditions that impact the WRM performance. In addition, the output variable is defined as a result gained from the input variables. One of the major benefits of the data-driven model is that different kinds of inputs and outputs are allowed to be included in the model without having special relationships. Moreover, all of the input variables have a similar opportunity to affect the road conditions. Therefore, here, air temperature, surface temperature, ice layer, snow layer, water thickness, and snow height were chosen as input variables and RSFC was chosen as the output variable. Historical data of these variables were measured every 10 min and collected from the Swedish Transport Administration's RWIS station on a European road at test site E18 in February 2019. The test site E18 is located in Sweden, Northern Europe, between Enköping and Västerås, the latitude and longitude are approximately 59.724 and17.029 [24], and the type of pavement was asphalt. The road weather station measured air temperature. Optical sensors measured ice layer (mm), snow layer (mm) (new snow), and RSFC. A road-mounted sensor measured surface temperature (°C), snow height (mm) (both new and old snow), and water thickness (mm). Table 1 shows the statistical description of the dataset.

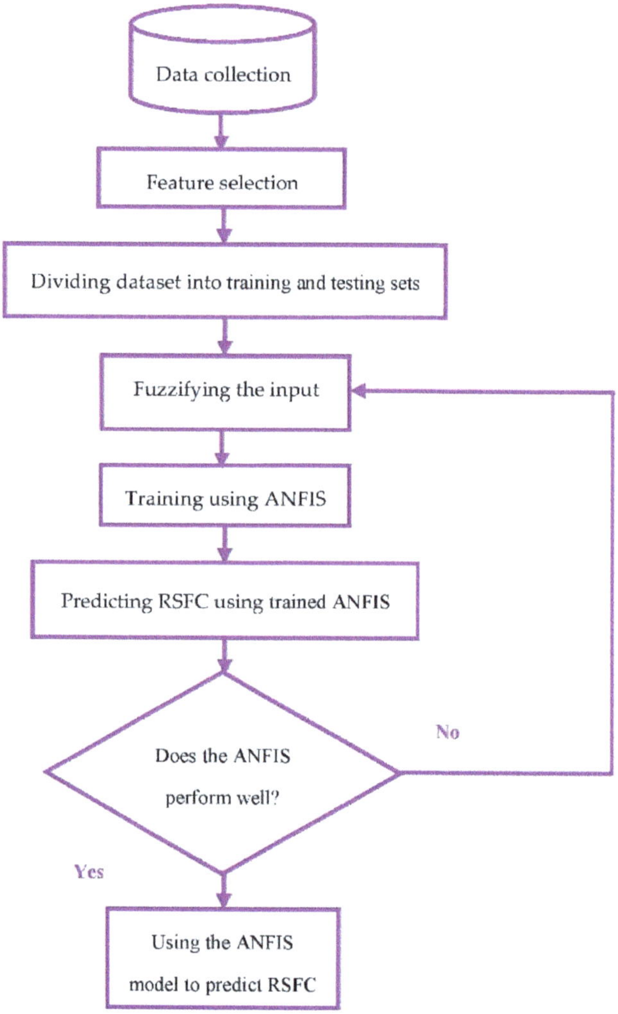

Figure 1. The framework used this study.

Table 1. Statistical description of the dataset.

Variables	Count	Mean	Std	Min	25%	50%	75%	Max
Ice layer	3847	0.019	0.059	0.000	0.000	0.000	0.000	0.510
Snow layer	3847	0.037	0.146	0.000	0.000	0.000	0.000	1.040
Water thickness	3847	0.060	0.135	0.000	0.000	0.030	0.060	1.880
Snow height	3847	2.562	5.341	0.000	0.000	0.000	2.000	47.000
Surface temperature	3847	0.607	4.627	−14.600	−1.500	1.100	3.300	14.200
Air temperature	3847	0.813	4.978	−20.000	−0.900	1.900	3.800	10.400
RSFC (output)	3847	0.750	0.149	0.110	0.780	0.810	0.820	0.820

In Table 1, the first column shows the number of observations, which are equal for all variables. The second and third columns illustrate the mean value and standard deviation of observations, respectively. The fourth and eighth columns are the minimum and maximum values for each variable. The fifth, sixth, and seventh columns demonstrate the 25th percentile (the lower or first quartile), 50th percentile (the median), and 75th percentile (the upper or third quartile), respectively.

3.2. Feature Selection

In the previous step, variables influencing RSFC were initially chosen. However, reducing the number of input variables decreases the model complexity and enhances the training process, which can lead to enhancing the model accuracy. Therefore, we used the Pearson correlation coefficient to select the most significant predictors. Table 2 shows the absolute value of correlation between the input variables and RSFC. Out of six input variables, four variables (ice layer, snow layer, water thickness, and snow height) were highly correlated with RSFC. Thus, these four input variables were used to design an RSFC prediction model.

Table 2. Pearson correlation coefficients between input variables and RSFC.

Input	Absolute Value of Correlation between Input and RSFC
Ice layer	0.88
Snow layer	0.69
Water thickness	0.65
Snow height	0.61
Surface temperature	0.29
Air temperature	0.27

3.3. Dividing the Dataset into Training and Testing Sets

The dataset needed to be divided into training and testing sets. The training dataset optimizes the parameters of the model, and the test dataset evaluates the model performance to predict RSFC. In this study, 70% of the observations were considered for training the ANFIS model and the rest of the observations were applied to test the model, since the testing set needs to be large enough to lead to meaningful statistical results. Table 3 shows the statistical information of the testing set.

Table 3. Statistical description of the testing set.

Variables	Mean	Std	Min	Max
Ice layer	0.016	0.047	0.000	0.380
Snow layer	0.015	0.053	0.000	0.830
Water thickness	0.045	0.135	0.000	1.880
Snow height	0.067	0.099	0.000	1.890
RSFC (output)	0.756	0.133	0.120	0.820

3.4. Generating Basic Fuzzy Inference System

In this stage, input variables were fuzzified by using Genfis3 in Matlab software. Genfis3 generates a structure based on the fuzzy inference system (FIS) using the fuzzy c-means (FCM) clustering method by extracting some fuzzy rules, which model the data behavior. The number of clusters specifies the number of rules and membership functions. We selected the 'Sugeno' type because Sugeno is more flexible to design a system more precisely [20]. The number of clusters was five, and the clustering (FCM) options were selected according to the default values in Matlab. The types of the input and output MFs were Gaussian and Linear, respectively. The number of input and output MFs (clusters) was five, equal to the number of fuzzy rules.

3.5. Training Using ANFIS

The training epoch number was set as 200, the initial step size was 0.01 with a decrease rate of 0.9 and an increase rate of 1.1, and the hybrid method was selected as the optimization method [25]. Increasing and decreasing the step sizes balances the exploration and exploitation to enhance the convergence speed and drive the process from the local minimum solution.

3.6. Evaluating Performance of ANFIS

A total of 3847 data points were considered in this study, of which 2693 (70%) observations were for training and 1154 (30%) were for testing the model. Figure 2 and Table 4 depict the structure of the ANFIS network designed in this study to predict the RSFC in winter. In fact, five layers built the ANFIS model based on node functions. The first layer was the "if part", or fuzzification; the second layer was implications (rules); the third layer was normalization; the fourth layer was the "then part", or defuzzification; and the fifth layer was the summation part (output) [20]. According to the collected road dataset, the fuzzy clustering of the predictors for a one-month period is presented in Figure 3. The degree of membership was between 0 and 1. A degree of membership of 0 means that the value does not belong to the given fuzzy set. A degree of membership of 1 means the value certainly belongs to the given fuzzy set. However, if the value of membership is between 0 and 1, it demonstrates the degree of uncertainty with which the value belongs in the given fuzzy set. The information and parameters of the MFs for each input (i.e., mean and standard deviation) and output (coefficients and constant) are shown in Tables 5–7. We considered five clusters for each input, and the output based on trial and error, which demonstrated the best results.

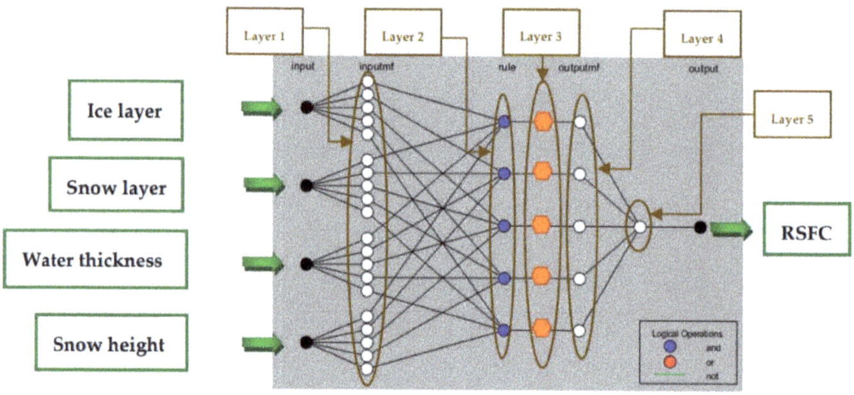

Figure 2. Structure of the ANFIS network applied in this study to predict the RSFC in winter.

Table 4. ANFIS network information used in this study.

Network Information	Number
Number of nodes	57
Number of linear parameters	25
Number of nonlinear parameters	40
Total number of parameters	65
Number of training data pairs	2693
Number of testing data pairs	1154
Number of fuzzy rules	5

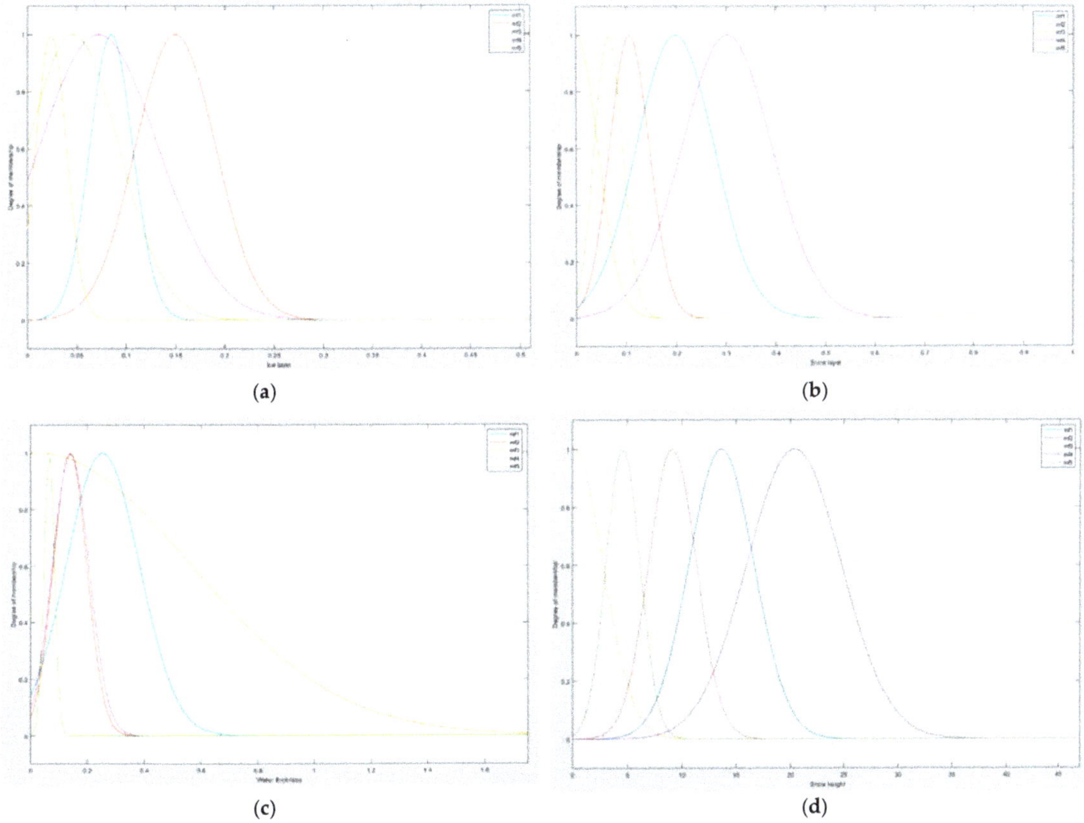

Figure 3. The fuzzy membership functions (Gaussian) selected for (**a**) ice layer, (**b**) snow layer, (**c**) water thickness, and (**d**) snow height.

Table 5. Information about selected inputs and output.

Variable	Range	Number of mf
Ice layer	[0, 0.51]	5
Snow layer	[0, 1]	5
Water thickness	[0, 1.75]	5
Snow height	[0, 47]	5
RSFC (output)	[0.11, 0.82]	5

Table 6. Parameters (Mean and Std values) of each Gaussian mf (cluster) for inputs.

mf	Ice Layer		Snow Layer		Water Thickness		Snow Height	
	Mean	**Std**	**Mean**	**Std**	**Mean**	**Std**	**Mean**	**Std**
mf 1	0.085	0.022	0.198	0.077	0.254	0.128	13.643	3.005
mf 2	0.150	0.040	0.106	0.040	0.139	0.059	9.121	2.202
mf 3	0.024	0.016	−0.001	0.043	0.030	0.530	0.087	2.666
mf 4	0.072	0.060	0.301	0.091	0.141	0.065	20.379	4.365
mf 5	0.046	0.046	0.064	0.028	0.065	0.018	4.593	1.551

Table 7. Parameters (coefficients and constant values) of each linear mf for the output.

mf	$Coeff_1$	$Coeff_2$	$Coeff_3$	$Coeff_4$	Constant
mf 1	−1.737	−0.284	−0.022	0.017	0.585
mf 2	0.598	−4.210	0.599	0.009	0.664
mf 3	−2.547	3.370	0.510	0	0.816
mf 4	−1.216	−0.237	−0.038	−0.001	0.689
mf 5	2.680	−0.026	−2.737	0.025	0.623

After building the base FIS, the model was trained by ANFIS. Figure 4 shows a 3D view of the relationship between the ice layer, snow layer, and RSFC. A 3D view of the relationship between parameters helps us to extract the relationship between effective variables to predict RSFC. For instance, in Figure 4, if the value of the ice layer is less than 0.3, the value of the snow layer has no measurable impact on the created value of the RSFC. The ANFIS rule viewer (for trained data) is shown in Figure 5. Each input column displays five Gaussian membership functions for each input variable and each row shows a particular rule. Hence, each membership function has a specific rule and maps the values of each input variable to rule input values. The output column indicates how various rules can be applied to the RSFC (output variable) [26].

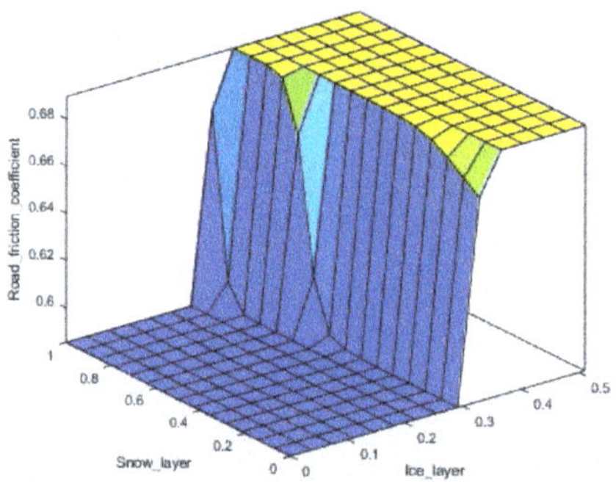

Figure 4. A 3D view of the relationship between the ice layer, snow layer and RSFC.

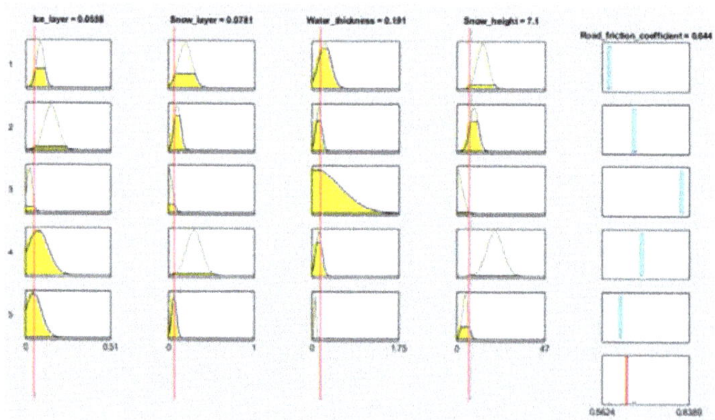

Figure 5. View of the fuzzy rule base for the designed intelligent fuzzy system for RSFC prediction (trained if-then rules).

Figures 6–10 visualize ANFIS performance for the training and test datasets. The graphs demonstrate that predicted values are close to the real values most of the time. Only a few numbers show obvious errors, which could be due to (i) these targets not being scientifically justifiable, or (ii) this method not being suitable to predict these targets. Figure 10 shows the residual plots that show the difference between real values and predicted values for both the training and testing datasets. As is clear, the value of 0 in the residual plots has the highest number and the residual plots are normally distributed, which means that ANFIS is the correct selection for our dataset. In addition, MSE and RMSE were selected as the evaluation metrics to evaluate the model performance (Table 8). RMSE values for the training and test datasets are 0.035 and 0.038, respectively. The low error of the test set indicates that the ANFIS model has a good generalization performance to effectively predict RSFC based on historical data for an unseen dataset.

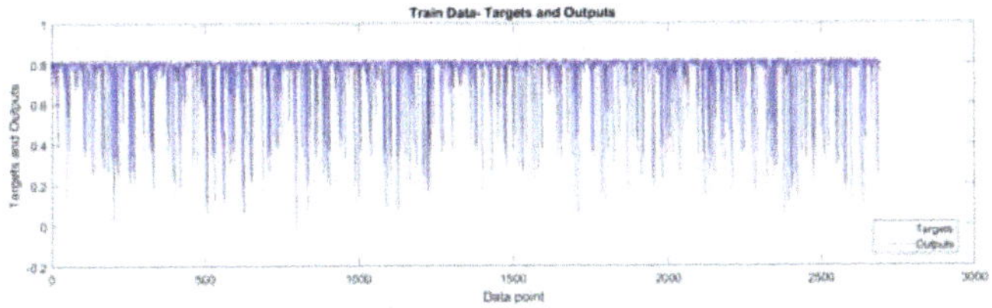

(a)

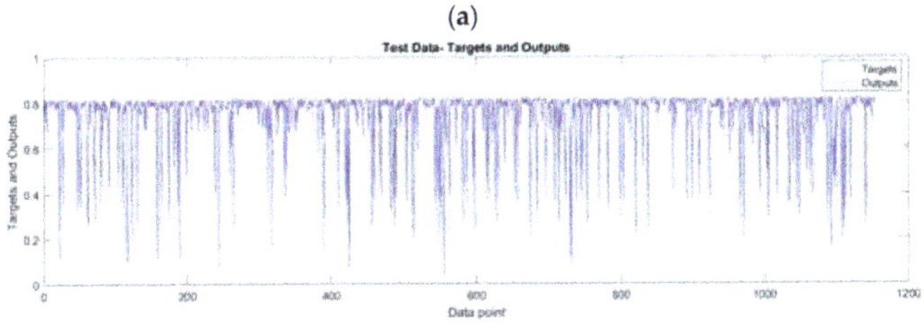

(b)

Figure 6. Comparison between real values (targets) and predicted values (outputs) for (**a**) training dataset, and (**b**) testing dataset.

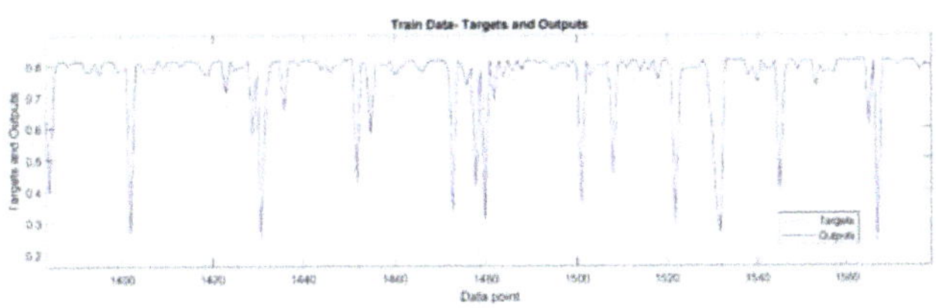

(a)

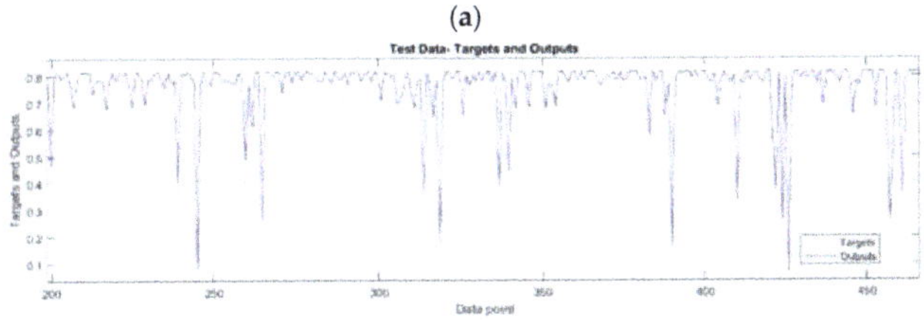

(b)

Figure 7. Comparison between real and predicted values of the special interval for (**a**) training dataset, and (**b**) testing dataset.

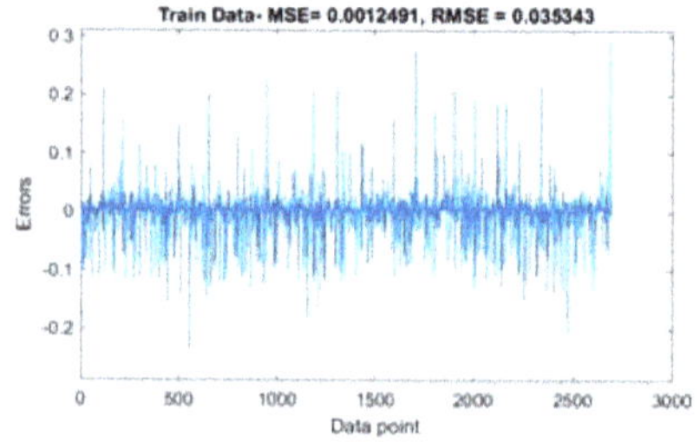

(**a**)

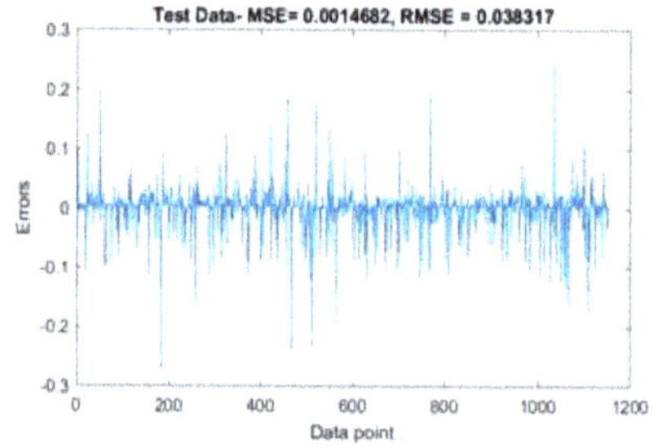

(**b**)

Figure 8. (**a**) Training errors, and (**b**) testing errors by the ANFIS model with Gaussian membership functions.

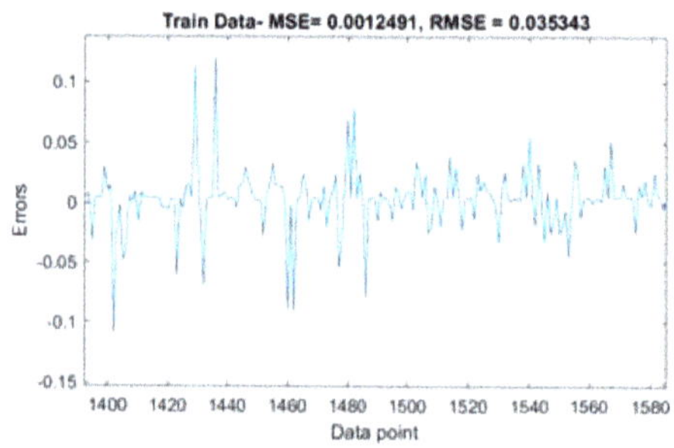

(**a**)

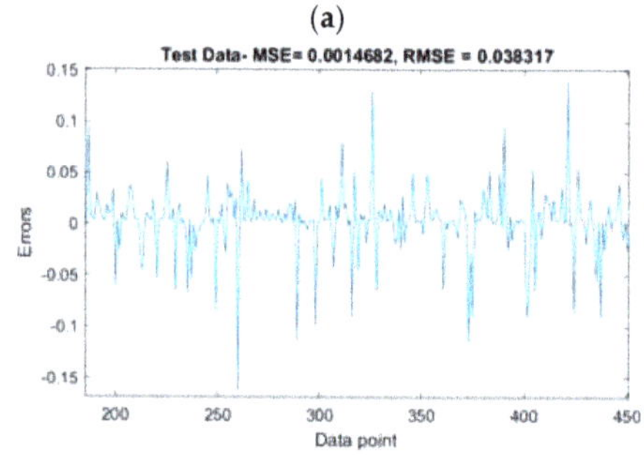

(**b**)

Figure 9. (**a**) Training errors, and (**b**) testing errors for the special interval.

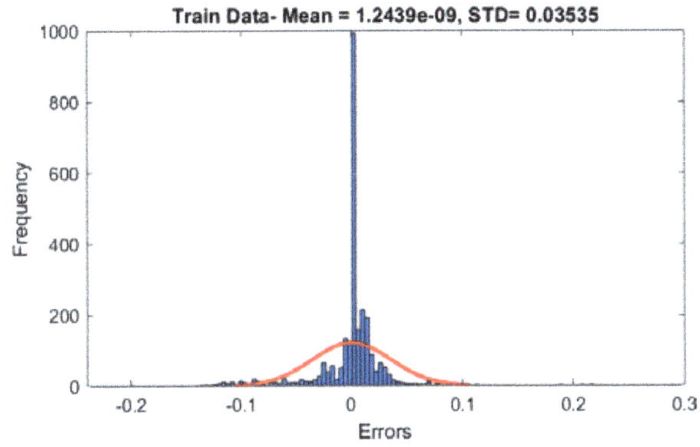

(a)

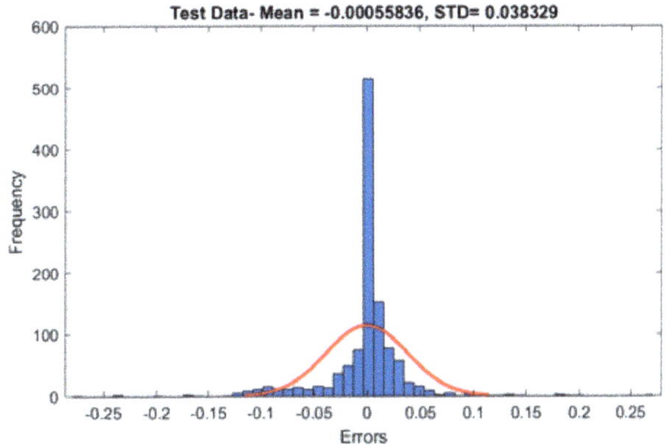

(b)

Figure 10. Residual distribution plot for (**a**) training set, and (**b**) testing set.

Table 8. MSE and RMSE values achieved by the ANFIS model for both training and testing datasets.

Evaluation Metric	Training Set	Testing Set
MSE	0.0012	0.0015
RMSE	0.0350	0.0380

4. Analytic Results

Analysis of the variables affecting the RSFC prediction model enables us to drive future insights to accurately predict different road surface conditions at a particular time. The RSFC prediction model helps us to discover the relationship between variables and eventually leads to an improvement in decision-making procedures. We utilized the most informative scatter chart (Figure 11) to plot the RSFC, ice layer, and the amount of chemicals used for WRM to extract valuable findings.

Generally, driving conditions are divided into the following three categories: (i) normal road conditions (RSFC $\geq$ 0.3), (ii) bad conditions (0.15 < RSFC < 0.3), and (iii) very bad conditions (RSFC $\leq$ 0.15). When the friction coefficient is under 0.15, the rate of accidents can be four times higher than in conditions with a friction coefficient of 0.35–0.44 [27]. In the previous figure, the data points are shown based on different values of the friction coefficient. It is clear that, with an increase in the thickness of the ice layer on the road surface, the RSFC drops sharply. If no chemicals (e.g., salt) are used on the road surface, this leads to a drastic reduction in road safety. Therefore, the RSFC prediction model contributes to detecting these dangerous situations in advance and taking action to both prevent dangerous vehicle accidents on the road and mitigate their associated severe consequences. Moreover, when the ice layer is thinner than 0.2 mm, using a small amount of salt contributes to increasing friction on the road surface. When the ice layer is almost 0 mm, using a high quantity of chemicals (salt) on the ground leads to extra expense (including materials, trucks, and truck drivers). Chemicals (salt) are not only the main reason for rust and corrosion on vehicles, but also exacerbate the harm to road infrastructure such as concrete bridges. Furthermore, salt has negative impacts on the environment, caused by melting into rivers, lakes, and into soil, damaging vegetation.

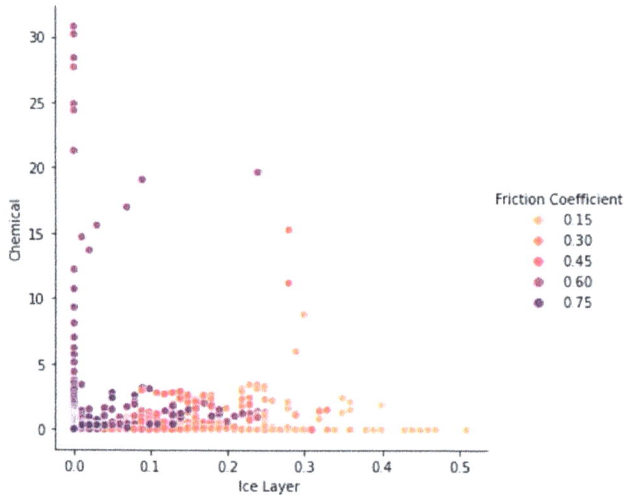

Figure 11. Scatter plot for the ice layer, chemicals, and RSFC.

5. Conclusions

In this paper, ANFIS was used to design a data-driven model to accurately manage the uncertainty hidden in historical data and predict the road surface friction coefficient in winter. The model was implemented in MATLAB software using real data, measured by a road weather information system, optical sensors, and road-mounted sensors at test site E18 in Sweden in February 2019. The graphical and numerical results of ANFIS modeling demonstrate the high reliability and accuracy of the model in handling uncertainty and predicting the road surface friction coefficient. This model can be considered as a main computational component in decision support systems, to assist decisions made about the type and time of winter road maintenance in a quantitative manner. Thus, the findings of this paper can be used to develop a winter road maintenance strategy for both pre-disaster and post-disaster periods. This accurate prediction model can help decision makers to make plans in advance, which will lead to optimizing the level of service. Preparing the optimal number of trucks and materials in real-time to treat snowy and icy roads leads to improved road transportation safety (by increasing the friction between tires and road surface), traffic flow (by removing snow and ice on the road), and economic productivity (by avoiding the use of extra materials and trucks). However, ANFIS demands computational power, and its performance is significantly dependent on data quantity and quality and specifying the number of member functions for input and output variables. Hence, in future, researchers should search for alternative mathematical methods that are less dependent on data.

Author Contributions: Conceptualization, M.H.; methodology, M.H.; software, M.H.; validation, M.H.; formal analysis, M.H.; investigation, M.H.; resources, M.H.; data curation, J.C.; writing—original draft preparation, M.H.; writing—review and editing, M.H. and G.P.P.; visualization, M.H.; supervision, G.P.P. and J.C.; project administration, G.P.P. All authors have read and agreed to the published version of the manuscript.

Funding: This research was funded by Ministry of Education and Research, Norway, grant number 470079.

Data Availability Statement: We have got the data from the Swedish transport administration's RWIS station at Test site E18. https://www.trafikverket.se/resa-och-trafik/forskning-och-innovation/aktuell-forskning/transport-pa-vag/testsite-e18--en-vagforskningsstation/ (accessed on 1 January 2020).

Conflicts of Interest: The authors declare no conflict of interest.

References

1. Feng, F.; Fu, L. Winter Road surface condition forecasting. *J. Infrastruct. Syst.* **2014**, *21*, 04014049. [CrossRef]
2. Strong, C.; Shi, X. Benefit-cost analysis of weather information for winter maintenance: A case study. *Transp. Res. Rec.* **2008**, *2055*, 119–127. [CrossRef]
3. Shao, J.; Lister, P.J. An automated nowcasting model of road surface temperature and state for winter road maintenance. *J. Appl. Meteorol. Climatol.* **1996**, *35*, 1352–1361. [CrossRef]
4. Mohseni, A. LTPP Data Analysis: Improved Low Pavement Temperature Prediction. *FHWA Contract* **1998**, *73*, 285–2730.
5. Kangas, M.; Heikinheimo, M.; Hippi, M. RoadSurf: A modelling system for predicting road weather and road surface conditions. *Meteorol. Appl.* **2015**, *22*, 544–553. [CrossRef]
6. Ye, Z.; Shi, X.; Strong, C.; Larson, R. Vehicle-based sensor technologies for winter highway operations. *IET Intell. Transp. Syst.* **2012**, *6*, 336–345. [CrossRef]
7. Ewan, L.; Al-Kaisy, A.; Veneziano, D. Remote Sensing of Weather and Road Surface Conditions: Is technology mature for reliable intelligent transportation systems applications? *Transp. Res. Rec.* **2013**, *2329*, 8–16. [CrossRef]
8. Feng, F.; Fu, L. *Evaluation of Two New Vaisala Sensors for Road Surface Conditions Monitoring*; HIIFP-054; Department of Civil & Environmental Engineering, University of Waterloo: Toronto, ON, Canada, 2008.
9. Ahabchane, C.; Trépanier, M.; Langevin, A. Street-segment-based salt and abrasive prediction for winter maintenance using machine learning and GIS. *Willey Trans. GIS* **2018**, *23*, 48–69. [CrossRef]
10. Pan, G.; Fu, L.; Yu, R.; Muresan, M.L. Winter Road surface condition recognition using a pre-trained deep convolutional neural network. In Proceedings of the Transportation Research Board 97th Annual Meeting, Washington, DC, USA, 7–11 January 2018; pp. 838–855.
11. Liu, B.; Yan, S.; You, H.; Dong, Y.; Li, Y.; Lang, J.; Gu, R. Road surface temperature prediction based on gradient extreme learning machine boosting. *Comput. Ind.* **2018**, *99*, 294–302. [CrossRef]
12. Roychowdhury, S.; Zhao, M.; Wallin, A.; Ohlsson, N.; Jonasson, M. Machine Learning Models for Road Surface and Friction Estimation using Front-Camera Images. In Proceedings of the 2018 International Joint Conference on Neural Networks (IJCNN), Rio de Janeiro, Brazil, 8–13 July 2018; pp. 1–8.
13. Panahandeh, G.; Ek, E.; Mohammadiha, N. Road friction estimation for connected vehicles using supervised machine learning. In Proceedings of the Intelligent Vehicles Symposium (IV), Los Angeles, CA, USA, 31 July 2017; pp. 1262–1267. [CrossRef]
14. Pu, Z.; Liu, C.; Shi, X.; Cui, Z.; Wang, Y. Road surface friction prediction using long short-term memory neural network based on historical data. *J. Intell. Transp. Syst.* **2020**, *26*, 34–45. [CrossRef]
15. Song, S.; Min, K.; Park, J.; Kim, H.; Huh, K. Estimating the maximum road friction coefficient with uncertainty using deep learning. In Proceedings of the 21st International Conference on Intelligent Transportation Systems (ITSC), Maui, HI, USA, 10 December 2018; pp. 3156–3161. [CrossRef]
16. Matuško, J.; Petrović, I.; Perić, N. Neural network based tire/road friction force estimation. *Eng. Appl. Artif. Intell.* **2008**, *21*, 442–456. [CrossRef]
17. Kim, H.M.; Park, S.H.; Han, S.I. Precise friction control for the nonlinear friction system using the friction state observer and sliding mode control with recurrent fuzzy neural networks. *Mechatronics* **2009**, *19*, 805–815. [CrossRef]
18. Ross, T.J. *Fuzzy Logic with Engineering Applications*; JWS: Hoboken, NJ, USA, 2005.
19. Jang, J.S.R. ANFIS: Adaptive-network-based fuzzy inference system. *IEEE Trans. Syst. Man Cybern.* **1993**, *23*, 665–685. [CrossRef]
20. Pourdaryaei, A.; Mokhlis, H.; Illias, H.A.; Kaboli, S.H.A.; Ahmad, S. Short-Term Electricity Price Forecasting via Hybrid Backtracking Search Algorithm and ANFIS Approach. *IEEE Access* **2019**, *7*, 77674–77691. [CrossRef]
21. Elbaz, K.; Shen, S.; Sun, W.; Yin, Z.; Zhou, A. Prediction Model of Shield Performance During Tunneling via Incorporating Improved Particle Swarm Optimization Into ANFIS. *IEEE Access* **2020**, *8*, 39659–39671. [CrossRef]
22. Shekarian, E.; Gholizadeh, A.A. Application of adaptive network based fuzzy inference system method in economic welfare. *Knowl. Based Syst.* **2013**, *39*, 151–158. [CrossRef]

23. Yousefi, M.; Hajizadeh, A.; Soltani, M.N. A comparison study on stochastic modeling methods for home energy management systems. *IEEE Trans. Industr. Inform.* **2019**, *15*, 4799–4808. [CrossRef]
24. Trafikverket. Available online: https://www.trafikverket.se/trafikinformation/vag/?TrafficType=personalTraffic&map=3%2F50315918%2F6763671.79%2F&Layers=RoadCondition%2BRoadWeather%2B (accessed on 12 December 2019).
25. MATLAB. *Version 9.6.0.1072779 (R2019a)*; The MathWorks Inc.: Natick, MA, USA, 2019. Available online: https://www.mathworks.com/help/fuzzy/neuro-adaptive-learning-and-anfis.html (accessed on 1 April 2019).
26. Khan, A.; Pahwa, V. Design and Implementation of ANFIS Based Controller on Variable Speed Isolated Wind-Diesel Hybrid System for Better Performance. *Am. J. Electr. Electron.* **2017**, *5*, 172–178. [CrossRef]
27. Wallman, C.G.; Åström, H. *Friction Measurement Methods and the Correlation between Road Friction and Traffic Safety: A Literature Review*; Swedish National Road and Transport Research Institute: Linköping, Sweden, 2001.

healthcare

MDPI

Article

The Service Capability of Primary Health Institutions under the Hierarchical Medical System

Shuo Liu, Jintao Lin, Yiwen He and Junfang Xu *

School of Public Health, Zhejiang University School of Medicine, Hangzhou 310058, China; a1147465914@163.com (S.L.); ljt181151104@163.com (J.L.); 3190104273@zju.edu.cn (Y.H.)
* Correspondence: xujf2019@zju.edu.cn

Abstract: Background: Primary health institutions (PHIs) are the foundation of the whole health system and the basic link to achieve the goal of all people enjoying primary health care. However, the service capability of primary health institutions is not under the hierarchical medical system. Method: Data were collected from the *China Health Statistics Yearbook* between 2014 and 2020. PHIs included community health centres, community health stations, and township hospitals in our study. The service capability of primary health institutions was analysed from the perspective of structure, process, and results. Structure capability was evaluated using the number of beds, number of personnel, number of health technicians, and proportion of the number of personnel in PHIs accounting for the total number of health personnel. Process capability was evaluated using the number of general practitioners. The number of outpatients and inpatients, medical income, the proportion of drug income, and the average number of patients and beds served by physicians in PHIs per day were employed to evaluate the resulting capability. Results: From 2014 to 2020, the number of community health service centres/stations increased, while the number of township health centres decreased. In the aspect of structure capability, the total number of personnel and health technicians in community health centres/stations and township hospitals both increased during 2014 and 2020. However, the increasing rate in PHIs was a little bit less than that of general medical institutions. The proportion of male health technicians in community health centres and township hospitals both decreased, while the proportion of female technicians in both increased. From 2014 to 2020, the number of beds in PHIs also increased from 138.12×10^4 to 164.94×10^4. However, the proportion of beds in PHIs accounting for the total number of beds in medical institutions decreased. For the resulting capability, from 2014 to 2019, the proportion of diagnosis and treatment times in PHIs decreased from 57.41% to 51.96%, although it increased in 2020. The proportion of inpatients in PHIs decreased from 20.03% to 16.11%. From 2014 to 2020, the utilisation rate of hospital beds in PHIs decreased (from 55.6% to 34% for community health centres and 60.5% to 53.6% for township hospitals). The average daily bed days of doctors in township hospitals was higher than that of doctors in community health service centres. However, the average medical cost of outpatients and the per capita medical cost of inpatients in community health service centres were higher than in township hospitals. Conclusion: In recent years, although the service capability showed an increasing trend in PHIs, the growth rate was lower than the general health institutions. The utilisation rates of PHIs, including beds and physicians, were decreased. Among PHIs, the utilisation in township hospitals was higher than in community health centres with a relatively low price. Under the hierarchical medical system and normalisation period of the COVID-19 epidemic, it is important to improve the service capability to achieve its goal of increasing PHI utilisation and decreasing secondary and tertiary hospital utilisation.

Keywords: primary health institution; service capability; hierarchical medical system

Citation: Liu, S.; Lin, J.; He, Y.; Xu, J. The Service Capability of Primary Health Institutions under the Hierarchical Medical System. *Healthcare* **2022**, *10*, 335. https://doi.org/10.3390/healthcare10020335

Academic Editors: Amir Khorram-Manesh and Krzysztof Goniewicz

Received: 24 December 2021
Accepted: 5 February 2022
Published: 10 February 2022

1. Introduction

Chronic diseases have become the biggest disease burden in China in the past 30 years. The primary goal of China's health system is to prevent and control chronic diseases, especially among the elderly. This reflects the urgency of speeding up the capacity-building of primary health institutions (PHIs) [1,2] as the foundations of the whole health system, which undertake the responsibility of providing basic health services, including public health, to people [1]. The ageing and growing burden of chronic diseases in China also highlights the need for a continuous and coordinated system based on primary health services [2]. To improve the health service level of the hierarchical health system, health resources should be effectively provided to the primary institutions, so as to promote the optimisation and adjustment of the structure, function, and layout of the health system as a whole.

The importance of primary healthcare has also been highlighted after the pandemic of COVID-19 [3]. For example, more than 4 million personnel from PHIs across the country participated in preliminary screening, diagnosis, and referral, which has greatly alleviated the pressure faced by general hospitals [4]. In addition, the importance of PHIs is not only to be reflected in the public health of disease prevention, but also in the diagnosis and treatment of some common diseases, especially during the pandemic. Currently, during the epidemic normalisation period, all the patients with a fever can be found in time through the PHIs. The fever patients can be transferred to the fever clinics at the higher-level hospitals to receive timely and effective treatment, which has played a positive role in the effective control of COVID-19. Although the application of tiered medical services in the prevention and control of sudden epidemic situations is quite effective, some problems have also emerged, such as the capability of PHIs in China.

Continuous monitoring and health management of COVID-19 patients after they are discharged from the hospital are carried out by PHIs. The COVID-19 epidemic is a huge test for the construction of medical alliances encouraged by China in recent years, which fully exposes the weak service level of PHIs. Since the outbreak of the epidemic, a considerable number of PHIs have been confronted with problems such as insufficient medical supplies, insufficient manpower and skills, and loopholes in public information systems. They are basically not equipped with screening and isolation capabilities, making it difficult to implement screening and classified isolation for community residents.

The Chinese government has recently issued a series of policies to improve primary health care. On 4 December 2020, the National Health Commission of China issued the notice on deepening the "Internet plus Health", and encouraged the development of the information system for PHIs [5]. On 24 May 2021, the State Council issued the 2021 key tasks for deepening the reform of the health system. One of the tasks is to accelerate the improvement of the basic infrastructure of community health centres and township hospitals [4]. It can be seen that the hierarchical medical system attaches unprecedented importance to the construction of the service capability of PHIs. At the same time, the implementation of a two-way referral policy, which requires the first diagnosis at PHIs, provides another chance to improve primary health care. The service capability of PHIs is directly related to the construction of the hierarchical health system and universal health coverage. Moreover, it also influences the social satisfaction of residents as a result of it often being difficult and expensive to see a doctor in China [6].

However, the current status of PHIs' service capability or the impacts of hierarchical medical system construction on PHIs' capability are unclear; for example, whether the capability of PHIs is increasing and in line with the goals of the hierarchical medical system. Scholars have performed a lot of research on the improvement paths of the medical service capacity of PHIs in China. However, most studies used one place or several indicators; the analysis of the change of the medical service capacity of PHIs from a comprehensive and national perspective is limited. To find the problems existing in the service of PHIs in China and provide evidence for improving the capability of primary health care, we aim to analyse the capability of PHIs from 2014 to 2020 from structural, process, and result perspectives.

2. Methods

2.1. Data Source

The related data of PHIs were collected from the *China Health Statistics Yearbook* [7] from 2014 to 2020, respectively, which included number of PHIs, personnel including health technicians in PHIs, number of health technicians in PHIs, beds and equipment above 10,000 yuan in medical institutions and PHIs, general practitioners in China, number of diagnoses and treatment times in PHIs, utilisation rate of hospital beds in PHIs, income of PHIs averaged by number of doctors' visits per day in PHIs, average daily bed days of doctors in PHIs, and medical expenses of patients.

2.2. Measurement of Service Capability

In the study, PHIs included community health centres, community health stations, and township hospitals. The service capability of PHIs was divided into structural service capability, process service capability, and result service capability. The indexes measuring structural service capability included the number of health technicians in China, the number of primary health technicians, the proportion of primary health technicians (the number of primary health technicians in PHIs to the number of health technicians in total medical institutions), the number of beds in PHIs, the proportion of beds in PHIs (the number of beds in PHIs to the number of beds in total medical institutions), and the utilisation rate of beds in PHIs. Number of general practitioners was used to evaluate the process service capability of PHIs. The indexes of result service capability contained the number of outpatients and inpatients in PHIs, medical income of PHIs, the proportion of drug income (the income of drugs in PHIs to the total drug income of total medical institutions), and the average number of patients and beds served by physicians in PHIs per day.

2.3. Statistical Analysis

Descriptive statistical analysis (i.e., frequency and percentage) was used to analyse the structure, process, and outcome service capability indicators of PHIs from 2014 to 2020. The trend and comparative analysis of the service capability of PHIs from 2014 to 2020 were also conducted. All data analysis was based on the statistical software SPSS 23.0 (IBM, Armonk, NY, USA). Variables with $p < 0.05$ were considered as statistically significant.

3. Results

3.1. Structure Service Capability in PHIs from 2014 to 2020

The number of community health service centres/stations increased from 34,238 in 2014 to 35,365 in 2020, while the number of township health centres decreased from 36,902 in 2014 to 35,762 in 2020 (Figure 1).

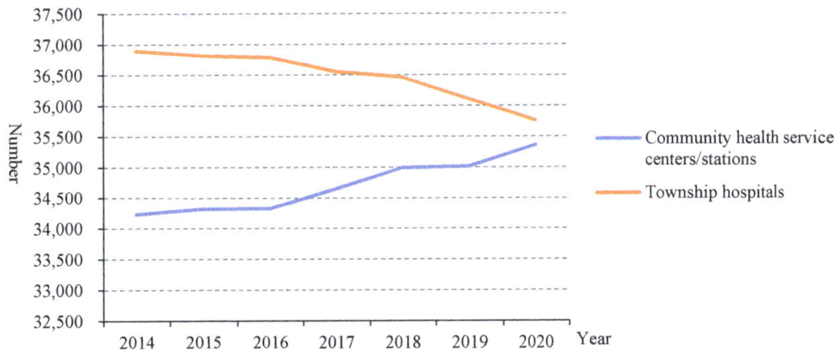

Figure 1. The number of PHIs in China from 2014 to 2020.

From 2014 to 2020, the total number of personnel and the number of health technicians in community health centres/stations both increased (Figure 2). The proportion of health technicians accounting for the total number of personnel in community health centres/stations remained almost unchanged before 2020 and increased slightly in 2020 (86.12%) compared to 2014 (85.42%). Similarly, the total number of personnel and the number of health technicians in township hospitals also increased, and the proportion of health technicians accounting for the total number of personnel in township hospitals remained almost unchanged before 2020, and increased slightly to 85.55% in 2020 compared to 84.45% in 2014.

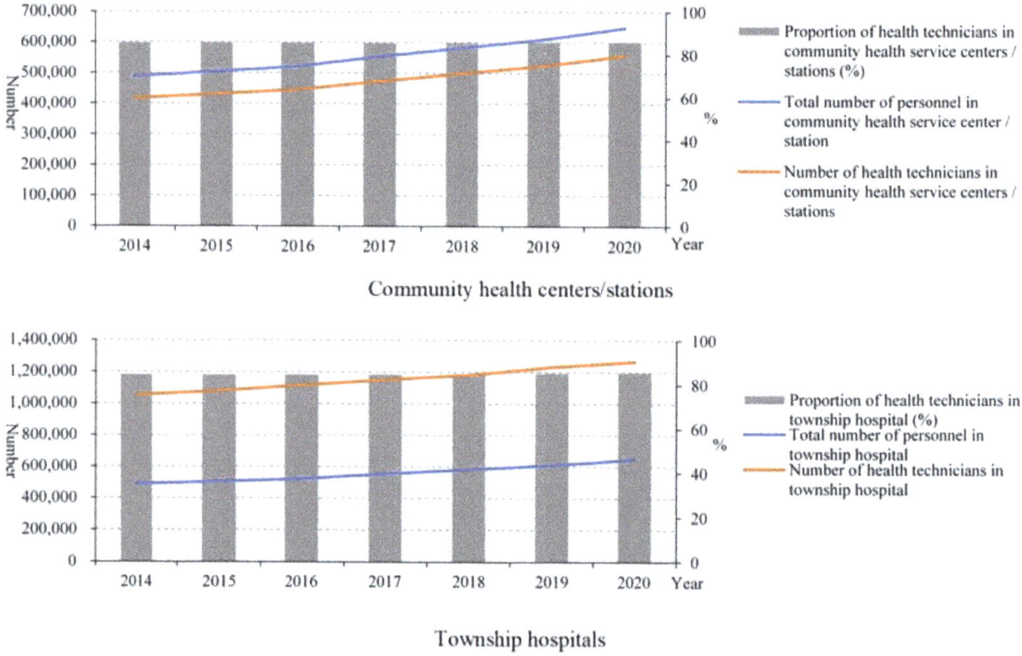

Figure 2. Personnel including health technicians in PHIs.

From Figure 3, we can see that the number of health technicians younger than 45 years old was reduced, and the proportion of male health technicians in PHIs, including community health centres and township hospitals, also showed a decreasing trend, while the proportion of females increased. Moreover, most health technicians (~60%) had an education level lower than undergraduate.

Although the number of beds in PHIs also increased to 164.94×10^4 in 2020 from 138.12×10^4 in 2014, the proportion of beds in PHIs accounting for the total number of beds in medical institutions decreased from 20.92% in 2014 to 18.12% in 2020. The equipment valued above 10,000 RMB showed a similar trend with beds in the number and proportion (Figure 4).

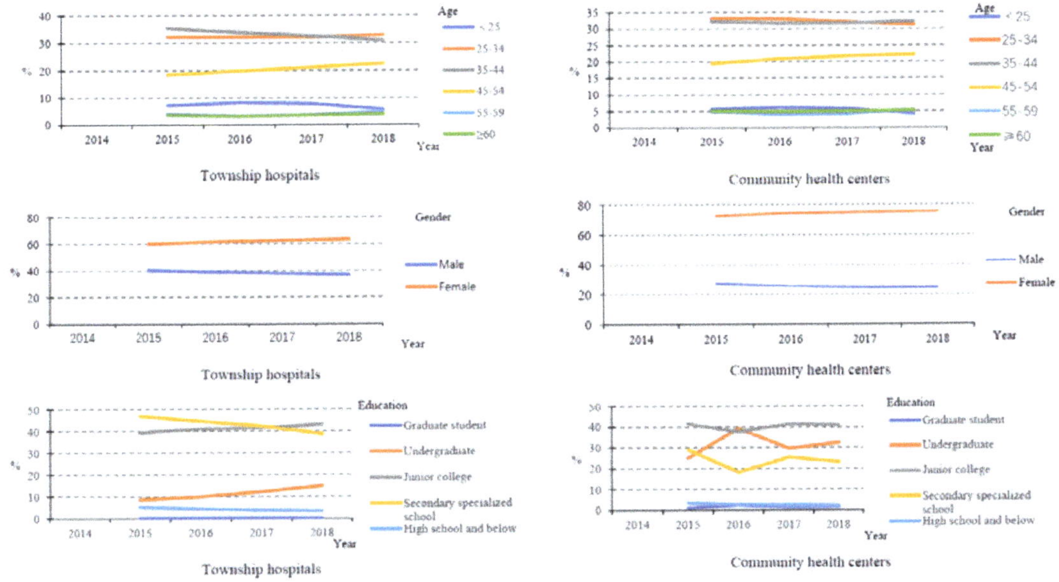

Figure 3. The characteristics of health technicians in PHIs.

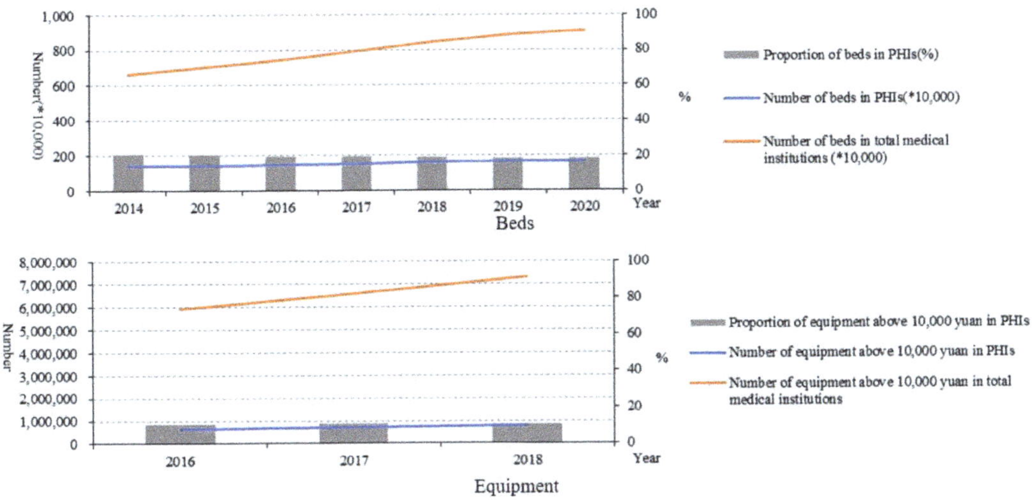

Figure 4. Beds and equipment above 10,000 yuan in medical institutions and PHIs.

3.2. Process Service Capability of PHIs

The number of general practitioners in China increased from 172,597 in 2014 to 308,740 in 2018 (Figure 5), as did the number of general practitioners per 10,000 people (1.26 in 2014 to 2.22 in 2018).

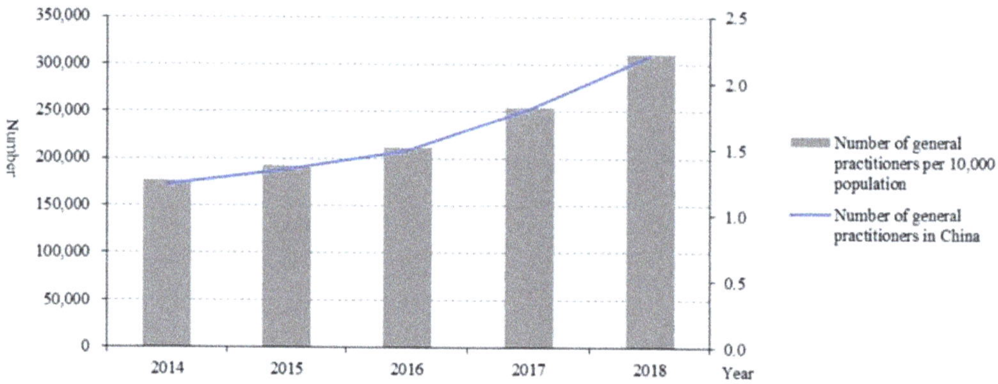

Figure 5. General practitioners in China from 2014 to 2018.

3.3. *Result Service Capability of PHIs*

From 2014 to 2019 (Figure 6), the number of diagnoses and treatment times by total medical institutions increased from 760,186.6 (10,000 person-times) to 872,000 (10,000 person-times), but it decreased to 774,000 (10,000 person-times) in 2020. For PHIs, the number of diagnoses and treatment declined from 453,087.1 (10,000 person-times) to 412,000 (10,000 person-times). Among PHIs, the number of diagnoses and treatment times in township hospitals was much higher than that of community health centres.

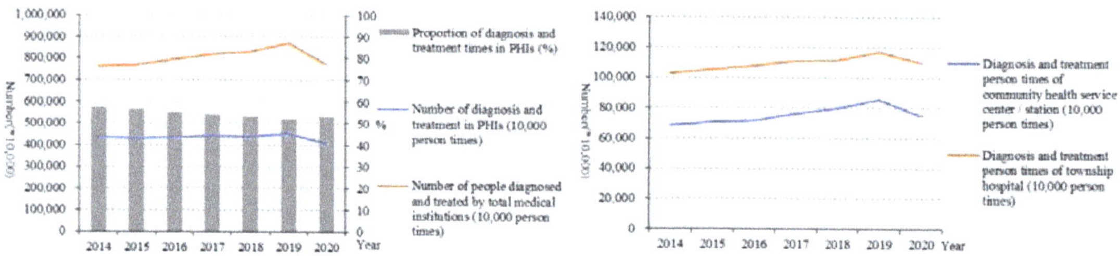

Figure 6. Number of diagnoses and treatments in PHIs (10,000 person-times).

From 2016 to 2018, the income of PHIs increased from 48,293,753 (10,000 yuan) to 61,246,366 (10,000 yuan), and the proportion of the income of PHIs accounting for the total income in medical institutions increased slightly from 14.56% to 14.9%. Among PHIs, the income in township hospitals was higher than that of community health centres. Moreover, the medical income in PHIs was much higher than government subsidies (Figure 7).

Figure 8 shows that the utilisation of beds in township hospitals was also higher than that of community health centres. However, both showed a decreasing trend during 2014 and 2020. The bed days per doctor's service also had a similar trend. The medical expenses per patient in PHIs were much lower than those of general medical institutions, and compared with community health centres, they were lower in township hospitals. However, the medical expenses per patient in PHIs increased in the last six years.

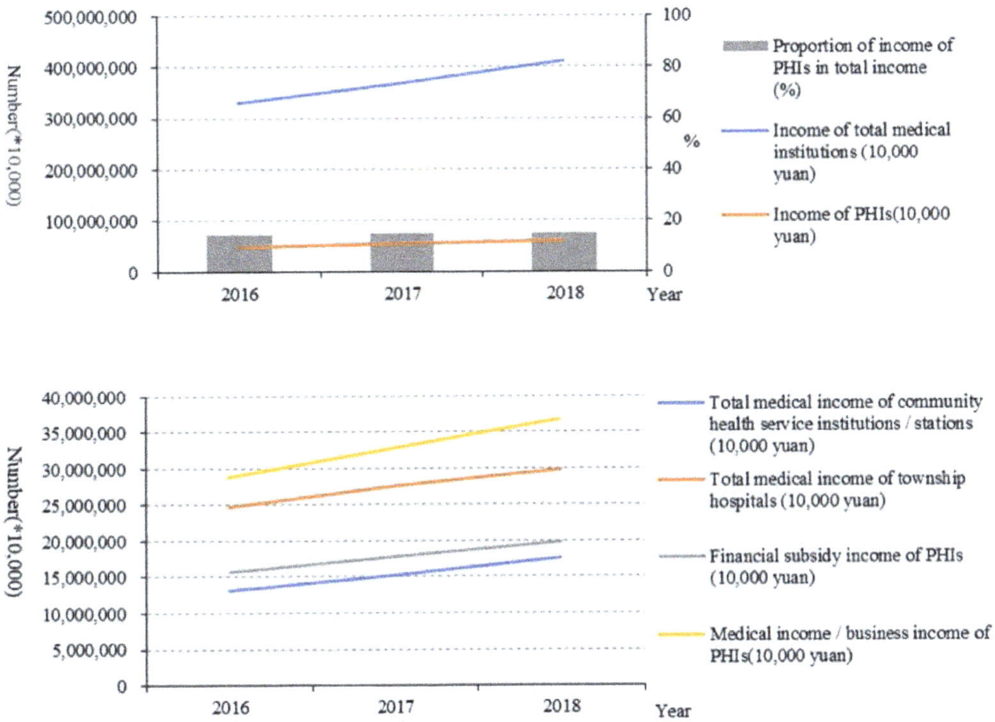

Figure 7. Income of PHIs (10,000 yuan).

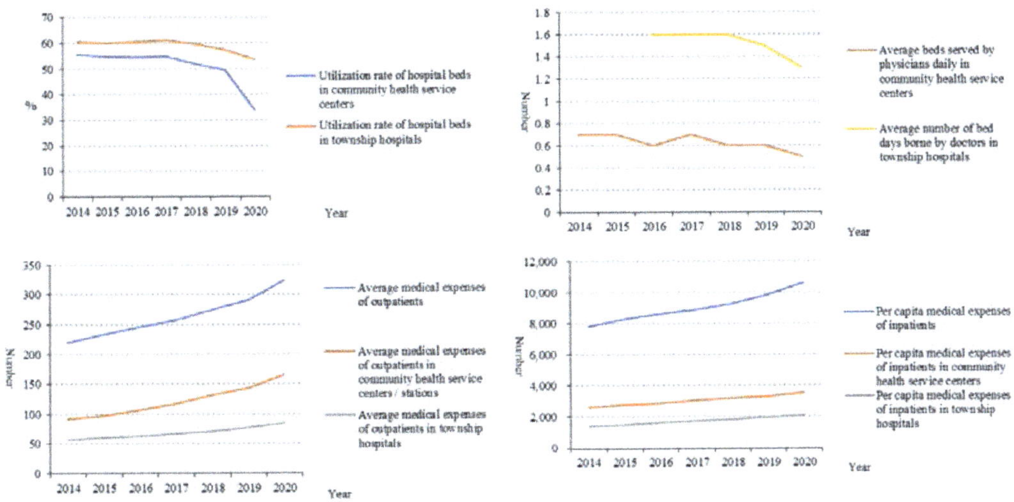

Figure 8. Beds utilisation, days served by doctors, and medical expenses of patients in PHIs.

4. Discussion

Since the implementation of the new medical reform, the service capability of PHIs has been improved, especially by the structure service capability. In the number of PHIs, community health service centres increased, while the number of township hospitals decreased. This is related to the fast urbanisation, which means many rural areas turned to urban areas and rural populations migrated to cities in China in recent years [8]. From the point of view of the structural service capability of the PHIs, the structural service capability of the PHIs in China has been improved as a whole. From 2015 to 2020, the number of health technicians in PHIs gradually increased, but the proportion of health technicians remained almost unchanged. This is because the number of total staff in PHIs also increased. In addition, from 2015 to 2018, the health technicians in community health service centres mainly had junior college degrees and undergraduate degrees, and the health technicians in township health centres mainly had secondary school degrees and junior college degrees, while there were very few with graduate degrees, suggesting that the construction of the talent teams in PHIs urgently needs to be improved [9]. From 2014 to 2020, the number of beds in PHIs also increased year by year, but the proportion of beds in PHIs decreased year by year. Moreover, the proportion of equipment above 10,000 RMB in PHIs remained almost unchanged. The number of health technicians younger than 35 years old was reduced, which may be due to the number of young people choosing to be health technicians reducing gradually. The proportion of male health technicians in PHIs also showed a decreasing trend, while the proportion of females increased. This may be related to safe working practices and low salaries in primary health facilities. Such characteristics make women who need more care for their families choose this job. These results indicated that the government should pay more attention to the resource allocation of PHIs. Moreover, reviewing the course of the COVID-19 epidemic, we can also find that the improvement of PHIs is the "most economical and effective" measure to control infectious diseases. The capability of PHIs is also the key to realising tiered diagnosis and treatment. To sum up, the structural service capability of PHIs in China has been improved as a whole, but there are still deficiencies that need to be improved.

As the gatekeeper of primary medical care, the number of general practitioners in China increased. The first consultation system of general practitioners is the key to realising the function of the gatekeeper [10]. The establishment of the first consultation system of general practitioners can give full play to the core role of rational allocation and effective utilisation of health resources [11]. General practitioners guide patients to seek medical treatment in a scientific and orderly manner and on-demand [12]. This also showed that under the hierarchical health system, primary healthcare and its capabilities were gradually improved. However, due to the lack of data, it is temporarily impossible to analyse the contract services of general practitioners in PHIs.

From the point of result service capability, the progress of the result service capability of the PHIs in China was not strong, and the utilisation of diagnoses and treatment at the PHIs level was low, although evidence has shown that 80% of diseases can receive effective treatment in the PHIs. From 2014 to 2019, the number of diagnoses and treatment times in PHIs almost remained the same and decreased in 2020. In addition, from 2019 to 2020, the number of diagnoses and treatment times by total medical institutions decreased, too. This has to do with the fact that COVID-19 has kept people indoors [13]. In addition, the proportion of diagnoses and treatment times in PHIs accounting for the total also decreased. The low utilisation of PHIs may also affect whether the COVID-19 epidemic can be effectively controlled. The main reason for the low utilisation may be the relatively low capacity in PHIs. In addition, the development of PHIs still lags behind the development of general hospitals, and the relatively weak situation of PHIs has not been substantially improved, which has been clearly shown in our results regarding service capability.

Among PHIs, the number of diagnoses and treatment times in township hospitals was much higher than that of community health centres. One explanation is that people in rural areas are more likely to choose township hospitals over large urban hospitals due to traffic constraints [6]. What is more, the average daily bed days of doctors in PHIs also did not increase. These indicated that patients tended to seek treatment in the general hospitals rather than PHIs. The government financial subsidy income and medical income both increased year by year, which showed that the new medical reform attaches enough importance to the financial support of PHIs and has achieved initial results [14]. Although the income of PHIs in China has improved, in order to achieve long-term development, PHIs need to make good use of this income, improve service capability, and create more value [15]. All in all, the outcome service capability of PHIs in China has been improved on the whole, but the effect is weak, and the reform efforts need to be further strengthened [16–19]. On the one hand, they should promote the effective integration of medical resources and improve the sharing system of medical resources in the region to strengthen the ability of PHIs. On the other hand, they should improve the helper mechanism of an integrated health care system by encouraging hospital professionals working in the PHIs regularly.

This study was subjected to some limitations. First, some aspects may benefit a lot from a qualitative study rather than quantitative research. Second, considering the significant difference in geography and economic levels, the service capability of PHIs are different within China, but this study lacks regional analysis. Third, due to the lack of some data, the process service capability cannot be analysed in depth. Moreover, future studies may benefit from a deep statistics analysis.

5. Conclusions

Under the hierarchical health system and normalisation period of the COVID-19 epidemic, to improve the capability of primary health services, many measures have been issued, including PHIs' functional orientation, talent team construction and financial compensation mechanism, structural service capability, process service ability, and the result service ability. These were improved, but on the whole, failed to achieve the expected effect, and some indicators even showed a downward trend, showing the weakening of medical service capabilities and the shrinking of medical service scope. This may significantly affect the carrying out of high-quality and effective health systems, as well as the emergency management of infectious diseases.

Author Contributions: All authors were responsible for the structure of this paper. J.L. drafted the paper and Y.H. and S.L. contributed the data collection and literature review. J.X. contributed to the study's conception and design, interpretation of the data, and critical revisions of the paper. All authors have read and agreed to the published version of the manuscript.

Funding: This work was supported by the Zhejiang Soft Science Program (No. 2021C35015).

Institutional Review Board Statement: Not applicable.

Informed Consent Statement: Not applicable.

Data Availability Statement: All of the main data have been included in the results. Additional materials with details may be obtained from the corresponding author.

Conflicts of Interest: The authors declare no conflict of interest.

References

1. Gao, L. *Research on Primary Medical Service Capability in Zhejiang Province under the Background of New Medical Reform*; Zhejiang University: Hangzhou, China, 2016.
2. Xiao, N.; Long, Q.; Tang, X.; Tang, S. A community-based approach to non-communicable chronic disease management within a context of advancing universal health coverage in China: Progress and challenges. *BMC Public Health* **2014**, *14* (Suppl. S2), S2. [CrossRef]
3. Khorram-Manesh A. Flexible surge capacity-public health, public education, and disaster management. *Health Promot. Perspect.* **2020**, *10*, 175–179.
4. General Office of the State Council. Circular of The General Office of the State Council on Printing and Distributing Key Tasks of Deepening the Reform of the Medical and Health System in 2021. Available online: http://www.gov.cn/zhengce/content/2021-06/17/content_5618799.htm (accessed on 1 December 2021).
5. General Office of the State Council. Notice on Furthering the "Internet + Medical and Health" and "Five One" Service Action. 2020. Available online: http://www.gov.cn/zhengce/zhengceku/2020-12/10/content_5568777.htm (accessed on 1 December 2021).
6. Fang, L. Understanding the dilemma of "New Medical reform": Review of the "Twelfth Five-Year plan" medical reform. *J. China Natl. Sch. Adm.* **2016**, *2*, 77–81. [CrossRef]

7. National Bureau of Statistics. *China Statistical Yearbook, 2014–2020*; China Statistics Press: Beijing, China, 2020.
8. Zhang, W.; Ung, C.O.L.; Lin, G.; Liu, J.; Li, W.; Hu, H.; Xi, X. Factors Contributing to Patients' Preferences for Primary Health Care Institutions in China: A Qualitative Study. *Front. Public Health* **2020**, *8*, 414. [CrossRef] [PubMed]
9. Hou, J.; Michaud, C.; Li, Z.; Dong, Z.; Sun, B.; Zhang, J.; Cao, D.; Wan, X.; Zeng, C.; Wei, B.; et al. Transformation of the education of health professionals in China: Progress and challenges. *Lancet* **2014**, *384*, 819–827. [CrossRef]
10. Shi, L.; Lee, D.C.; Liang, H.; Zhang, L.; Makinen, M.; Blanchet, N.; Kidane, R.; Lindelow, M.; Wang, H.; Wu, S. Community health centers and primary care access and quality for chronically-ill patients-a case-comparison study of urban Guangdong Province, China. *Int. J. Equity Health* **2015**, *14*, 90. [CrossRef] [PubMed]
11. Li, W.; Gan, Y.; Dong, X.; Zhou, Y.; Cao, S.; Kkandawire, N.; Cong, Y.; Sun, H.; Lu, Z. Gatekeeping and the utilization of community health services in Shenzhen, China: A cross-sectional study. *Medicine* **2017**, *96*, e7719. [CrossRef] [PubMed]
12. Shi, J.; Jin, H.; Shi, L.; Chen, C.; Ge, X.; Lu, Y.; Zhang, H.; Wang, Z.; Yu, D. The quality of primary care in community health centers: Comparison among urban, suburban and rural users in Shanghai, China. *BMC Fam. Pract.* **2020**, *21*, 178. [CrossRef] [PubMed]
13. Zhu, M.; Li, H.; Wei, Q. Research on the role of hierarchical medical system in coping with public health emergencies. *Chin. Health Leg. Syst.* **2021**, *29*, 7–11, 35. [CrossRef]
14. Dong, E.; Liu, S.; Chen, M.; Wang, H.; Chen, L.W.; Xu, T.; Wang, T.; Zhang, L. Differences in regional distribution and inequality in health-resource allocation at hospital and primary health centre levels: A longitudinal study in Shanghai, China. *BMJ Open* **2020**, *10*, e035635. [CrossRef] [PubMed]
15. Wang, H.H.; Wang, J.J.; Wong, S.Y.; Wong, M.C.; Mercer, S.W.; Griffiths, S.M. The development of urban community health centres for strengthening primary care in China: A systematic literature review. *Br. Med. Bull.* **2015**, *116*, 139–153. [CrossRef] [PubMed]
16. Li, L.; Fu, H. China's health care system reform: Progress and prospects. *Int. J. Health Plan. Manag.* **2017**, *32*, 240–253. [CrossRef] [PubMed]
17. Chen, J.; Xu, S.; Gao, J. The Mixed Effect of China's New Health Care Reform on Health Insurance Coverage and the Efficiency of Health Service Utilisation: A Longitudinal Approach. *Int. J. Environ. Res. Public Health* **2020**, *17*, 1782. [CrossRef] [PubMed]
18. Wang, S. *Current Situation Research and Policy Suggestions of Health Human Resources at Grass-Roots Level in China*; Capital Medical University: Beijing, China, 2016.
19. Zhou, W. Current situation, Problems and Suggestions of grassroots health talents. *Chin. Gen. Pract.* **2010**, *13*, 685–688.

International Journal of
Environmental Research and Public Health

MDPI

Article

Effect of the Strategic Thinking, Problem Solving Skills, and Grit on the Disaster Triage Ability of Emergency Room Nurses

Jina Yang [1] and Kon Hee Kim [2,*]

[1] Emergency Room, Myongji Hospital, Ilsan 10475, Korea; yang.jina119@gmail.com
[2] College of Nursing, Ewha Womans University, Seoul 03760, Korea
* Correspondence: konhee@ewha.ac.kr; Tel.: +82-2-3277-4489

Abstract: In this descriptive study, we aimed to identify factors related to emergency room nurses' disaster triage ability. A total of 166 nurses who worked for emergency departments of general hospitals completed a structured questionnaire consisting of the Disaster Triage Ability Scale (DTAS), the Strategic Thinking Scale (STS), the Problem-Solving Inventory (PSI), and the Original Grit Scale (Grit-O). The data were analyzed using SPSS/WIN 25.0 by means of descriptive statistics, *t*-test, one-way ANOVA, the Scheffé post hoc test, Pearson's correlation coefficients, and stepwise multiple regression. Participants' DTAS averaged 14.03 ± 4.28 (Range 0–20) and showed a statistically significant difference according to their experience of triage education ($t = 2.26$, $p = 0.022$) as a disaster triage-related attribute. There were significant correlations among DTAS and confidence in the PSI ($r = 0.30$, $p < 0.001$), the approach-avoidance style in the PSI ($r = -0.28$, $p < 0.001$), and futurism in the STS ($r = 0.19$, $p = 0.019$). The strongest predictor was confidence in the PSI; in addition, 14.1% of the DTAS was explained by confidence in the PSI, approach-avoidance in the PSI, and futurism in the STS. Emergency room nurses who received triage education showed a higher level of the DTAS and their DTAS could be explained by problem-solving skills and strategic thinking. Therefore, it is necessary to develop and implement triage education programs integrated with stress management to improve the approach-avoidance style to ensure better problem-solving skills and to utilize various training methods to enhance confidence to improve problem-solving skills and futurism as part of strategic thinking.

Keywords: thinking; problem-solving; grit; triage; nurse

Citation: Yang, J.; Kim, K.H. Effect of the Strategic Thinking, Problem Solving Skills, and Grit on the Disaster Triage Ability of Emergency Room Nurses. *IJERPH* **2022**, *19*, 987. https://doi.org/10.3390/ijerph19020987

Academic Editors: Amir Khorram-Manesh and Krzysztof Goniewicz

Received: 22 December 2021
Accepted: 13 January 2022
Published: 16 January 2022

1. Introduction

Disasters are no longer uncommon. In the case of a disaster with multiple casualties, severity classification is essential for efficient use of limited manpower and resources [1]. Nurses are mainly responsible for the triage role in the clinical setting. Rapid information collection and accurate decision-making—that is, clinical reasoning ability—are essential for severity classification. In order to acquire this ability, continuous and systematic education is needed, and for the development and application of severity classification education programs, it is necessary to investigate the degree of nurses' severity classification abilities and their influencing factors.

Understanding and implementing severity classification in disasters with mass-casualty incidents is vital in order to disperse any limited resources among victims with the highest possibility of survival. Recent previous mass-casualty incident studies have found that improper first aid and victim transfer distribution results in re-transfer due to inadequate severity classifications at the mass-casualty incident site [2,3]. Therefore, it is essential to perform proper severity classification in mass-casualty incident situations because it directly affects the decline of resources and the health of casualties.

The individual who performs a severity classification at the disaster site must be a competent medical professional who can identify the incident site, allocate resources, set priorities, and transfer the victims according to patient severity [4]. Emergency room triage nurses (ERTNs) are exemplar healthcare professionals who can perform such tasks [5]. Research has revealed that more than 90% of the medical professionals who perform severity classification using the Korea Triage and Acuity Scale (KTAS) are nurses. Taken together, these data suggest that ERTNs are the ideal medical professionals to make the most appropriate choices according to victim health problems and the amount of resources available in disastrous situations.

Severity classification requires strategic thinking, which involves deciding upon new and appropriate actions based on existing methods and facts learned from specific situations in order to achieve the best goal in a given situation [6]. Strategic thinking provides indisputable facts through formal analysis and refers to making a choice among different solutions that systematically minimizes the risk factors when damage occurs to an organization [7]. One study revealed that classification strategies affect severity classifications and, subsequently, the health outcomes of patients in disastrous pediatric events [8]. Therefore, strategic thinking is required in order to determine the method and range of severity classifications using the type and disaster scales and assessing the health state of casualties.

Severity classification requires an understanding of the overall situation of a disaster, resource availability, the number and condition of victims, the classification of skills based on strategic and critical thinking, and professional medical knowledge, which must be used in a timely manner. Problem-solving skills in nursing refer to the ability to resolve health issues promptly through critical thinking, based on knowledge and experience [9,10]. Problem-solving skills require self-confidence, approach-avoidance style, and control. Confidence has a positive effect on the problem-solving process and outcome. Approach-avoidance style refers to the approach style of working hard to avoid bad things, and it is similar to coping with stress. In the process of solving problems, control over one's consciousness and behavior is required [11]. In severity classifications, problem solving skills are essential and affect accuracy through strategic and critical thinking. A previous study has shown that problem-solving skills improve the accuracy of severity classifications [12].

In a disastrous situation that is full of uncertainty, personal characteristics such as passion, persistency, and courage in spite of failure are required in those who perform severity classification. Grit refers to the characteristic of courage or determination that is required for successful goal achievement [13]. It does not mean simply passion and perseverance, but also includes the courage and persistence necessary to do the job in spite of failures without being discouraged [14]. Previous study results have shown high levels of stress in ERTNs who performed severity classification in mass-casualty incident simulation training. Therefore, grit is necessary to perform severity classification accurately in a stressful disaster situation.

Disaster triage ability (DTA) includes making the most appropriate choice for the best outcome according to the health issues of the victims and limited resources, and demonstrating courage, passion, and persistence in order to practice successful leadership. Furthermore, severity classification results influence the disaster cycle in relation to recovery; therefore, there is a need for ERTNs to have DTA that is based on specialized knowledge and skills in emergency situations. In this study, we investigated strategic thinking, problem-solving skills, grit, and DTA in ERTNs. Additionally, we examined these factors' relationships and influences on DTA, and aimed to provide a data-based framework for the development of severity classification training.

2. Materials and Methods

2.1. Design

This study was a descriptive study that sought to demonstrate the effects of strategic thinking, problem solving skills, and grit on DTA.

2.2. Participants

The participants were chosen from ERTNs in general hospitals located in metropolitan areas who had a minimum of 1 year of experience, who could efficiently and promptly classify patients based on emergency medical knowledge [15,16]. The sample size was calculated using G*Power 3.1.9.4 under the conditions of a significance level (α) of 0.05 and power ($1 - \beta$) of 0.80 for multiple regression analysis [17]. According to the Cohen criterion, the medium effect size (f^2) and predictors were set to 0.15 and 22, respectively, to calculate the number of samples required, which was 163. Considering the dropout rate, 195 questionnaires were distributed and 86.6% (169) copies were collected [18]. Three insufficient responses were excluded. Consequently, 166 responses from ERTNs were used in this study.

2.3. Measurements

2.3.1. General and Severity Classification-Related Characteristics

A questionnaire assessing the general (gender, year of birth, education level, clinical experience, and ER experience) and severity-classification-related (disaster education participation, disaster triage education participation, disaster triage experience, KTAS qualification) characteristics were used.

2.3.2. Strategic Thinking

The Strategic Thinking Scale (STS), which was developed by Salavati et al. [7], was translated and used in this study, with the authors' permission. Translation was conducted according to the WHO translation guidelines [19], in the following sequence: forward translation; expert panel back translation; pre-testing and cognitive interviewing; and the final version. Briefly, a bilingual United States registered nurse with over ten years of ER experience conducted the forward translation. The tool translated into Korean was then back-translated by a professional translator with a PhD in translation (Korean-English). To determine culturally different expressions and the degree of correspondence between the original tool and the translated version, a panel supervised the document. This panel included a nurse with at least ten years of ER clinical experience, a professional translator with a PhD in Korean-English translation, and an English native speaker. Their opinion indicated that there were no cultural differences; however, some word changes were required and the tool was modified accordingly. Next, pre-testing was conducted on five nurses with at least one year of ER experience. The final tool was approved through cognitive interviewing, which confirmed that the content was appropriate and did not contain any issues in understanding and responding. This five-point Likert scale had four sub-areas with 26 items: system thinking, conceptual thinking, futurism, and intelligent opportunism. Higher scores indicated a higher strategic thinking ability. Cronbach's α was 0.85 when the tool was developed [7], and was 0.71 in this study.

2.3.3. Problem-Solving Skills

Problem-solving skills (PSS) was measured using the Problem Solving Inventory (PSI) developed by Heppner and Petersen [20], translated by Jeon [21]. The tool, a five-point Likert scale, consisted of 21 items with three sub-areas: confidence, approach-avoidance style, and person control. The higher the score, the higher the PSS. Cronbach's α was 0.89 when the tool was developed [20], 0.90 in the research of Jeon [21], and 0.86 in this study.

2.3.4. Grit

The Original Grit Scale (Grit-O), which was developed by Duckworth et al. [14] and translated by Lee and Son [22], was used in this study. This five-point Likert scale consists of two sub-areas with twelve items: consistency of interests and perseverance of efforts. Higher scores indicated higher grit. Cronbach's α was 0.81 when the tool was developed [14], 0.79 in the research of Lee and Son [22], and 0.86 in this study.

2.3.5. Disaster Triage Ability

With the authors' permission, 20 items were extracted, revised, and supplemented from the Disaster Triage Education in Korea Disaster Life Support—Basic (KDLS-Basic) scale, which was developed by the Central Emergency Medical Center [23]. The content validity was verified by five experts (two emergency medicine specialists, two emergency structural science professors, and one ER specialist nurse) using the Content Validity Index (CVI) with a four-point Likert scale. The questions were adopted after confirming the minimal CVI of all 20 questions (0.99). Correct answers counted for one point, whereas incorrect answers obtained zero points. Higher scores indicated higher DTA, with a perfect score of 20.

2.4. Data Collection

During May 2019, following the Institutional Review Board (IRB) approval, we explained the purpose and method of the study to the head of the institution, the nursing department, and emergency unit for approval. Next, consent forms and structured questionnaires were distributed to voluntary participants, who were informed of the study's purpose and method. Informed consent forms and questionnaires were collected in separate collection boxes and small souvenirs were offered to the participants.

2.5. Data Analysis

Data were analyzed with the SPSS/WIN 25.0 program, using descriptive statistics, the independent t-test, one-way ANOVA, and Scheffé post-hoc analysis. The correlations between ST, PSS, Grit, and DTA were analyzed using Pearson's correlation coefficients. The effects of ST, PSS, and Grit on DTA were analyzed using stepwise multiple linear regression analysis.

2.6. Ethical Consideration

This study was conducted following approval by the IRB (MJH 2019-04-010-001). To acquire permission for this survey, the author explained the purpose and methods of our study to the head of each institution and the research manager of the nursing department in all participating institutions. The purpose and methods of the study were explained to the voluntary study participants before the informed consent forms and questionnaires were distributed. It was explained to participants that they can withdraw their participation in the study at any time with no disadvantages. To protect their privacy, the study participants were not specified; the consent forms and questionnaire were collected autonomously. In addition, these collections occurred simultaneously. The completed questionnaires were stored in a locked personal drawer and will be discarded immediately upon completion of the study. Furthermore, the computerized data is encrypted and stored in a personal computer accessible only to the primary investigator and will be deleted after three years of storage period.

3. Results

3.1. General and Severity Classification-Related Characteristics

The mean age of ERTNs was 29.12 ± 4.81, and '36+' showed the highest proportion, at 13.9%. There were 89.2% females, and 85.5% possessed a Bachelor's degree or less. The mean clinical experience was 70.22 ± 66.33 months, and over half (58.4%) had '<5 years' of experience. The mean experience in the ER was 63.66 ± 56.15 months, and 59.6% had worked '<60 months' in ER. There were 64.5% and 51.8% of participants who had undertaken disaster and disaster triage education, respectively. Finally, 38.6% had severity classification experience, and 60.8% possessed a KTAS qualification (Table 1).

Table 1. Participants' general characteristics (*N* = 166).

Characteristics	Categories	N (%)	Mean ± SD	Disaster Triage Ability	
				Mean ± SD	t or F (*p*)
Age (year)	≤30 31–35 ≥36	112(73.5) 21(12.6) 23(13.9)	29.12 ± 4.81	13.71 ± 4.40 14.29 ± 4.99 15.48 ± 2.33	1.70 (0.186)
Gender	M F	18(10.8) 148(89.2)		14.89 ± 3.16 13.93 ± 4.40	0.90 (0.369)
Education	Bachelor's or less Master's or higher	142(85.5) 24(14.5)		13.89 ± 4.25 14.83 ± 4.49	−0.99 (0.322)
Total clinical experience (month)	≤59 60–119 ≥120	97(58.4) 42(25.3) 27(16.3)	70.22 ± 66.33 (Range 12–480)	14.11 ± 3.74 13.69 ± 5.13 14.26 ± 4.82	0.19 (0.829)
Emergency room experience (month)	≤59 60–119 ≥120	99(59.6) 42(25.3) 25(15.1)	63.66 ± 56.15 (Range 12–360)	14.18 ± 3.73 13.71 ± 5.13 13.96 ± 4.89	0.18 (0.837)
Disaster education	Yes No	107(64.5) 59(35.5)		14.12 ± 4.16 13.86 ± 4.53	0.33 (0.712)
Disaster triage education	Yes No	86(51.8) 80(48.2)		14.94 ± 4.13 13.13 ± 4.46	2.26 (0.022)
Disaster triage-related experience	Yes No	64(38.6) 102(61.4)		14.14 ± 3.43 13.96 ± 4.76	0.78 (0.867)
Korean Triage and Acuity Scale (KTAS) certificate	Yes No	101(60.8) 65(39.2)		14.25 ± 3.91 13.69 ± 4.82	0.81 (0.417)

3.2. Participants' Strategic Thinking, Problem-Solving Skills, Grit, and Disaster Triage Ability

The mean ST score was 3.23 ± 0.19 points. When measuring the sub-areas, intelligent opportunism had the highest score (3.53 ± 0.35), followed by futurism (3.26 ± 0.48), conceptual thinking (3.25 ± 0.24), and system thinking (2.86 ± 0.18). The mean PSS score was 3.41 ± 0.39, and by sub-areas, approach-avoidance style 3.60 ± 0.37, confidence 3.47 ± 0.52, and person control 2.83 ± 0.74. The mean grit score was 3.02 ± 0.47, and by sub-areas, perseverance of efforts was 3.13 ± 0.48 and consistency of interests was 2.85 ± 0.60. The mean DTA score was 14.03 ± 4.28 (range, 2–19; Table 2).

Table 2. Strategic thinking, problem-solving skills, grit, and disaster triage ability. (*N* = 166).

Variable	Mean ± SD	Min	Max	Range
Strategic Thinking	3.23 ± 0.19	2.62	3.92	1–5
Conceptual Thinking	2.86 ± 0.18	2.43	3.43	1–5
System Thinking	3.25 ± 0.24	2.67	3.67	1–5
Futurism	3.26 ± 0.48	1.83	5.00	1–5
Intelligent Opportunism	3.53 ± 0.35	2.71	4.43	1–5
Problem-Solving Skills	3.41 ± 0.39	2.67	4.57	1–5
Confidence	3.47 ± 0.52	2.29	4.86	1–5
Approach-avoidance style	3.60 ± 0.37	2.40	4.30	1–5
Person Control	2.83 ± 0.74	1.25	4.75	1–5
Grit	3.02 ± 0.47	2.00	4.36	1–5
Consistency of Interests	2.85 ± 0.60	1.50	4.33	1–5
Perseverance of Effort	3.13 ± 0.48	2.00	4.50	1–5
Disaster Triage Ability	14.03 ± 4.28	2.00	19.00	0–20

3.3. Association of Disaster Triage Ability with General and Severity Classification-Related Characteristics

There was no significant difference in DTA according to the general characteristics; however, there was a significant effect of disaster triage education on DTA (t = 2.26, $p = 0.022$); nurses who participated in disaster triage training had significantly higher DTA scores (Table 1).

3.4. Association between Strategic Thinking, Problem-Solving Skills, Grit, and Disaster Triage Ability

DTA had a positive correlation with futurism (r = 0.19, $p = 0.019$), a sub-area of STS. Additionally, there was a significant positive and negative correlation with confidence (r = 0.30, $p < 0.001$) and approach-avoidance style (r = −0.28, $p < 0.001$), which are sub-areas of PSI; however, this was only to a weak degree (Table 3).

Table 3. Correlations among strategic thinking, problem-solving skills, grit, and disaster triage ability (*N*= 166).

r(*p*)	DTA [1]	ST [2]					PSS [7]				Grit		
		Total	CT [3]	S [4]	F [5]	I [6]	Total	C [8]	AAS [9]	PC [10]	Total	CI [11]	PE [12]
DTA [1]	1												
ST [2]	−0.06 (0.452)	1											
CT [3]	0.01 (0.879)	0.07 (0.376)	1										
S [4]	−0.02 (0.827)	0.49 (<0.001)	−0.14 (0.078)	1									
F [5]	0.19 (0.019)	0.80 (<0.001)	−0.05 (0.548)	0.16 (0.035)	1								
I [6]	0.05 (0.514)	0.73 (<0.001)	−0.24 (0.002)	0.27 (<0.001)	0.36 (<0.001)	1							
PSS [7]	0.03 (0.742)	0.46 (<0.001)	−0.20 (0.008)	0.12 (0.120)	0.60 (<0.001)	0.26 (0.001)	1						
C [8]	0.30 (<0.001)	0.41 (<0.001)	−0.23 (0.003)	0.15 (0.057)	0.57 (<0.001)	0.19 (0.013)	0.83 (<0.001)	1					
AAS [9]	−0.28 (<0.001)	0.41 (<0.001)	−0.10 (0.214)	0.11 (0.171)	0.41 (<0.001)	0.32 (<0.001)	0.73 (<0.001)	0.32 (<0.001)	1				
PC [10]	−0.09 (0.253)	0.26 (0.001)	−0.16 (0.037)	0.02 (0.829)	0.44 (<0.001)	0.07 (0.353)	0.82 (<0.001)	0.64 (<0.001)	0.37 (<0.001)	1			
Grit	−0.02 (0.772)	0.32 (<0.001)	−0.15 (0.050)	0.16 (0.045)	0.41 (<0.001)	0.15 (0.058)	0.54 (<0.001)	0.55 (<0.001)	0.24 (0.002)	0.52 (<0.001)	1		
CI [11]	−0.05 (0.531)	0.14 (0.070)	−0.08 (0.314)	0.14 (0.069)	0.22 (0.004)	−0.02 (0.797)	0.32 (<0.001)	0.39 (<0.001)	0.01 (0.855)	0.37 (<0.001)	0.80 (<0.001)	1	
PE [12]	0.03 (0.689)	0.32 (<0.001)	−0.22 (0.005)	0.12 (0.139)	0.42 (<0.001)	0.19 (0.014)	0.56 (<0.001)	0.54 (<0.001)	0.32 (<0.001)	0.47 (<0.001)	0.89 (<0.001)	0.53 (<0.001)	1

[1] Disaster triage ability. [2] Strategic thinking. [3] Conceptual thinking. [4] System thinking. [5] Futurism. [6] Intelligent opportunism. [7] Problem-solving skills. [8] Confidence. [9] Approach-avoidance style. [10] Person control. [11] Consistency of interests. [12] Perseverance of efforts.

3.5. Factors Influencing Disaster Triage Ability

Multiple regression analysis was conducted to identify the factors influencing DTA in ERTNs. Futurism, confidence, and approach-avoidance style were used as independent variables. Multicollinearity between tolerance limits and independent variables, as well as mutual independence between residuals, were identified. Tolerance was 0.55–0.88, the variance inflation factor (VIF) was <10 (range, 1.14–1.81). This confirmed the low correlation between independent variables without multicollinearity. The Durbin–Watson coefficient was closed to two (range, 1.91–2.01) [20], confirming the independence of the residuals.

The factors influencing DTA were identified as the approach-avoidance style, a sub-area of PSI (β = −0.27, p < 0.001); confidence, a sub-area of PSI (β = 0.22, p = 0.004); and futurism, a sub-area of STS (β = 0.17, p = 0.030). These variables explained 14.1% of the DTA. Among these three factors, approach-avoidance style was the most significant factor. Consequently, the DTA of ERTNs was considered higher when individuals reported lower approach-avoidance styles and higher confidence in PSI, and higher futurism in STS (Table 4).

Table 4. Influencing factors on disaster triage ability among emergency room nurses (N = 166).

Variables		Disaster Triage Ability					
		B	β	t	p	Tolerance	VIF [1]
(constant)		12.00		2.88	0.005		
Problem-Solving Skills	Approach-avoidance style	−3.67	−0.27	−3.22	<0.001	0.88	1.14
	Confidence	2.16	0.22	2.16	0.004	0.58	1.73
Strategic Thinking	Futurism	1.20	0.17	1.55	0.030	0.55	1.81
		R^2 = 0.150, Adjusted R^2 = 0.141, F = 8.91, p < 0.001					

[1] VIF: variance inflation factor.

4. Discussion

Interest in disaster medical care has increased and related activities due to the occurrence of various disaster accidents. This demand has strengthened the need for severity classification abilities, which influence the success and failure of response results. ERTNs are ideal medical professionals to make appropriate severity classification choices because of their experiences identifying the severity of casualties according to health issues and resource availability. This descriptive survey study sought to provide a new basis for the educational intervention for improved DTA in ERTNs by identifying the degrees of strategic thinking, problem-solving skills, grit, and disaster triage ability in ERTNs. We found that the mean DTA score of ERTNs was 14.03, which can be converted to over 70.15 points in a 100-point scale. A novel tool was used to measure DTA in this study; therefore, we converted the points calculated to a 100-point scale for comparison and analysis with previous studies. The result of this study was similar to a study with Canadian ERTNs, who had a mean DTA score of 72.2 points [24]. This study used a KTAS based on the Canada Triage and Acuity Scale (CTAS) and ERTNs were assessed using similar classification tools to those in the present study. Interestingly, a previous domestic severity classification study reported different results; DTA was lower in domestic military nursing personnel (63.5 points) [25] and higher in 119 paramedics (75.7 points) [26]. This indicates that nurses who perform different occupational duties show differences in their DTA.

A previous study reported that the mean DTA scores of 119 paramedics, which included nurses, were different according to age, clinical experience, and job title [27]. In contrast, there was no difference in DTA scores associated with general characteristics in this study. However, a direct comparison was difficult, as previous studies did not investigate general characteristics [24] or did not consider their relationship to DTA, although age, clinical experience, and job title have been investigated [28]. A previous study confirmed a significant difference in DTA according to the general characteristics, such as age, clinical experience, and job title of the ERTNs [29]. Taken together, these data suggest that a follow-up study assessing the relationship between DTA and general characteristics is required. These differences are significant for the development of DTA educational programs.

This study confirmed the significant difference in DTA according to the presence of disaster triage education; higher DTA scores were associated with disaster triage education participation. This result is similar to a study on US ERTNs, which showed a significant DTA improvement after a video simulation education course [28], and a study on 119 paramedics and public health care emergency teams, which revealed improvements in timing and DTA after education [30]. According to findings of the National Disaster Health Medical Education [31], opportunities for severity classification education are relatively limited because there are no separately operated severity classification courses, and these skills are only included as a part of disaster-related education. Therefore, specialized disaster triage education courses and programs are required.

Our results revealed that a higher DTA score was associated with enhanced confidence in PSI, higher futurism in STS, and a lower level of the approach-avoidance style. These results were similar to those of a previous study showing that higher confidence and job performance was correlated with a higher DTA score in ERTNs in US general hospitals [28]. Confidence in PSI refers to the ability to choose and apply a solution among various options [20]. It is dependent on basic knowledge and performance frequency [31]. This suggests that education should combine theory and practice. Futurism in STS refers to the future assessment ability and is improved through practice [7]. Approach-avoidance style refers to stress-coping skills, which are dependent on stress defense mechanisms [11]. Research has indicated that enhanced DTA is associated with a well-formed approach-avoidance style, which suggests the need for an approach-avoidance style-forming programs. Furthermore, our results differ from research showing that other emergency medical professionals who use appropriate approach-avoidance style defense mechanisms are healthier in disaster situations [11]. This may be due to a limitation of the appropriate approach-avoidance style defense mechanisms in ERTNs due to constant exposure to emergency situations. Hence, the application of appropriate approach-avoidance style defense mechanism formation education in ERTNs is necessary.

The explanatory power of the factors influencing DTA in ERTNs assessed in this study (approach-avoidance style and confidence in PSI, futurism in STS) was 14.1%. Similarly, previous study results have revealed that confidence in PSI [32] and futurism in STS [33] significantly influence DTA. In contrast to our results, mass-casualty incident simulation training of ERTNs has shown that stresses associated with the approach-avoidance style alone significantly affect DTA [34]. DTA aims to distribute medical resources to casualties with higher probabilities of survival. It is responsible for evaluating patients, communicating with and between professionals; providing initial first aid; allocating medical resources; and monitoring, reassessing and managing the flow of the patient treatment [16]. A study on Swedish ERTNs analyzed the skills and influential factors relating to DTA and confirmed that confidence for PSI [32] and futurism in STS enabled the best choices in regard to future situations [33]. Furthermore, another study assessed mass-casualty incident situation training of nurses, doctors, and other healthcare workers from general hospitals in Thailand. They found that severity classification stress was significantly influenced by individual approach-avoidance style [34], which is in contrast with our study. Taken together, our study and previous data highlight that enhanced confidence in PSI, futurism in STS, and the influence of the approach-avoidance style in PSI can improve DTA.

This study confirmed that the influence of an approach-avoidance style and confidence in PSI, futurism in STS, and disaster triage education affect DTA. The approach-avoidance style in PSI is affected by stress coping skills, and confidence in PSI and futurism in STS are affected by education and practice; therefore, this study has provided data that can be used to develop further strategic thinking education programs.

There are some limitations of this study. We sought participation in a limited area; therefore, generalization is limited. Follow-up studies that use national random data are suggested. Furthermore, repeated research through objective data collection, such as measuring DTA using impartial observers, is suggested because it is difficult to exclude subjective effects with self-report-oriented data collection, as used in this study. Moreover, this study identified approach-avoidance style and confidence on PSI and futurism on STS as significant influencing factors; however, there was a low level of explanatory power. We suggest a follow-up study to elucidate the other influencing factors in DTA.

5. Conclusions

This study was conducted in order to provide data on the requirements for the development of DTA in ERTNs who play a major role in severity classification in emergency situations. This was performed by identifying the degree and influential factors on DTA in current ERTNs. Our data revealed at least an intermediate level of DTA in ERTNs, which was significantly increased with disaster triage education. Approach-avoidance style and confidence, sub-areas of PSI, and futurism, a sub area of STS, affected DTA, with an explanatory power of 14.1%.

When developing and applying an educational intervention for DTA, it is important to promote the approach-avoidance style as part of a stress coping program. The preparation and application of stress-coping programs such as mindfulness, meditation, relaxation, and so on, may be considered for ERTNs. Furthermore, the use of learning methods such as conceptual guidance, theory, and task-based learning are crucial. Education increases DTA; therefore, the continuous development and application of disaster triage education programs will be most efficient. It is also necessary to provide an opportunity to maintain and improve nurses' severity classification ability through repeated learning using virtual reality, augmented reality, and extended reality, and to verify the effectiveness of this approach. Additionally, as a follow-up study, the authors suggest an analysis of patient outcomes and medical costs according to the number of triage experiences and their success or failure. Considering the rapid nurse turnover rate due to the shortage of nursing manpower, we suggest a study to verify the effectiveness of severity classification education according to the period of clinical experience.

Author Contributions: Conceptualization, J.Y. and K.H.K.; methodology, J.Y. and K.H.K.; software, J.Y. and K.H.K.; validation, J.Y. and K.H.K.; formal analysis, J.Y. and K.H.K.; investigation, J.Y.; resources, J.Y. and K.H.K.; data curation, J.Y. and K.H.K.; writing—original draft preparation, J.Y. and K.H.K.; writing—review and editing, K.H.K.; visualization, J.Y. and K.H.K.; supervision, K.H.K.; project administration, K.H.K. All authors have read and agreed to the published version of the manuscript.

Funding: This research did not receive any specific grant from funding agencies in the public, commercial, or not-for-profit sectors.

Institutional Review Board Statement: The study was conducted according to the guidelines of the Declaration of Helsinki and approved by the Institutional Review Board of Myongji Hospital (MJH 2019-04-010-001, 30 April 2019).

Informed Consent Statement: Informed consent was obtained from all participants involved in the study. Written informed consent was obtained from the participants to publish this paper.

Data Availability Statement: The data presented in this study are not publicly available due to participants' privacy.

Acknowledgments: The authors thank each of the participants in this study.

Conflicts of Interest: The authors declare no conflict of interest.

References

1. McCoy, C.E.; Chakravarthy, B.; Lotfipour, S. Guidelines for field triage of injured patients: In conjunction with the morbidity and mortality weekly report published by the Center for Disease Control and Prevention. *West J. Emerg. Med.* **2013**, *14*, 69–76. [CrossRef] [PubMed]
2. Woo, J.H.; Lee, G.; Cho, J.S.; Yang, H.J.; Lim, Y.S.; Kim, J.J.; Park, W.B.; Jang, J.Y.; Jang, J.H.; Hyun, S.Y.; et al. Disaster medical responses to the disaster scene of long-distance on highway-field triage and disaster communication by social media for 106-vehicle chain collision in Yeong-Jong grand bridge. *Korean Soc. Emerg. Med.* **2015**, *26*, 449–457.
3. Cha, M.I.; Kim, G.W.; Kim, C.H.; Choa, M.; Choi, D.H.; Kim, I.; Wang, S.J.; Woo, I.S.; Yoon, H.D.; Lee, K.H.; et al. A study on the disaster medical response during the Mauna Ocean resort gymnasium collapse. *Korean J. Emerg. Med.* **2017**, *28*, 97–108. [CrossRef] [PubMed]
4. Wang, S.J. Development of a national disaster medical manual. *J. Korean Soc. Disaster Prev. Saf.* **2016**, *9*, 39–45. [CrossRef]

5. Lee, E.N.; Kim, B.J.; Kim, S.S.; Kang, K.H.; Kim, Y.S. Development of an in-service education program for emergency room nurses according to their career ladders. *Clin. Nurs. Res.* **2018**, *14*, 99–111.
6. Randolph, S.A. Strategic thinking. *Workplace Health Saf.* **2013**, *61*, 52. [CrossRef] [PubMed]
7. Salavati, S.; Veshareh, E.J.; Safari, H.; Veysian, A.; Amirnezhad, G. Strategic thinking and its related factors in a medical science university in Iran. *Electron. Physician* **2017**, *9*, 4332–4340. [CrossRef] [PubMed]
8. Kelen, G.D.; Troncoso, R.; Trebach, J.; Levin, S.; Cole, G.; Delaney, C.M.; Jenkins, J.L.; Fackler, J.; Sauer, L. Effect of reverse triage on creation of surge capacity in a pediatric hospital. *JAMA Pediatrics* **2017**, *171*, e164829. [CrossRef]
9. Lee, S.J.; Jang, G.S. The effects of action learning on nurses' problem solving, communication, emotional creativity and innovation behavior. *J. Korean Soc. Health Med. Ind.* **2014**, *8*, 73–87. [CrossRef]
10. Kim, H.S.; Han, S.J. The survey on the influence of clinical nurse's critical thinking disposition, problem-solving skill and self-efficacy on patients' safety competencies. *J. Korea Ind.-Acad. Technol. Soc.* **2016**, *17*, 598–608. [CrossRef]
11. Arble, E.; Arnetz, B.B. A model of first-responder coping: An approach/avoidance bifurcation. *Stress Health* **2017**, *33*, 223–232. [CrossRef] [PubMed]
12. Follmann, A.; Ohligs, M.; Hochhausen, N.; Beckers, S.K.; Rossaint, R.; Czaplik, M. Technical support by smart glasses during a mass casualty incident: A randomized controlled simulation trial on technically assisted triage and telemedical app use in disaster medicine. *J. Med. Internet Res.* **2019**, *21*, e11939. [CrossRef]
13. Lee, S.B.; Bae, E.H.; Son, Y.W.; Lee, S.R. Grit as a buffer against negative feedback: The effect of grit on emotional responses to negative feedback. *J. Korean Psychol. Assoc. Soc. Personal.* **2016**, *30*, 25–45.
14. Duckworth, A.L.; Peterson, C.; Matthews, M.D.; Kelly, D.R. Grit: Perseverance and passion for long-term goals. *J. Personal. Soc. Psychol.* **2007**, *92*, 1087–1101. [CrossRef]
15. Oh, J.H. How to use the Korean Emergency Patient Classification Tool (KTAS)?: A survey for classifiers at 1 year after the project. In Proceedings of the 2017 Korean Society of Emergency Medicine Spring Conference, Gwangju, Korea, 20–21 April 2017.
16. Korean Society of Emergency Medicine (K-EM). *In Korean Emergency Patient Classification Tool. Korean Severity Classification System: Participant Manual*; The Korean Society of Emergency Medicine: Seoul, Korea, 2014.
17. Kang, H.C.; Yeon, G.P.; Han, S.T. Consideration of the use of effect size in nursing research. *Korean J. Nurs.* **2015**, *45*, 641–649. [CrossRef] [PubMed]
18. Cohen, J. *Statistical Power Analysis for the Behavioral Sciences*, 2nd ed.; Lawrence Erlbaum Associates: Hillsdale, NJ, USA, 1989.
19. World Health Organization. *Process of Translation and Adaptation of Instruments [Internet]*; WHO: Geneva, Switzerland, 2016. Available online: https://www.who.int/substance_abuse/research_tools/translation/en/ (accessed on 20 March 2019).
20. Heppner, P.; Petersen, C. The development and implications of a personal problem solving inventory. *J. Couns. Psychol.* **1982**, *29*, 66–75. [CrossRef]
21. Jeon, S.G. Social skills training program for social adaptation of schizophrenic patients. *Ment. Health Soc. Work* **1995**, *2*, 33–50.
22. Lee, S.; Son, Y.W. What are the strong predictors of academic achievement?—Deliberate practice and grit. *Korean J. Sch. Psychol.* **2013**, *10*, 349–366.
23. Central Emergency Medical Center. *Korean Disaster Medical Support Basic Curriculum (KDLS-Basic) Materials*; Ministry of Health and Welfare: Sejong, Korea, 2017.
24. Curran, S.G.; Franc, J.M. A pilot study examining the speed and accuracy of triage for simulated disaster patients in an emergency department setting: Comparison of a computerized version of Canadian Triage Acuity Scale (CTAS) and Simple Triage and Rapid Treatment (START) methods. *Can. J. Emerg. Med.* **2017**, *19*, 364–371. [CrossRef] [PubMed]
25. Park, J.Y.; Choi, S.M. A study of the triage performance of military nurses and related factors using a mass casualty scenario, paper exercise. *Gunjin Nurs. Res.* **2012**, *30*, 128–142.
26. Lee, H.J.; Cho, G.J. Comparison of knowledge level of triage in 119 EMTs. *J. Korean Emerg. Rescue Soc.* **2014**, *18*, 43–54. [CrossRef]
27. Kim, Y.S. The Influence of Severity Classification Education Program on the Accuracy of Severity Classification: Focusing on 119 Paramedics and Quick Response Teams at Public Health Centers. Master's Thesis, Korea National Transportation University, Uiwang, Korea, 2018.
28. Dubovsky, S.L.; Antonius, D.; Ellis, D.G.; Ceusters, W.; Sugarman, R.C.; Roberts, R.; Kandifer, S.; Phillips, J.; Daurignac, E.C.; Leonard, K.E.; et al. A preliminary study of a novel emergency department nursing triage simulation for research applications. *BMC Part Springer Nat.* **2017**, *10*, 15. [CrossRef] [PubMed]
29. No, Y.S. Relation between Ability of Clinical Decision Making of Nurse in Emergency Room with Performing Nursing Work. Master's Thesis, Ajou University, Suwon, Korea, 2010.
30. Yu, H.I.; Lee, S.H.; Wang, S.J. Status of health medical education program for disaster victims. *Korean Soc. Disaster Inf. Conf.* **2018**, *11*, 240–241.
31. Jung, A.H.; Moon, M.Y. A study on the clinical competence, problem solving ability according to frequency of fundamental nursing skill performance, confidence of core fundamental nursing skill performance during clinical practice in nursing students. *Asia-Pac. J. Multimed. Serv. Converg. Art Humanit. Sociol.* **2018**, *8*, 451–463. [CrossRef]
32. Andersson, A.K.; Omberg, M.; Svedlund, M. Triage in the emergency department: A qualitative study of the factors which nurses consider when making decisions. *Nurs. Crit. Care* **2006**, *11*, 136–145. [CrossRef] [PubMed]

33. Archibald, M.M.; Barnard, A. Futurism in nursing: Technology, robotics and the fundamentals of care. *J. Clin. Nurs.* **2018**, *11–12*, 2473–2480. [CrossRef]
34. Kuhls, D.A.; Chestovich, P.J.; Coule, P.; Carrison, D.M.; Chua, C.M.; Wora-Urai, N.; Kanchanarin, T. Basic Disaster Life Support (BDLS) training improves first responder confidence to face Mass-Casualty Incidents in Thailand. *Prehospital Disaster Med.* **2017**, *32*, 492–500. [CrossRef] [PubMed]

healthcare

MDPI

Article

Can a Healthcare Quality Improvement Initiative Reduce Disparity in the Treatment Delay among ST-Segment Elevation Myocardial Infarction Patients with Different Arrival Modes? Evidence from 33 General Hospitals and Their Anticipated Impact on Healthcare during Disasters and Public Health Emergencies

Na Li [1,2], Junxiong Ma [1,2], Shuduo Zhou [1,2], Xuejie Dong [1,2], Mailikezhati Maimaitiming [3], Yinzi Jin [1,2,*] and Zhijie Zheng [1,2]

1 Department of Global Health, School of Public Health, Peking University, Beijing 100871, China; lina2021@bjmu.edu.cn (N.L.); junxiongma@bjmu.edu.cn (J.M.); zhoushuduo@pku.edu.cn (S.Z.); dongxj@bjmu.edu.cn (X.D.); zhengzj@bjmu.edu.cn (Z.Z.)
2 Institute for Global Health and Development, Peking University, Beijing 100871, China
3 School of Health Humanities, Peking University, Beijing 100871, China; maili@bjmu.edu.cn
* Correspondence: yzjin@bjmu.edu.cn; Tel.: +86-15-00108-1989; Fax: +86-10-8280-2144

Citation: Li, N.; Ma, J.; Zhou, S.; Dong, X.; Maimaitiming, M.; Jin, Y.; Zheng, Z. Can a Healthcare Quality Improvement Initiative Reduce Disparity in the Treatment Delay among ST-Segment Elevation Myocardial Infarction Patients with Different Arrival Modes? Evidence from 33 General Hospitals and Their Anticipated Impact on Healthcare during Disasters and Public Health Emergencies. *Healthcare* **2021**, *9*, 1462. https://doi.org/10.3390/healthcare9111462

Academic Editors: Amir Khorram-Manesh and Krzysztof Goniewicz

Received: 7 September 2021
Accepted: 26 October 2021
Published: 28 October 2021

Abstract: (1) Background: Chest pain center accreditation has been associated with improved timelines of primary percutaneous coronary intervention (PCI) for ST-segment elevated myocardial infarction (STEMI). However, evidence from low- and middle-income regions was insufficient, and whether the sensitivity to improvements differs between walk-in and emergency medical service (EMS)-transported patients remained unclear. In this study, we aimed to examine the association of chest pain center accreditation status with door-to-balloon (D2B) time and the potential modification effect of arrival mode. (2) Methods: The associations were examined using generalized linear mixed models, and the effect modification of arrival mode was examined by incorporating an interaction term in the models. (3) Results: In 4186 STEMI patients, during and after accreditation were respectively associated with 65% (95% CI: 54%, 73%) and 71% (95% CI: 61%, 79%) reduced risk of D2B time being more than 90 min (using before accreditation as the reference). Decreases of 27.88 (95% CI: 19.57, 36.22) minutes and 26.55 (95% CI: 17.45, 35.70) minutes in D2B were also observed for the during and after accreditation groups, respectively. The impact of accreditation on timeline improvement was greater for EMS-transported patients than for walk-in patients. (4) Conclusions: EMS-transported patients were more sensitive to the shortened in-hospital delay associated with the initiative, which could exacerbate the existing disparity among patients with different arrival modes.

Keywords: chest pain center accreditation; healthcare quality improvement; door-to-balloon time; arrival mode; ST-segment elevation myocardial infarction

1. Introduction

ST-segment elevation myocardial infarction (STEMI) is the deadliest and most time-sensitive acute cardiac event. Primary percutaneous coronary intervention (PCI) is the typically recommended treatment for STEMI cases. The door-to-balloon time, also referred to as the in-hospital delay, which denotes the interval from the patient's arrival at the emergency department to the first inflation of an angioplasty balloon in the occluded coronary artery, is widely used to assess the timeliness of primary PCI [1]. A door-to-balloon time of 90 min or less is given as the Class I (highest level) recommendation according to the American College of Cardiology/American Heart Association (ACC/AHA) and European Society of Cardiology (ESC) guidelines [2,3]. Despite the widespread promulgation and endorsement of the guideline, their translation into clinical practice remains suboptimal. In China, only 32.6% of STEMI patients receive primary PCI within 90 min of arrival [4]. Moreover, there is a very pronounced gap in the door-to-balloon time between walk-in and emergency medical service (EMS)-transported STEMI patients undergoing primary PCI [5–8]. Therefore, implementation of a healthcare quality improvement initiative, ensuring that hospitals provide timely guideline-recommended clinical practice, is warranted to reduce the in-hospital delay.

A growing strand of studies indicate that accreditation of chest pain centers can facilitate the implementation of strategies to improve healthcare quality for STEMI. Accredited chest pain centers should follow the criteria according to the recommended guideline, accompanied with a number of quality improvement activities (e.g., establishing a standardized monitor system of healthcare performance, carrying out healthcare performance review and feedback). For instance, the United States and Germany have witnessed improvements in the management and clinical outcomes of STEMI patients after an extensive adoption of nationwide programs for chest pain center professional society accreditation [9–12]. Positive empirical evidence in developed countries has shown that chest pain center accreditation is associated with shortened in-hospital delay for STEMI care [10,13]. However, two key questions remained unanswered: First, does the positive effect of chest pain center accreditation on the in-hospital delay found in other settings apply to China, where the proportion of cases receiving guideline-recommended treatments remains low [4]? Second, given the large disparity in the in-hospital delay among patients with different arrival modes [5,6,8,14,15], is the association between chest pain center accreditation and the in-hospital delay different between walk-in and EMS-transported cases? If so, is chest pain center accreditation widening or narrowing the existing disparities in in-hospital delay? Furthermore, integration of prehospital and hospital care is one of the dimensions of chest pain center accreditation criteria in China. It requires that hospitals should establish a regional collaborative healthcare delivery system that integrates prehospital emergency systems and in-hospital green passages, coordination and division of labor between different hospital departments, and connections between hospitals and community healthcare centers. This also plays a key role in optimizing the capacity of public health infrastructure and/or systems to respond at times of public health emergencies and disasters. Therefore, if chest pain center accreditation is beneficial to timeliness for STEMI patients and other acute cardiac events, it would also contribute to the promptness of triage, transfer, and treatment at times of public health emergencies and disasters.

2. Materials and Methods

2.1. Study Design and Population

For this study, we utilized data from all the accredited hospitals with PCI capabilities in Beijing during January 2016 to June 2019. For our study, we recruited STEMI patients who met the following criteria:

(1) A discharged diagnosis of STEMI, according to ischemic symptoms, ECG, or positive cardiac markers;
(2) Underwent primary PCI;
(3) Arrived at hospital by either of arrival modes: directly by self or transported via EMS.

Patients were excluded if they had an unknown mode of arrival ($N = 15$), missing hospital arrival time, or implausible door-to-balloon time, such as a negative value or time exceeding 24 h ($N = 37$).

2.2. Measurement

2.2.1. Accreditation Status

Hospitals' accreditation status was authenticated by the National Health Commission of China in April 2018. Chest pain center accreditation is made available to all hospitals in Beijing, and hospitals voluntarily continue to apply for the accreditation in a staggered manner. To June 2019, there were a total of 33 hospitals with accredited chest pain centers in Beijing. Thus, not every hospital had enrolled chest pain patients for 18 months. It takes months to receive accreditation, which is based on a review of information from multiple sources, including self-assessment statements, data reports, and field surveys, jointly led by the National Health Commission of China and a specialist team. Data on individual patients were extracted from the electronic medical systems of each hospital, regarding the data elements which were selected based on the ACC/AHA clinical practice guideline [2]. The accreditation statuses of hospital were grouped as 'before accreditation' (had not applied for accreditation), 'during accreditation' (were applying for accreditation), and 'after accreditation' (had been accredited). Patients who were admitted to hospitals before, during, and after the corresponding date of accreditation were, respectively, classified into the 'before accreditation' group, the 'during accreditation' group, and the 'after accreditation' group.

2.2.2. Outcomes

The primary outcome was the in-hospital delay, measured by the door-to-balloon time and the percentage of cases with door-to-balloon time of more than 90 min. Door-to-balloon time was defined as the interval from the STEMI patient's arrival at the hospital to inflation of the balloon to restore flow.

2.2.3. Covariates

The EMS-transported patients were defined as patients transported to the hospital by EMS services. Walk-in patients were defined as those arriving at the hospital by self- or private transportation, taxi, public transportation, or walking to the hospital.

Patient-level covariates included age, sex (male or female), and signs and symptoms at presentation: whether the patient had sustainable chest pain (refers to the onset of chest pain that lasts more than 30 min and cannot be relieved by rest), intermittent chest pain (refers to chest pain that lasts a few minutes at a time and can be relieved by rest or elimination of the triggers), chest pain relief, abdominal pain, dyspnea, cardiogenic shock, heart failure, malignant arrhythmia, receiving prehospital cardiopulmonary resuscitation or not, heart rate (beats/min), blood pressure (mmHg), and Killip class (I to IV) [16]. Hospital-level characteristics included time of day of arrival (8:00 a.m. to 16:59 p.m., 17:00 p.m. to 11:59 p.m., 12:00 a.m. to 7:59 a.m.), weekday or off-day arrival (off-days include weekends and Chinese official holidays), hospital level, and region of hospital (urban or suburb). Hospital levels in China are divided into several levels according to the scale, facilities, and ability of hospitals: grade III A, B, and C; grade II A, B, and C; and grade I, with grade IIIA being the highest level. Hospitals of grade IIIA have high-level capacity for primary PCI, and the number of PCIs meets certain requirements, ensuring that emergency PCI operations are performed 24 h a day.

2.3. Data Analysis

The characteristics of patients and hospitals and the in-hospital delay were compared between walk-in and EMS-transported patients, with the use of the chi-square test for categorical variables and the *Kruskal–Wallis* test for continuous variables. Categorical variables are presented as counts and percentages. Quantitative variables are expressed as means $\pm$ standard deviations (SDs) or medians and interquartile ranges. p values of less than 0.05 were considered to indicate statistical significance. We describe the median of door-to-balloon times and the percentage of patients for whom door-to-balloon times were 90 min or more across arrival modes and accreditation status.

To account for clustering of patients within hospitals, we employed generalized linear mixed models with a random effect term for the hospital to examine the associations of arrival mode and accreditation status with in-hospital delay (Model 1). The logistic regression was performed for the percentage of cases with door-to-balloon time of more than 90 min, and the effect estimates are reported as odds ratios (ORs) and 95% CI. For the door-to-balloon time, the effect estimates were calculated from the linear regression and reported as changes in minutes. Variables included in the models were selected based on their physiological relevance and potential to be associated with outcomes. We initiated the model development with a crude model (no adjustment) and then added a range of covariates into the regression models based on previous studies in the literature [14,17–19]. All the models were adjusted for sex, age, signs and symptoms at presentation, heart rate, blood pressure and Killip class, arrival mode, time of day of arrival, day of arrival, class of hospital, region of hospital, and accreditation status. To examine the modification effect of arrival mode in the association of accreditation status with the in-hospital delay, an interaction term of arrival mode and accreditation status was incorporated into the model (Model 2). All the models were adjusted for covariates, with $p < 0.05$ considered the level of statistical significance. Hospital was added as a random effect term in the models to adjust for unobserved hospital-level factors. All statistical analyses were performed using R software.

3. Results

3.1. Characteristics of Patients and Hospitals

A total of 4186 STEMI patients undergoing PCI from 33 hospitals were enrolled in this study, including 1284 (30.7%) EMS-transported patients and 2902 (69.3%) walk-in patients. The overall median age of the patients was 60 years, and 80.5% were men. The patients admitted to hospitals before, during, and after accreditation accounted for 43.2%, 13.7, and 43.1%, respectively. A comparison of patient- and hospital-level characteristics by arrival mode is presented in Table 1. In general, compared with walk-in patients, EMS-transported patients had lower heart rate (73.5 versus 75.9 beats/min, $p < 0.001$), lower systolic blood pressure (122.7 versus 132.5 mmHg, $p < 0.001$), lower diastolic blood pressure (76 versus 81.3 mmHg, $p < 0.001$), and lower rate of Killip I status (81.3% versus 89.7%, $p < 0.001$). Regarding hospital-level characteristics, 72.2% of EMS-transported patients arrived at urban hospitals, slightly larger than the proportion of walk-in patients (67.1%, $p < 0.001$).

Table 1. Patient- and hospital-level characteristics of participants.

Characteristics	Overall	Arrival Mode		*p* Value
		EMS-Transported	Walk-In	
Number of admissions, *n* (%)	4186 (100)	1284 (30.7)	2902 (69.3)	
Patient-level				
Sex, *n* (%)				
Male	3368 (80.5)	1025 (79.8)	2343 (80.7)	0.521
Female	818 (19.5)	259 (20.2)	559 (19.3)	
Age, median (q1, q3)	60 (52, 69)	61 (53, 70)	60 (51, 69)	0.010
Sustainable chest pain, *n* (%)	2385 (57.0)	858 (66.8)	1527 (52.6)	<0.001
Intermittent chest pain, *n* (%)	545 (13.0)	136 (10.6)	409 (14.1)	0.001
Chest pain relief, *n* (%)	27 (0.6)	10 (0.8)	17 (0.6)	0.008
Abdominal pain, *n* (%)	34 (0.8)	6 (0.5)	28 (1.0)	0.182
Dyspnea, *n* (%)	38 (0.9)	9 (0.7)	29 (1.0)	0.644
Shock, *n* (%)	31 (0.7)	21 (1.6)	10 (0.3)	<0.001
Heart failure, *n* (%)	15 (0.4)	10 (0.8)	5 (0.2)	0.007
Malignant arrhythmia, *n* (%)	33 (0.8)	22 (1.7)	11 (0.4)	<0.001
CPR, *n* (%)	17 (0.4)	13 (1.0)	4 (0.1)	<0.001
Heart rate (beats/min), mean (SD)	75.1 (18.0)	73.5 (19.2)	75.9 (17.3)	<0.001
Systolic blood pressure (mm Hg), mean (SD)	129.5 (27.7)	122.7 (27.5)	132.5 (27.3)	<0.001
Diastolic blood pressure (mm Hg), mean (SD)	79.6 (18.0)	76.0 (18.4)	81.3 (17.6)	<0.001
Killip class, *n* (%)				
I	3324 (87.1)	974 (81.3)	2350 (89.7)	<0.001
II	334 (8.8)	136 (11.4)	198 (7.6)	
III	39 (1.0)	24 (2.0)	15 (0.6)	
IV	120 (3.1)	64 (5.3)	56 (2.1)	

Table 1. *Cont.*

Characteristics	Overall	Arrival Mode		*p* Value
		EMS-Transported	Walk-In	
Hospital-level				
Region, *n* (%)				
Urban	2875 (68.7)	927 (72.2)	1948 (67.1)	0.001
Suburb	1311 (31.3)	357 (27.8)	954 (32.9)	
Hospital level, *n* (%)				
Grade III A	3262 (77.9)	985 (76.7)	2277 (78.5)	0.223
Non-grade III A	924 (22.1)	299 (23.3)	625 (21.5)	
Day of arrival, *n* (%)				
Weekday	2788 (66.6)	856 (66.7)	1932 (66.6)	0.982
Off-day	1398 (33.4)	428 (33.3)	970 (33.4)	
Time of day of arrival, *n* (%)				
8 a.m. to 16:59 p.m.	1861 (45.6)	588 (46.1)	1273 (45.3)	0.726
17 p.m. to 11:59 p.m.	1113 (27.3)	351 (27.5)	762 (27.1)	
12 a.m. to 7:59 a.m.	1110 (27.2)	336 (26.4)	774 (27.6)	
Accreditation status, *n* (%)				
Before	1809 (43.2)	576 (44.9)	1233 (42.5)	<0.001
During	574 (13.7)	217 (16.9)	357 (12.3)	
After	1803 (43.1)	491 (38.2)	1312 (45.2)	

Abbreviations: EMS, emergency medical service; CPR, cardiopulmonary resuscitation; q1, the first quartile; q3, the third quartile; SD, standard deviation. Notes: Sustainable chest pain refers to the onset of chest pain that lasts more than 30 min and cannot be relieved by rest. Intermittent chest pain refers to chest pain that lasts a few minutes at a time and can be relieved by rest or elimination of the triggers.

The in-hospital delay also varied in the two groups of patients (Table 2) and by different status (Figure S1 and Table S1). The median door-to-balloon time (70 versus 85 min, $p < 0.001$) and the percentage of cases with door-to-balloon time more than 90 min (26.7% versus 43.9%, $p < 0.001$) in EMS-transported patients were lower than those in walk-in patients.

Table 2. Door-to-balloon time in patients with different arrival modes.

Outcome	Overall	Arrival Mode		*p* Value
		EMS-Transported	Walk-In	
Door-to-balloon time (minutes), median (q1, q3)	81 (62, 105)	70 (52, 90)	85 (67, 111)	<0.001
Door-to-balloon time >90 min, *n* (%)				
No	2568 (61.3)	941 (73.3)	1627 (56.1)	<0.001
Yes	1618 (38.7)	343 (26.7)	1275 (43.9)	

Abbreviations: EMS, emergency medical service; q1, the first quartile; q3, the third quartile.

3.2. Association between Accreditation Status and In-Hospital Delay

Figure 1 shows the results of generalized linear mixed models of the likelihood of door-to-balloon time being more than 90 min. According to the full adjustment model, compared with the 'before accreditation' group, the risk of the door-to-balloon time being more than 90 min was significantly lower in both the 'during accreditation' group (OR: 0.35, 95% CI: 0.27, 0.46) and the 'after accreditation' group (OR: 0.29, 95% CI: 0.21, 0.39). Arrival by EMS was associated with a lower risk of the door-to-balloon time being more than 90 min, compared with arrival by self (OR: 0.49, 95% CI: 0.41, 0.58). The results generated by crude models are presented in Table S2.

Figure 2 shows the results of generalized linear mixed models of the door-to-balloon time. Compared with the 'before accreditation' group, we observed significant decreases of 27.88 (95% CI: −36.22, −19.57) minutes and 26.55 (95% CI: −35.70, −17.45) minutes for the 'during accreditation' group and 'after accreditation' group, respectively. Those transported by EMS exhibited a 21.62 (95% CI: −27.27, −16.11) minute decrease in door-to-balloon time compared with walk-in patients. The results generated by crude models are presented in Table S3.

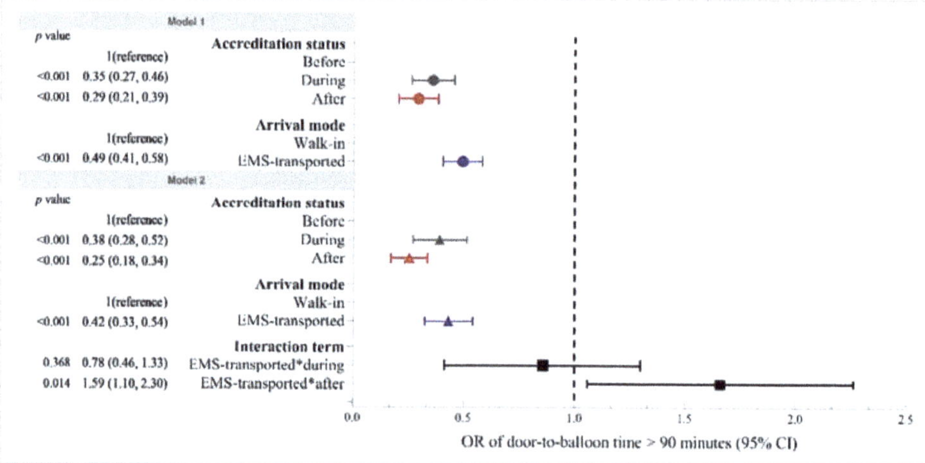

Figure 1. Associations of in-hospital delay (door-to-balloon time of >90 min) with accreditation status and arrival mode. Abbreviations: 95% CI, 95% confidence interval; EMS, emergency medical service. Notes: Both Models 1 and 2 were adjusted for sex, age, signs and symptoms at presentation, heart rate, blood pressure and Killip class, arrival mode, time of day of arrival, day of arrival, class of hospital, region of hospital, and accreditation status. Model 1 did not contain an interaction term. Model 2 included an interaction term of arrival mode and accreditation status. The OR value of the interaction term indicates that the decreased likelihood of door-to-balloon time being more than 90 min associated with accreditation status for EMS-transported patients was $(OR - 1) * 100\%$-more than that for walk-in patients.

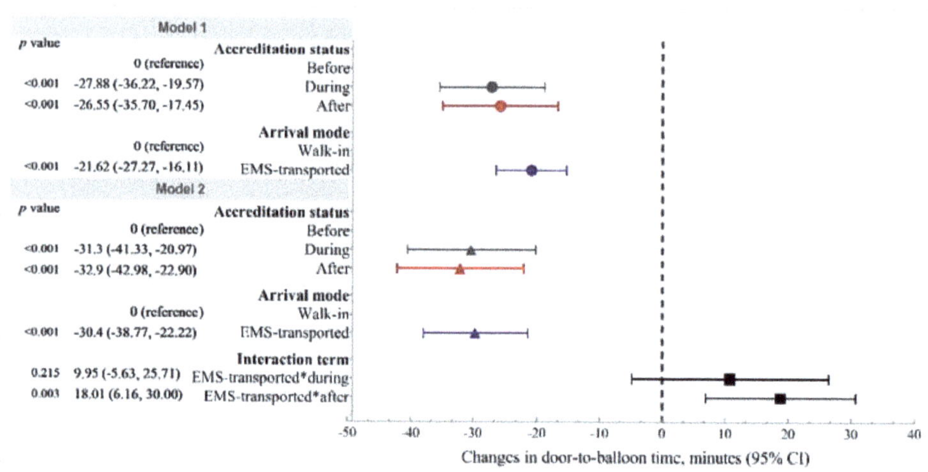

Figure 2. Associations of door-to-balloon time with accreditation status and arrival mode. Abbreviations: 95% CI, 95% confidence interval; EMS, emergency medical service. Notes: Both Model 1 and 2 were adjusted for sex, age, signs and symptoms at presentation, heart rate, blood pressure and Killip class, arrival mode, time of day of arrival, day of arrival, class of hospital, region of hospital, and accreditation status. Model 1 did not contain an interaction term. Model 2 included an interaction term of arrival mode and accreditation status. The β value of the interaction term indicates that the decrease in door-to-balloon time associated with accreditation status for EMS-transported patients was β minutes more than that for walk-in patients.

3.3. Association between Accreditation Status and Disparity of In-Hospital Delay across Arrival Modes

After adding the interaction term between accreditation status and arrival by EMS, the negative associations between 'after accreditation' status and in-hospital delay remained statistically significant and had larger coefficient sizes in the likelihood of door-to-balloon time being more than 90 min (OR: 0.25, 95% CI: 0.18, 0.34) and the door-to-balloon time (β: −32.90, 95% CI: −42.98, −22.90). In terms of differences in arrival mode, the coefficient sizes of arrival by EMS were also larger in the in-hospital delay: the likelihood of door-to-balloon time being more than 90 min (OR: 0.42, 95% CI: 0.33, 0.54) and the door-to-balloon time (β: −30.40, 95% CI: −38.77, −22.22).

The OR of the interaction term of arrival by EMS and 'during accreditation' was statistically insignificant, suggesting that arrival by EMS did not modify the effect of accreditation process on in-hospital delay. The OR of the interaction term of arrival by EMS and 'after accreditation' was 1.59 (95% CI: 1.10, 2.30), indicating that completed accreditation widened the disparity in the in-hospital delay between walk-in and EMS-transported patients. The impact of completed accreditation on the likelihood of door-to-balloon time being more than 90 min for EMS-transported patients was 59% greater than that for walk-in patients (Figure 1). Similar patterns were also found for the door-to-balloon time. A β value of 18.01 was found for the interaction term of arrival by EMS and 'after accreditation', suggesting that the reduction in the door-to-balloon time associated with completed accreditation for EMS-transported patients was 18.01 min more than that for walk-in patients (Figure 2).

4. Discussion

To the best of our knowledge, this was the first study to identify the modifying role of arrival mode in associations of chest pain center accreditation with in-hospital delay. Our results reflect an overall significant reduction in the in-hospital delay among STEMI patients after hospitals were accredited; however, the improvement was inconsistent between walk-in and EMS-transported patients. Our findings suggest that the healthcare quality improvement initiative may widen the disparity in treatment delay for patients with different arrival modes, providing implications for the optimization of implementation strategies for the continuous quality improvement of healthcare for acute chest pain.

Our results showed that compared with 'before accreditation', both 'during accreditation' and 'after accreditation' statuses were associated with lower prevalence of in-hospital delay among STEMI patients undergoing primary PCI. This finding is generally consistent with studies conducted in other regions, which indicated that chest pain center accreditation was associated with improved processes and outcomes for patients with STEMI [9,12,20]. Generally, chest pain center accreditation is a hospital-based, multifaceted, continuous quality improvement initiative from a multidisciplinary approach; it can be an efficient way to improve the in-hospital process and is of great significance to shortening the treatment time for STEMI patients. Furthermore, the negative associations of completed accreditation ('after accreditation' status) with in-hospital delay were more pronounced among EMS-transported patients than among walk-in patients.

There are several potential explanations for the observed disparity in sensitivity to chest pain center accreditation efforts. First, establishment of a regional collaborative healthcare network from a multiagency approach was emphasized in the current practice for achieving chest pain center accreditation criteria. Delivery of EMS always occurs across multiple sectors, including emergency departments, centers for prehospital care, ambulance stations, and day care or primary healthcare centers, and it requires at least two different services, with each service provided by different settings. Care coordination is critical for the delivery of EMS to ensure that healthcare professionals interact with each other to provide timely and efficient healthcare. A large number of studies have also shown that the transmission of prehospital electrocardiogram and prehospital diagnosis is the primary basis for a hospital to decide whether to bypass the emergency department and cardiac care unit, which can reduce the in-hospital delay for EMS-transported STEMI patients [21–23]. Pre-hospital ECGs going directly to the hospital by bypassing the emergency department and even coronary care unit is a general practice for achieving this objective. The EMS-transported patients also had greater and significantly faster receipt of initial reperfusion therapies [24]. Second, the condition of patients who are transported to hospital by ambulance is generally considered to be more urgent and more severe. They are given more attention and a higher medical priority when arriving at emergency departments. As soon as the ambulance arrives, prompt diagnosis, triage, and treatment are provided by healthcare professionals who are on stand-by in advance. Third, for walk-in patients, they have to undergo the normal medical procedures after arriving at the hospital, such as consulting, registering, paying, and even waiting for treatment. They cannot get the rapid and priority healthcare that patients transported by EMS can have. As a result, the time interval between their arrival at the gate of the hospital and initiation of reperfusion is extended.

In addition to the integration of prehospital and hospital care, implementation measurements required by the chest pain center accreditation criteria could also provide a plausible explanation for the mitigation of in-hospital delay among STEMI patients requiring primary PCI. Accredited hospitals continuously report data on individual patients for quality monitoring and assessment. The indicators for measuring clinical performance quarterly and annually are reported, and a ranking is calculated based on the percentile of each indicator and a weighted composite score. In terms of auditing and feedback regarding clinical performance, an improvement in adherence to the guideline recommendations is facilitated through monthly and quarterly hospital-specific performance feedback reports. The hospital-specific data are compared against a variety of internal and external benchmarks, including the temporal trend in performance and comparison points to regional or national performance thresholds, led by the National Health Commission of China. A series of regular meetings and case management and case study meetings are carried out at least once every quarter to share 'best practice' clinical support tools in hospitals. Regarding educational outreach to clinicians, routine educational programs are organized, and the contents of training include rules and guidelines for chest pain center construction, clinical skills for the diagnosis and treatment of STEMI cases, and standardization and guidelines for real-time data reporting. These dimensions of implementation measurements required by the chest pain center accreditation criteria could also benefit the development of public health capacity and capability to respond to public health emergencies by saving resources for triage, promoting efficiency of transfer, and optimizing timeliness of treatment.

The current findings suggest that some attention should be channeled to walk-in patients in order to eliminate the inequality of the implementation effect of the healthcare quality improvement between patients with different arrival modes. The strategies to deal with this disparity might include, but are not restricted to, the following suggestions. From the patient level, health education on recognition of the onset symptoms of STEMI and awareness of seeking treatment by calling EMS should be encouraged and perhaps conducted by community healthcare centers and hospital-based chest pain centers. The existing evidence indicates that wider use of EMS by patients with acute chest pain may offer a considerable opportunity for improvement in public health [14,21,22,25,26]. From the level of healthcare professionals, physicians, general practitioners, and nurses in emergency department should pay close attention to walk-in patients whose main complaint is chest pain. On the one hand, healthcare professionals should improve capacity for rapid diagnostics and triage of STEMI requiring primary PCI. On the other hand, the hospital could set up a green channel to optimize the ambulatory treatment process for them so as to buy time for healthcare professionals. From the hospital level, it is warranted to reinforce the information sharing and communication between the emergency and cardiology departments and establish a multidisciplinary coordinated team of healthcare professionals for comprehensive triage, treatment, and transfer of STEMI cases.

There were some limitations to this study. First, the nature of the cross-sectional design of this study restricted us to making causal inferences between the chest pain center accreditation and decreased in-hospital delay. Rather, the associations found in the present study underscore the need for research to capitalize on chest pain center accreditation to mitigate in-hospital delay. Second, this study included patients who were undergoing PCI; therefore, the results cannot be generalized to all patients with STEMI. Third, we were unable to adjust for medical history and socioeconomic indicators (e.g., income, educational attainment, marriage status, etc.) due to the unavailability of relevant data for the patients. However, a previous publication suggested that these variables are not associated with in-hospital delay but might be associated with pre-hospital delay and mortality [27]. Moreover, in terms of measuring the effect on the in-hospital delay rather than clinical outcomes, we adjusted for Killip classification, which is positively associated with medical history of patients [16,28] and could account for the partial confounding effect of medical history. Finally, although our analysis included all 33 centers accredited during January 2016 to June 2019 in Beijing, it is inevitable to introduce heterogeneity regarding the quality of data collection. Voluntary participation of hospitals made it difficult for us to compare with those not seeking accreditation.

5. Conclusions

Among STEMI patients undergoing primary PCI, EMS-transported patients were more sensitive to the shortened in-hospital delay associated with chest pain center accreditation efforts. This effect might exacerbate the existing disparity in in-hospital delay among patients with different arrival modes. Thus, more attention should be paid to walk-in patients and more strategies for increasing the utilization of EMS should be considered in further healthcare quality improvement.

Supplementary Materials: The following are available online at https://www.mdpi.com/article/10.3390/healthcare9111462/s1, Figure S1: Median and interquartile range of door-to-balloon time by accreditation status and arrival mode. Table S1: Median and interquartile range of door-to-balloon time (minutes) by accreditation status and arrival mode. Table S2: Odds ratio (OR) and 95% confidence interval (95% CI) of in-hospital delay associated with accreditation status and transfer mode. Table S3: Changes in door-to-balloon time and 95% confidence interval (95% CI) associated with accreditation status and transfer mode. Table S4: Odds ratio (OR) and 95% confidence interval (95% CI) of in-hospital delay associated with accreditation status by arrival mode. Table S5: Changes in door-to-balloon time and 95% confi-dence interval (95% CI) associated with accreditation status by arrival mode. Table S6: Odds ratio (OR) and 95% confidence interval (95% CI) of covariates obtained from fully adjusted models. Table S7: Changes in door-to-balloon time (minutes) and 95% confidence interval (95% CI) of co-variates obtained from fully adjusted models.

Author Contributions: Conceptualization, Y.J. and Z.Z.; Data curation, J.M., X.D. and M.M.; Formal analysis, N.L.; Funding acquisition, Y.J.; Investigation, S.Z.; Methodology, N.L. and Y.J.; Project administration, Y.J.; Software, N.L.; Supervision, Y.J. and Z.Z.; Validation, Z.Z.; Visualization, N.L.; Writing—original draft, N.L.; Writing—review and editing, Y.J. All authors have read and agreed to the published version of the manuscript.

Funding: This research was funded by Natural Science Foundation of Beijing Municipality, grant number 9204025 and the National Natural Science Foundation of China, grant number 71904004.

Institutional Review Board Statement: The study was conducted according to the guidelines of the Declaration of Helsinki and approved by the Institutional Review Board of Peking University Institutional Review Board (IRB000001052-21020).

Informed Consent Statement: Informed consents were obtained from hospitals for research approval to collect data without requiring individual patient informed consent. Patient confidentiality is protected in the following ways: (1) data are de-identified before their use in research and (2) the use of data for these purposes is closely overseen by the accredited hospitals and the Beijing Chest Pain Center Alliance.

Data Availability Statement: The data presented in this study are available on request from the corresponding author. The data are not publicly available due to privacy.

Conflicts of Interest: The authors declare no conflict of interest. The funders had no role in the design of the study; in the collection, analyses, or interpretation of data; in the writing of the manuscript, or in the decision to publish the results.

References

1. Moscucci, M.; Eagle, K.A. Reducing the door-to-balloon time for myocardial infarction with ST-segment elevation. *N. Engl. J. Med.* **2006**, *355*, 2364–2365. [CrossRef] [PubMed]
2. Krumholz, H.M.; Anderson, J.L.; Brooks, N.H.; Fesmire, F.M.; Lambrew, C.T.; Landrum, M.B.; Weaver, W.D.; Whyte, J.; Bonow, R.O.; Bennett, S.J.; et al. ACC/AHA clinical performance measures for adults with ST-elevation and non-ST-elevation myocardial infarction: A report of the American College of Cardiology/American Heart Association Task Force on Performance Measures (Writing Committee to Develop Performance Measures on ST-Elevation and Non-ST-Elevation Myocardial Infarction). *Am. J. Coll. Cardiol.* **2006**, *47*, 236–265.
3. Ibanez, B.; James, S.; Agewall, S.; Antunes, M.J.; Bucciarelli-Ducci, C.; Bueno, H.; Caforio, A.L.; Crea, F.; Goudevenos, J.A.; Halvorsen, S.; et al. 2017 ESC Guidelines for the management of acute myocardial infarction in patients presenting with ST-segment elevation: The Task Force for the management of acute myocardial infarction in patients presenting with ST-segment elevation of the European Society of Cardiology (ESC). *Eur. Heart J.* **2018**, *39*, 119–177. [PubMed]
4. The Writing Committee of the Report on Cardiovascular Health and Diseases in China. Report on cardiovascular health and diseases in China 2019: An updated summary. *Chin. Circ. J.* **2020**, *35*, 833–854.
5. Bansal, E.; Dhawan, R.; Wagman, B.; Low, G.; Zheng, L.; Chan, L.; Newton, K.; Swadron, S.P.; Testa, N.; Shavelle, D.M. Importance of hospital entry: Walk-in STEMI and primary percutaneous coronary intervention. *West. J. Emerg. Med.* **2014**, *15*, 81–87. [CrossRef] [PubMed]
6. Canto, J.G.; Zalenski, R.J.; Ornato, J.P.; Rogers, W.J.; Kiefe, C.I.; Magid, D.; Shlipak, M.G.; Frederick, P.D.; Lambrew, C.G.; Littrell, K.A.; et al. Use of emergency medical services in acute myocardial infarction and subsequent quality of care: Observations from the National Registry of Myocardial Infarction 2. *Circulation* **2002**, *106*, 3018–3023. [CrossRef] [PubMed]
7. Callachan, E.L.; Alsheikh-Ali, A.A.; Nair, S.C.; Bruijns, S.; Wallis, L.A. Outcomes by mode of transport of ST elevation MI patients in the United Arab Emirates. *West. J. Emerg. Med.* **2017**, *18*, 349–355. [CrossRef] [PubMed]
8. So, D.Y.; Ha, A.C.; Turek, M.A.; Maloney, J.P.; Higginson, L.A.; Davies, R.F.; Ryan, S.C.; le May, M.R. Comparison of mortality patterns in patients with ST-elevation myocardial infarction arriving by emergency medical services versus self-transport (from the Prospective Ottawa Hospital STEMI Registry). *Am. J. Cardiol.* **2006**, *97*, 458–461. [CrossRef] [PubMed]
9. Jollis, J.G.; Al-Khalidi, H.R.; Roettig, M.L.; Berger, P.B.; Corbett, C.C.; Doerfler, S.M.; Fordyce, C.B.; Henry, T.D.; Hollowell, L.; Magdon-Ismail, Z.; et al. Impact of regionalization of ST-segment–elevation myocardial infarction care on treatment times and outcomes for emergency medical services–transported patients presenting to hospitals with percutaneous coronary intervention. *Circulation* **2018**, *137*, 376–387. [CrossRef]
10. Jollis, J.G.; Al-Khalidi, H.R.; Roettig, M.L.; Berger, P.B.; Corbett, C.C.; Dauerman, H.L.; Fordyce, C.B.; Fox, K.; Garvey, J.L.; Gregory, T.; et al. Regional systems of care demonstration project: American Heart Association mission: Lifeline STEMI systems accelerator. *Circulation* **2016**, *134*, 365–374. [CrossRef]
11. Scholz, K.H.; Maier, S.K.; Jung, J.; Fleischmann, C.; Werner, G.S.; Olbrich, H.G.; Ahlersmann, D.; Keating, F.K.; Jacobshagen, C.; Moehlis, H.; et al. Reduction in treatment times through formalized data feedback: Results from a prospective multicenter study of ST-segment elevation myocardial infarction. *JACC Cardiovasc. Interv.* **2012**, *5*, 848–857. [CrossRef] [PubMed]
12. Scholz, K.H.; Lengenfelder, B.; Jacobshagen, C.; Fleischmann, C.; Moehlis, H.; Olbrich, H.G.; Jung, J.; Maier, L.S.; Maier, S.K.G.; Bestehorn, K.; et al. Long-term effects of a standardized feedback-driven quality improvement program for timely reperfusion therapy in regional STEMI care networks. *Eur. Heart J. Acute Cardiovasc. Care* **2021**, *10*, 397–405. [CrossRef] [PubMed]
13. Ross, M.A.; Amsterdam, E.; Peacock, W.F.; Graff, L.; Fesmire, F.; Garvey, J.L.; Kelly, S.; Holmes, K.; Karunaratne, H.; Toth, M.; et al. Chest pain center accreditation is associated with better performance of centers for medicare and medicaid services core measures for acute myocardial infarction. *Am. J. Cardiol.* **2008**, *102*, 120–124. [CrossRef]
14. Mathews, R.; Peterson, E.D.; Li, S.; Roe, M.T.; Glickman, S.W.; Wiviott, S.D.; Saucedo, J.F.; Antman, E.M.; Jacobs, A.K.; Wang, T.Y. Use of emergency medical service transport among patients with ST-segment-elevation myocardial infarction: Findings from the national cardiovascular data registry acute coronary treatment intervention outcomes network registry-get with the guidelines. *Circulation* **2011**, *124*, 154–163. [CrossRef] [PubMed]
15. Lin, Q.; Xu, X.; Zhang, Y.; Wang, F.; Gu, J.; Xu, Y.; Zhu, Y.; Li, J. Assessed influencing factors of reperfusion time and outcome in ST segment elevation myocardial infarction patients with different prehospital transfer pathways to the hospital. *Chin. J. Emerg. Med.* **2020**, *29*, 921–928.
16. O'gara, P.T.; Kushner, F.G.; Ascheim, D.D.; Casey, D.E.; Chung, M.K.; de Lemos, J.A.; Ettinger, S.M.; Fang, J.C.; Fesmire, F.M.; Franklin, B.A.; et al. 2013 ACCF/AHA guideline for the management of ST-elevation myocardial infarction: Executive summary: A report of the American College of Cardiology Foundation/American Heart Association Task Force on Practice Guidelines. *Am. Coll. Cardiol.* **2013**, *61*, e78–e140. [CrossRef]

17. Fan, F.; Li, Y.; Zhang, Y.; Li, J.; Liu, J.; Hao, Y.; Smith, S.C., Jr.; Fonarow, G.C.; Taubert, K.A.; Ge, J.; et al. Chest pain center accreditation is associated with improved in-hospital outcomes of acute myocardial infarction patients in China: Findings from the CCC-ACS project. *J. Am. Heart Assoc.* **2019**, *8*, e013384. [CrossRef]
18. Sun, P.; Li, J.; Fang, W.; Su, X.; Yu, B.; Wang, Y.; Li, C.; Chen, H.; Wang, X.; Zhang, B.; et al. Effectiveness of chest pain centre accreditation on the management of acute coronary syndrome: A retrospective study using a national database. *BMJ Qual. Saf.* **2020**, *30*, 867–875. [CrossRef]
19. Ma, J.; Dong, X.; Jin, Y.; Zheng, Z.J. Health care quality improvement for ST-segment elevation myocardial infarction: A retrospective study based on propensity-score matching analysis. *Int. J. Environ. Res. Public Health* **2021**, *18*, 6045. [CrossRef]
20. Montoy, J.C.C.; Shen, Y.C.; Brindis, R.G.; Krumholz, H.M.; Hsia, R.Y. Impact of ST-segment-elevation myocardial infarction regionalization programs on the treatment and outcomes of patients diagnosed with non-ST-segment-elevation myocardial infarction. *J. Am. Heart Assoc.* **2021**, *10*, e016932. [CrossRef]
21. Ducas, R.A.; Labos, C.; Allen, D.; Golian, M.; Jeyaraman, M.; Lys, J.; Mann, A.; Copstein, L.; Vokey, S.; Rabbani, R.; et al. Association of pre-hospital ECG administration with clinical outcomes in ST-segment myocardial infarction: A systematic review and meta-analysis. *Can. J. Cardiol.* **2016**, *32*, 1531–1541. [CrossRef] [PubMed]
22. Hutchison, A.W.; Malaiapan, Y.; Jarvie, I.; Barger, B.; Watkins, E.; Braitberg, G.; Kambourakis, T.; Cameron, J.D.; Meredith, I.T. Prehospital 12-lead ECG to triage ST-elevation myocardial infarction and emergency department activation of the infarct team significantly improves door-to-balloon times: Ambulance Victoria and MonashHEART acute myocardial infarction (MonAMI) 12-lead ECG project. *Circ. Cardiovasc. Interv.* **2009**, *2*, 528–534. [PubMed]
23. Kontos, M.C.; Gunderson, M.R.; Zegre-Hemsey, J.K.; Lange, D.C.; French, W.J.; Henry, T.D.; McCarthy, J.J.; Corbett, C.; Jacobs, A.K.; Jollis, J.G.; et al. Prehospital activation of hospital resources (PreAct) ST-segment-elevation myocardial infarction (STEMI): A standardized approach to prehospital activation and direct to the catheterization laboratory for STEMI recommendations from the American Heart Association's mission: Lifeline program. *J. Am. Heart Assoc.* **2020**, *9*, e011963.
24. Diercks, D.B.; Kontos, M.C.; Chen, A.Y.; Pollack, C.V.; Wiviott, S.D.; Rumsfeld, J.S.; Magid, D.J.; Gibler, W.B.; Cannon, C.P.; Peterson, E.D.; et al. Utilization and impact of pre-hospital electrocardiograms for patients with acute ST-segment elevation myocardial infarction: Data from the NCDR (National Cardiovascular Data Registry) ACTION (Acute Coronary Treatment and Intervention Outcomes Network) registry. *J. Am. Coll. Cardiol.* **2009**, *53*, 161–166. [CrossRef]
25. Afolabi, B.A.; Novaro, G.M.; Pinski, S.L.; Fromkin, K.R.; Bush, H.S. Use of the prehospital ECG improves door-to-balloon times in ST segment elevation myocardial infarction irrespective of time of day or day of week. *Emerg. Med. J.* **2007**, *24*, 588–591. [CrossRef] [PubMed]
26. Coyne, C.J.; Testa, N.; Desai, S.; LaGrone, J.; Chang, R.; Zheng, L.; Kim, H. Improving door-to-balloon time by decreasing door-to-ECG time for walk-in STEMI patients. *West. J. Emerg. Med.* **2015**, *16*, 184–189. [CrossRef] [PubMed]
27. Kauppi, W.; Herlitz, J.; Karlsson, T.; Magnusson, C.; Palmér, L.; Axelsson, C. Pre-hospital predictors of an adverse outcome among patients with dyspnoea as the main symptom assessed by pre-hospital emergency nurses—A retrospective observational study. *BMC Emerg. Med.* **2020**, *20*, 1–12. [CrossRef]
28. DeGeare, V.S.; Boura, J.A.; Grines, L.L.; O'Neill, W.W.; Grines, C.L. Predictive value of the Killip classification in patients undergoing primary percutaneous coronary intervention for acute myocardial infarction. *Am. J. Cardiol.* **2001**, *87*, 1035–1038. [CrossRef]

International Journal of
Environmental Research and Public Health

MDPI

Article

Development and Validation of an Instrument to Measure Work-Related Stress among Rescue Workers in Traumatic Mass-Casualty Disasters

Yu-Long Chen [1,2], Wen-Chii Tzeng [3], En Chao [4] and Hui-Hsun Chiang [3,*]

1 Department of Emergency Medicine, Taipei Tzu Chi Hospital, Buddhist Tzu Chi Medical Foundation, New Taipei City 231, Taiwan; yulong0129@tzuchi.com.tw
2 School of Medicine, Tzu Chi University, Hualien 970, Taiwan
3 School of Nursing, National Defense Medical Center, Taipei 114, Taiwan; wctzeng@mail.ndmctsgh.edu.tw
4 Department of Medical Affairs, SongShan branch, Tri-Service General Hospital, Taipei 105, Taiwan; fajohnny@g.ukn.edu.tw
* Correspondence: huihsunchiang@mail.ndmctsgh.edu.tw; Tel.: +886-2-87923100 (ext. 18761); Fax: +889-2-87923109

Abstract: Rescue workers are a population at high-risk for mental problems as they are exposed to work-related stress from confrontation with traumatic events when responding to a disaster. A reliable measure is needed to assess rescue workers' work-related stress from their surveillance of a disaster scene to help prevent severe PTSD and depressive symptoms. The purpose of this study was to develop and validate the Work-Related Stress Scale (WRSS) designed to measure stress in rescue workers after responding to traumatic mass-casualty events. An exploratory sequential mixed methods procedure was employed. The qualitative phase of the item generation component involved in-depth interviews of 7 experienced rescue workers from multiple specialties who had taken part in 1 or 2 mass-casualty events: the 2018 Hualien earthquake or the 2016 Tainan earthquake. In the quantitative phase, a modified Delphi approach was used to achieve consensus ratings by the same 7 raters on the items and to assess content validity. Construct validity was determined by confirmatory factor analysis using a broader sample of 293 rescue workers who had taken part in 1 of 2 mass-casualty events: the 2018 Hualien earthquake or the 2021 Hualien train derailment. The final WRSS consists of 16 items total and 4 subscales: Physical Demands, Psychological Response, Environmental Interruption, and Leadership, with aggregated alphas of 0.74–0.88. The WRSS was found to have psychometric integrity as a measure of stress in rescue workers after responding to a disaster.

Keywords: work-related stress; disaster rescue workers; traumatic events; mass-casualty incidents; disaster management

Citation: Chen, Y.-L.; Tzeng, W.-C.; Chao, E.; Chiang, H.-H. Development and Validation of an Instrument to Measure Work-Related Stress among Rescue Workers in Traumatic Mass-Casualty Disasters. *IJERPH* **2021**, *18*, 8340. https://doi.org/10.3390/ijerph18168340

Academic Editor: Paul B. Tchounwou

Received: 21 July 2021
Accepted: 5 August 2021
Published: 6 August 2021

1. Introduction

Traumatic disasters with mass casualties incur major human and healthcare costs in countries such as Taiwan that provide many opportunities for such events to occur [1]. The effects of these catastrophes are experienced not only by the victims at the disaster site; they also create a high risk of long-term negative psychological consequences in the rescue workers [2–4]. Rescue workers, especially firefighters, are first responders who provide immediate support to victims at a disaster site. Those who work with multiple other professionals on a rescue team (e.g., in a search and rescue operation) have been found to experience several specific physical–psychosocial–environmental–organizational challenges, such as problems related to food and drink, job-related conflicts with the control tower, lack of cooperation from other team members, confusion about who has what duties, and harsh work environments that require observing and identifying very badly damaged bodies of children and adults [5,6]. Despite these multiple challenges, there are no instruments designed to measure stress surveillance in rescue workers after deployment to traumatic disasters [7].

Rescue workers, especially first responders, are at a high risk for experiencing high levels of psychosocial work stress and depression [8]. In this population, these psychosocial factors appear to be more complex and multifaceted than the environmental factors and the physical and mental strain evoked by work-related accidents [9]. Rescue workers must confront mass-fatality incidents involving many dead bodies and/or body parts as well as emotional involvement with the deceased victims, at times under the threat of injury to themselves [10]. Greater physical strain has been associated with unfair distribution of work tasks, and greater psychological strain has been associated with frequent differences of opinion with other workers or supervisors that interfere with the work [8]. Other research on the stress experienced by rescue workers has shown these stressors to include environmental factors and ineffective cooperation with team members or those in the control tower in the aftermath of a disaster [5]. Direct or indirect exposure to such work environments plays an important role in creating negative psychological consequence in rescue workers when the circumstances are extreme and inhumane and the emotional reactions toward the victims are overwhelming [11].

Work-related stress has been significantly associated with depressive symptoms, burnout, and PTSD symptoms among rescue workers [11,12]. They are at a high risk for physical and mental problems, as they are confronted with traumatic events and endure work-related stress exposure [13]. It is important to develop an instrument for assessing work-related stress specifically for rescue workers who experience physical and psychological impairment after responding to a disaster [14]. The measures of work-related stress currently available have been criticized for the heterogeneous nature of the populations to which they have been applied and their non-specificity re disaster-related events [15,16], especially traumatic mass-casualty events [13]. Our aim was to fill this knowledge gap by developing and evaluating the psychometric integrity of a measure of work-related stress designed specifically for rescue workers.

2. Methods and Results

We developed and validated the WRSS across different cultures and types of traumatic mass-casualty disasters, using a succession of qualitative and quantitative methods. In so doing, we followed the recommendations of Zhou [17], who proposed a mixed methods model that features application of both factor analysis and application of mixed-methods integration procedures to culture-relevant data obtained through qualitative interviews to assess the construct validity of a test instrument.

2.1. Item Generation for the WRSS

2.1.1. Participant Recruitment and Eligibility Criteria

The original sample for the scale construction consisted of 7 disaster rescue personnel (2 females and 5 males) with various search and rescue (SAR) backgrounds: logistics, search, rescue, SAR dog controller, security officer, and commander. Each had taken part in the response to one of two traumatic mass-casualty events in Hualien, Taiwan: an earthquake on 6 February 2018 or a train derailment on 2 April 2021. The earthquake measured 6.4 on the momentary magnitude scale. It claimed at least 17 dead and 285 injured, and featured bodily mutilations [18]. The train derailment claimed 49 dead, most featuring bodily mutilation or body parts, and a further 247 injured and requiring medical treatment [19]. Both traumatic disasters had the potential to cause members of the SAR team to experience physical–psychological stress at the time and psychological and emotional trauma later [14]. The demographic data for the rescue workers are presented in Appendix A Table A1.

2.1.2. The Interview (Qualitative Component)

Qualitative data were collected through in-depth face-to-face semi-structured interviews of the above 7 rescue workers, all of whom who agreed to be interviewed. The focus of the interviews was first on participants' experiences of their most recent SAR operation and on how they experienced the work-related stress and the effects of the SAR procedures on them (see Appendix A Table A2). The interviews lasted 45 to 90 min.

The qualitative analysis of the interview data included several steps. In the first step, the researcher analyzed the verbatim transcriptions of the audio-taped interviews using thematic analysis [20]. The transcripts were first read to obtain a general sense of the topic and bring it into focus. There was no sorting or coding of the data in the first step. In the second step the transcripts were reread, and descriptive phrases were extracted. In the third step, the relevant phrases were coded, keeping the codes as similar to the participants' meanings as possible. In the fourth step, the researcher developed categories from the codes by aggregating similar codes. The codes and categories were examined and compared within and across items to identify relevant relationships. The researcher's inferences were analyzed and compared with those from the 7 interviewees using a form of peer debriefing.

The four thematic categories of the causes of the traumatic stress identified by the researcher in the third step of the analysis were: physiological demands (of the stress), psychological response (to the stress), leadership (by the team leader), and environmental interruption (at the disaster site). The researcher then generated the 69 original items of the WRSS so they would correspond to these themes.

2.1.3. The Modified Delphi Approach (Quantitative Component)

The 69 items were further evaluated to achieve consensus from the same 7 rescue workers (raters) using a modified four-stage Delphi method [21]. In this study, the Delphi process required three rounds of item selection and modification. In Round 1, the judges were asked to independently rate each of the 69 statements on whether they agreed that it is a good measure of traumatic stress using a 5-point Likert scale ("strongly agree", "agree", "adequate but needs modification", "disagree", "strongly disagree") in the context of responding to a disaster. It has been demonstrated that 5-point scales produce stable findings in modified Delphi studies [22]. The raters were also provided an opportunity to elaborate or explain their ratings and contribute further ideas for each category through responses to open-ended questions provided by the researcher. Using this information, the researcher eliminated 35 items in which there was less than 70 percent of inter-rater agreement and reworded some of the remaining 34. The rescue workers then rated these 34 items in Round 2. The Round 1 process was repeated, which led the researcher to eliminate 6 more items according to the previous criterion. The entire process was repeated in Round 3, leading to the elimination of 9 more items. The ratings of each of the remaining 19 items met the criterion for consensus, defined as >70% of participants affirming the good quality of the item by choosing the response "agree" or "strongly agree". This definition of consensus has been considered appropriate in previous Delphi studies [23]. Results from the modified Delphi procedure are reported in Appendix A Table A3.

2.2. *Content Validity of the WRSS*

Content validity is the degree to which an instrument covers the conceptual domain of the construct it is intended to measure [24]. The content validity of the 19-item WRSS was assessed by a panel of 3 judges with professional expertise in disaster rescue and emergency management. All were instructors with the Disaster Medical Assistance Team (DMAT) and had personally witnessed several catastrophic disasters in Taiwan. They rated each item on whether it reflected traumatic stress using a 4-point Likert scale with the following response options: "agree very much", "agree", "agree a little bit", and "not agree at all". The content validity of the scale was found to be 0.94 by using the content validity index (CVI) to detect the validity of the items.

2.3. Construct Validity of the WRSS

2.3.1. Participant Recruitment and Eligibility Criteria

Using an online sample-size calculator for structural equation models, it was estimated that 305 participants would be required to detect a moderate effect ($\rho = 0.23$) of high work-related stress for rescue workers who had a high workload [13]. This allowed for 5 latent variables, 19 observed variables, power of 0.8, and alpha of 0.05 [25].

Purposive sampling was used to recruit the participants from March 2018 to May 2021. A sample of 305 rescue workers who were engaged with the 2018 Hualien earthquake or the 2021 Hualien train derailment disasters agreed to participate in the study after the purpose and procedure had been explained by the researchers, who were referred by the occupational nurse. Participants were assured that their participation was anonymous and would not influence their work. Of the 305 rescue workers recruited, 12 were unable to complete the questionnaire because of work-shift rotation problems. Data from the remaining 293 rescue workers were used for the analyses.

2.3.2. Procedure and Data Analysis

After signing the consent form, it took about 15–20 min for the participants to complete the questionnaire in a quiet room in a comfortable environment. The questionnaire consisted of the 19-item WRSS and items requesting the same demographic information obtained from the rescue workers who participated in the 2018 Hualien earthquake or the 2021 Hualien train derailment disasters. We used two separate boxes to collect the consent forms and questionnaires to assure anonymity.

Table 1 presents the demographic characteristics of the sample. To summarize, most participants were men ($n = 283$, 96.6%), were married ($n = 191$, 65.2%), and were between 31–40 years old ($n = 175$, 59.7%). Most reported that their SAR experience was less than or equal to 5 years ($n = 236$, 80.5%), and that their service as firemen was less than 5 years ($n = 200$, 68.3%).

Table 1. Demographics of the rescue workers and differences in their WRSS scores ($n = 293$).

			Work-Related Stress		
	n	%	M	SD	p [a]
Age					0.82
≤30	79	27.0	43.22	8.77	
31–40	175	59.7	43.26	8.29	
>40	39	13.3	42.20	13.32	
Gender					0.15
Female	10	3.4	38.78	10.24	
Male	283	96.6	43.26	9.09	
Marital status					0.31
Single	102	34.8	43.87	8.77	
Married	191	65.2	42.71	9.35	
Firefighting service (years)					0.14
≤5	200	68.3	43.29	7.86	
>5	93	31.7	43.70	10.95	
SAR service (years)					0.77
≤5	236	80.5	43.30	8.72	
>5	57	19.5	42.40	10.92	

Note. [a] from independent t test or ANOVA; SAR: search and rescue.

Following the recommendations of Zhou [17], confirmatory factor analysis (CFA) was employed, without a prior exploratory factor analysis, to examine the construct-based validity of the 19-item WRSS using *Mplus* software version 8.2 [26]. The purpose was to confirm a common factor pattern and to determine whether the scale structure in fact corresponds to the four themes identified from the interviews. The determination of which items were to be retained for the final scale was based on their model fit with the factor pattern [27] and conformance to the guiding theoretical definitions of the work-related stress dimensions [2].

Results from the CFA indicated that a four-factor solution was best. After 3 items were removed from the scale because of cross-loadings of the variables, the remaining 16-items fell into four factors (or subscales) with appropriate names corresponding to the four themes derived from the interviews: (1) Environmental Interruption (four items); (2) Psychological Response (five items); (3) Leadership (four items); and (4) Physiological Demands (three items). Participants responded to each item on a four-point scale: (a) "not at all stressful"; (b) "a little bit stressful"; (c) "stressful"; and (d) "very stressful". Average variance extracted (AVE) was > 0.5 except for Psychological Response (0.43), but the composite reliability for this subscale was higher than the acceptable level of 0.6 [28]. Table 2 presents the CFA results for each item on each factor and Table 3 presents the items on the final scale.

Table 2. Summary of confirmatory factor analysis and reliability of Work-Related Stress Scale (n = 293).

Construct/Item	Factor Loading (T Value)	Cronbach's Alpha	AVE	Composite Reliability	Bootstrap 95% CI
PHY		0.85	0.66	0.85	
01 Hard to fall asleep because of poor sleep environment	0.84 (32.46)				1.00–1.00
02 Intermittent sleep	0.89 (38.25)				0.90–1.12
04 Enduring sleeplessness	0.70 (19.83)				0.71–0.98
PSY		0.78	0.43	0.79	
10 The victims are my relatives [a]	0.56 (11.44)	Deleted			
11 Seeing my team members get injured at work	0.61 (13.95)				1.00–1.00
13 Expressing my condolences to the victims and not allowing myself to be affected by negative emotions	0.70 (18.22)				0.78–1.26
14 Seeing bodily mutilation or severed body parts	0.69 (17.46)				0.95–1.62
16 Touching the dead body unexpectedly	0.73 (19.73)				0.91–1.47
18 Media interview requests	0.53 (10.88)				0.73–1.15
ENV		0.88	0.65	0.88	
21 No one can be searched and rescued [a]	0.69 (19.31)	Deleted			
22 Finding all the victims or remains [a]	0.71 (20.94)	Deleted			
24 Insufficient manpower	0.75 (24.33)				1.00–1.00
25 Safety of the SAR process not confirmed	0.84 (35.41)				0.97–1.22
26 Worry about the spread of infectious disease at the disaster site	0.83 (33.37)				0.89–1.15
27 Worry about potential harm to rescue workers during disaster rescue	0.80 (30.88)				1.02–1.32
LEAD		0.74	0.54	0.82	
30 Confusing commands or unclear dispatches from the commander	0.46 (8.93)				1.00–1.00
31 Forced to change the SAR route	0.72 (21.04)				0.71–0.96

Table 2. *Cont.*

Construct/Item	Factor Loading (*T* Value)	Cronbach's Alpha	AVE	Composite Reliability	Bootstrap 95% CI
33 Differences of opinion with team members	0.88 (39.85)				0.89–1.15
34 Chaotic workplace with dysfunctional command system	0.81 (30.16)				0.91–1.17

Note. PHY: physical demands; PSY: psychological response; ENV: environmental interruption; LEAD: leadership. Fit indices: $\chi^2(98) = 183.84$, $p \leq 0.001$; CFI = 0.96, TLI = 0.95; RMSEA = 0.06; SRMR = 0.05. CI: confidence interval; bootstrap = 1000; range: lower 2.5% to upper 2.5%. The criterion column refers to the raters' assessments and specifies how many of them classified each item as 1: strongly disagree; 2: disagree; 3: adequate but needs minor rewording; 4: agree; and 5: strongly agree. n = number of raters; %: percent of inter-rater agreement, defined as the percent of participants affirming the good quality of the item by choosing the response "agree" or "strongly agree"; *M*: mean rating assigned to each item. [a] deleted following confirmatory factor analysis; item 10: cross-loadings of ENV and PSY (MI = 52.47); item 21: cross-loadings of PSY and ENV (MI = 32.25); items 22: cross-loadings of ENV and PSY (MI = 15.65).

Table 3. Final items on the Work-Related Stress Scale and ratings from the modified Delphi method.

Subscale	Item #	Item	Rating 1	2	3	4	5	%	*M*
PHY	1	Hard to fall asleep because of poor sleep environment	0	0	2	3	2	0.71	4.00
	2	Intermittent sleep	0	0	1	3	3	0.86	4.29
	4	Enduring sleeplessness	0	0	1	3	3	0.86	4.29
PSY	11	Seeing my team members get injured at work	0	0	2	2	3	0.86	4.14
	13	Expressing my condolences to the victims and not allowing myself to be affected by negative emotions	0	0	1	5	1	0.86	4.00
	14	Seeing bodily mutilation or severed body parts	0	0	1	4	2	0.86	4.14
	16	Touching the dead body unexpectedly	0	0	2	3	2	0.71	4.00
	18	Media interview requests	0	0	1	5	1	0.86	3.86
ENV	24	Insufficient manpower	0	0	2	3	2	0.71	4.00
	25	Failure to confirm the safety of the SAR process	0	0	1	4	2	0.86	4.14
	26	Worry about the spread of infectious disease because of poor environment	0	0	2	3	2	0.71	4.00
	27	Worry about potential harm to rescue workers during disaster rescue	0	0	1	3	3	0.86	4.29
LEAD	30	Confused command of unclear dispatch from the commander	0	0	2	3	2	0.71	3.86
	31	Forced to change the SAR route	0	0	1	4	2	0.86	4.14
	33	Differences of opinion with team members	0	0	2	4	1	0.71	3.86
	34	Chaotic workplace with dysfunctional command system	0	0	2	3	2	0.71	4.00

Note. ENV: environmental interruption; PSY: psychological response; LEAD: leadership domain; PHY: physical demands; SAR: search and rescue.

2.4. Reliability of the WRSS

The reliability of the 16-item WRSS was assessed through internal consistency analysis.

Cronbach's alpha values for the four subscales ranged from 0.74 to 0.88 and the composite reliability values ranged from 0.79 to 0.88. For the total scale, Cronbach's alpha was 0.89 (see Table 2).

2.5. Ethical Considerations

In conformance to the ethics requirements, for each phase of scale construction and validation it was emphasized that participants' cooperation was voluntary and that their answers were confidential and would be used only for the purposes of this study. All participants provided their written informed consent. The Institutional Review Board of the Tri-Service General Hospital approved the study (Approval No. 1-107-05-061).

3. Results and Discussion

3.1. Main Results

The present study demonstrates that the WRSS has good psychometric integrity. The finding from the interviews that this work-related stress has four dimensions is noteworthy, and four subscales corresponding to these four dimensions (Physical Demands, Psychological Response, Environmental Interruption, and Leadership) were identified in the construct validation phase. We can thus conclude that the WRSS is a well-validated and reliable instrument that is suitable for assessing work-related stress in rescue workers responding to traumatic mass-casualty incidents.

Proper preparation has been shown to be crucial before experiencing the onset of a catastrophic event [13]. Our results indicate that rescue professionals and administrative officers need more specific information about the work-related stress that rescue workers experience and the associated challenges to prepare them to rescue and save the lives of victims. Moreover, in the interviews, the participants registered strong complaints against their administrative officers for not providing them with safety procedures and the necessary control of the environment during SAR events, as well as against the mass media. The findings of our research, which was specifically targeted to disasters, may provide information that will help rescue workers succeed in their rescue operations and improve the quality of disaster SAR. They therefore highlight the importance of developing a specific work-related stress measure for rescue workers.

3.2. Comparisons with the Literature

Our results are consistent with what has been found in previous studies that have explored the high physical and mental health risks faced by disaster responders [4,29]. In our interviews, participants expressed a lack of preparation for deployment, specifically a lack of rest and poor sleep quality. These results are consistent with previous research that has shown that rescue workers' health status, inability to fully regain energy, exhausted from disaster-support work, and perceived physical disturbances play an important role in the creation of work-related stress and aggravate the psychological burdens they face [30,31]. Unpredictable situations involving a threat to human life, such as those faced by disaster rescue workers, have been shown to cause an increase in cardiac sympathetic excitation [32].

High-quality team leadership has been shown to be significantly associated with a lowered risk of subsequent mental distress [33]. Good team leadership plays an important role in employee health and well-being as well as reducing burnout [34]. It is also an essential antecedent of occupational safety; rule-oriented leadership that formulates plans for future operations collaboratively with the workers improves the workers' motivation to comply with safety regulations and to participate in safety-promoting activities [35]. Our results indicate that rescue professionals and administrative officers need more specific information about the work-related stress that rescue workers experience and the associated challenges in order to prepare them for rescue missions and to save the lives of victims. The results of this study are consistent with those of a previous study demonstrating an increased risk of harmful consequences of simply being in the disaster environment; they include infectious disease, catastrophic injury to oneself or coworkers, severe burns, and psychological stress [36]. These results, as well as our own, call for increased attention to rescue workers' safety needs and the overall consequences of their work after the deployment.

3.3. Strengths and Limitations

Although the results of the present study are a valuable contribution to the literature, several limitations should be noted. Although the instrument has adequate overall psychometric integrity, the number of rescue workers available to serve as raters was small because there are so few catastrophic events that workers respond to. The resulting small sample size in the scale construction phase could have impacted the accuracy of the estimates from the measurement models. Likewise, the samples of raters in both phases may not have been representative of the population of workers who respond to traumatic mass-casualty disasters, because the period of data collection was small (2018 to 2021). Moreover, most of the raters were young men, few of whom were from an organization, and all of them were from just one culture. These factors limit the generalizability of the findings. Future research should use samples from different populations. Finally, previous empirical studies on work-related stress in disaster rescue, including our own study, have been retrospective rather than prospective; future research should include prediction of the consequences of work-related stress in disaster rescue. The strength of employing an exploratory sequential mixed methods approach for constructing the WRSS is that it provided a better understanding of the experiences of the participants because of the inclusion of a qualitative component. The weakness of our application of this approach is the lack of generalizability of the findings.

4. Conclusions

In this paper, the construction of a scale measuring work-related stress in rescue workers with good validity and trustworthiness was described. This 16-item, four-factor instrument, for which there is evidence of good content and construct validity, enables a fast, comprehensive, and systematic assessment of the stress suffered by rescue workers from responding to traumatic mass-casualty disasters. The results should increase understanding of rescue workers' needs and the stresses they experience while responding to traumatic events; paying attention to the outcomes of this research is likely to be important for improving the efficiency and safety of disaster rescue workers. Rescue professionals and administrative officers need to pay more attention to monitoring the work-related stress of rescue workers and the associated challenges to prepare them for SAR and to save the lives of victims.

Author Contributions: All authors contributed to this manuscript. Y.-L.C. contributed to the acquisition of quantitative data and reviewed the article critically. W.-C.T. contributed to the acquisition of qualitative data and reviewed the article critically. E.C. contributed to the acquisition of quantitative data, interpreted data, and reviewed the article critically. H.-H.C. conceptualizing and designed the study, acquired the data, analyzed the data, interpreted the data, and reviewed the article critically for important intellectual content. All authors have read and agreed to the published version of the manuscript.

Funding: This work was supported in part by the Ministry of the National Defense Medical Affairs Bureau, Taiwan (MND-MAB-110-050), the Ministry of Science and Technology, Taiwan (MOST 108-3111-Y-016-014) and Taipei Tzu Chi Hospital, Buddhist Tzu Chi Medical Foundation, Taiwan (TCRD-TPE-108-41).

Institutional Review Board Statement: The study was conducted according to the guidelines of the Declaration of Helsinki, and approved by the Institutional Review Board of Tri-Service General Hospital (protocol code: 1-107-05-021).

Informed Consent Statement: Informed consent was obtained from all subjects involved in the study.

Data Availability Statement: Datasets related to this article can be requested from corresponding author.

Acknowledgments: We are grateful to our participants for their time and effort. We are thankful to the New Taipei City Fire Department, the Taipei City Fire Department, and the Hualien County Fire Department for their cooperation in this study.

Conflicts of Interest: The authors declare no conflict of interest.

Appendix A

Table A1. Demographics of the qualitative interview raters (n = 7).

Variable	n (%)
Age (years)	
20–30	2 (28.6)
31–40	3 (42.9)
41–50	2 (28.6)
Gender (males) Marital status	5 (71.4)
Single or divorced	1 (14.3)
Married	6 (85.7)
Job specialties	
Logistics	1 (9.1)
Search and rescue	4 (36.4)
SAR dog controller	1 (9.1)
Security officer	3 (27.3)
Commander	2 (18.2)
SAR service (years)	
5–10	1 (14.3)
11–15	3 (42.9)
>15	3 (42.9)
Number of SAR disasters	
1–2	1 (14.3)
3–5	0
6–10	1 (14.3)
>10	5 (45.5)

Note. SAR: search and rescue.

Table A2. Semi-Structured Interview Guide.

Main Questions	Follow Up Topics If Necessary
What was your role in this disaster rescue?	
Can you please tell me about your most impressive disaster SAR experience?	Can you please tell me about your experience regarding:
	When, where, how, with whom?
	Why is this the most impressive experience for you?
	Can you please tell me about your experience regarding:
	Perceived challenges ahead?
	Feelings or perceptions?
	Subsequent effects?
Can you please tell me what is the most important stressor you noticed in your past disaster rescues	Can you please tell me about your experience regarding:
	When did you start work?
	Influences or impact?
	Present experience?
	Perceived challenges ahead?
	Late effects or impact?
	Specific challenges?
Can you please tell me how you deal with the effects of your experiences of disaster SAR?	Can you please tell me about your experience regarding:
	Influences on physical health?

Table A2. *Cont.*

Main Questions	Follow Up Topics If Necessary
	Goal achievement?
	Benefit from psychological support?
	Family relationships?
	Social activity?
	Sleep quality?
	Symptom interference?
	Specific challenges?

Note. SAR: search and rescue.

Table A3. Numbers of remaining items after rounds 1 to 3 of the Delphi procedure.

Factor	Original	Round 1	Round 2	Round 3
Physical Demands	13	7	5	3
Psychological Response	21	9	6	5
Environmental Interruption	20	12	12	7
Leadership	15	6	5	4
Total	69	34	28	19

References

1. Lin, C.H.; Chang, W.H.; Wu, C.L.; Pan, S.T.; Chi, C.H. Medical response to 2016 earthquake in Taiwan. *Lancet* **2016**, *388*, 129–130. [CrossRef]
2. Khatri, J.; Fitzgerald, G.; Chhetri, M.B.P. Health risks in disaster responders: A conceptual framework. *Prehosp. Disaster Med.* **2019**, *34*, 209–216. [CrossRef]
3. Beaglehole, B.; Mulder, R.T.; Boden, J.M.; Bell, C.J. A Systematic Review of the Psychological Impacts of the Canterbury Earthquakes on Mental Health. *Aust. N. Z. J. Public Health* **2019**, *43*, 274–280. [CrossRef]
4. Mao, X.; Fung, O.W.M.; Hu, X.; Loke, A.Y. Psychological impacts of disaster on rescue workers: A review of the literature. *Int. J. Disaster Risk Reduct.* **2018**, *27*, 602–617. [CrossRef]
5. Lee, K.; Lee, S.H.; Park, T.; Lee, J.Y. Stressors of Korean disaster relief team members during the Nepal Earthquake dispatch: A consensual qualitative research analysis. *J. Korean Med. Sci.* **2017**, *32*, 507–513. [CrossRef]
6. Nagamine, M.; Harada, N.; Shigemura, J.; Dobashi, J.; Yoshiga, M.; Esaki, N.; Tanaka, N.; Tanichi, M.; Yoshino, A.; Shimizu, K. The effects of living environment on disaster workers: A one-year longitudinal study. *BMC Psychiatry* **2016**, *16*, 358. [CrossRef] [PubMed]
7. Lee, J.Y.; Kim, S.W.; Bae, K.Y.; Kim, J.M.; Shin, I.S.; Yoon, J.S. Factors associated with posttraumatic stress disorder symptoms among community volunteers during the Sewol Ferry Disaster in Korea. *Compr. Psychiatry* **2017**, *77*, 38–44. [CrossRef]
8. Lunau, T.; Wahrendorf Müller, A.; Wright, B.; Dragano, N. Do resources buffer the prospective association of psychosocial work stress with depression? Longitudinal evidence from ageing workers. *Scand. J. Work. Environ. Health* **2018**, *44*, 183–191. [CrossRef] [PubMed]
9. Lusa, S.; Punakallio, A.; Luukkonen, R.; Louhevaara, V. Factors associated with changes in perceived strain at work among fire-fighters: A 3-year Follow-Up Study. *Int. Arch. Occup. Environ. Health* **2006**, *79*, 419–426. [CrossRef] [PubMed]
10. Benedek, D.M.; Fullerton, C.; Ursano, R.J. First responders: Mental health consequences of natural and human-made disasters for public health and public safety workers. *Annu. Rev. Public Health* **2007**, *28*, 55–68. [CrossRef]
11. Saijo, Y.; Ueno, T.; Hashimoto, Y. Job stress and depressive symptoms among Japanese fire fighters. *Am. J. Ind. Med.* **2007**, *50*, 470–480. [CrossRef]
12. Kawashima, Y.; Nishi, D.; Noguchi, H.; Usuki, M.; Yamashita, A.; Koido, Y.; Okubo, Y.; Matsuoka, Y.J. Post-traumatic stress symptoms and burnout among medical rescue workers 4 years after the Great East Japan Earthquake: A longitudinal study. *Disaster Med. Public Health Prep.* **2016**, *10*, 848–853. [CrossRef]
13. Gärtner, A.; Behnke, A.; Conrad, D.; Kolassa, I.-T.; Rojas, R. Emotion regulation in rescue workers: Differential relationship with perceived work-related stress and stress-related symptoms. *Front. Psychol.* **2019**, *9*, 2744. [CrossRef]
14. Kleim, R.; Westphal, M. Mental health in first responders: A review and recommendation for prevention and intervention strategies. *Traumatology* **2011**, *17*, 17–24. [CrossRef]
15. Geronazzo-Alman, L.; Eisenberg, R.; Shen, S.; Duarte, C.S.; Musa, G.J.; Wicks, J.; Fan, B.; Doan, T.; Guffanti, G.; Bresnahan, M.; et al. Cumulative exposure to work-related traumatic events and current post-traumatic stress disorder in New York City's first responders. *Compr. Psychiatry* **2017**, *74*, 134–143. [CrossRef]

16. Fjeldheim, C.B.; Nöthling, J.; Pretorius, K.; Basson, M.; Ganasen, K.; Heneke, K.R.; Cloete, K.J.; Seedat, S. Trauma exposure, posttraumatic stress disorder and the effect of explanatory variables in paramedic trainees. *BMC Emerg. Med.* **2014**, *14*, 11. [CrossRef]
17. Zhou, Y. A mixed methods model of scale development and validation analysis. *Measurement* **2019**, *17*, 38–47. [CrossRef]
18. Chen, P.F.; Chen, Y.L.; Su, P.L.; De Peng, Y.; Chen, L.F. Understanding the 6 February 2018, Hualien earthquake sequence through catalog compilation. *Terr. Atmos. Ocean. Sci.* **2019**, *30*, 399–409. [CrossRef]
19. Focus Taiwan CNA English News. Death Toll Revised to 50 in Train Crash as Human Remains Identified. 4 April 2021. Available online: https://focustaiwan.tw/society/202104040018 (accessed on 6 April 2021).
20. Hadi, M.A.; José Closs, S. Ensuring rigour and trustworthiness of qualitative research in clinical pharmacy. *Int. J. Clin. Pharm.* **2016**, *38*, 641–646. [CrossRef]
21. Brady, S.R. Utilizing and adapting the Delphi method for use in qualitative research. *Int. J. Qual. Methods* **2015**, *14*, 1–6. [CrossRef]
22. Schofield, R.; Chircop, A.; Baker, C.; Dietrich Leurer, M.; Duncan, S.; Wotton, D. Entry-to-practice public health nursing competencies: A Delphi method and knowledge translation strategy. *Nurse Educ. Today* **2018**, *65*, 102–107. [CrossRef]
23. Vogel, C.; Zwolinsky, S.; Griffiths, C.; Hobbs, M.; Henderson, E.; Wilkins, E. A Delphi study to build consensus on the definition and use of big data in obesity research. *Int. J. Obes.* **2019**, *43*, 2573–2586. [CrossRef] [PubMed]
24. Iyer, R.D. Developing and validating a questionnaire to measure some factors of school culture: A psychometric process. *Prabandhan Indian J. Manag.* **2017**, *10*, 7–18. [CrossRef]
25. Soper, D.S. A-Priori Sample Size for Structural Equation Models Software. 2021. Available online: https://www.danielsoper.com/statcal (accessed on 8 February 2020).
26. Muthén, L.K.; Muthén, B.O. *Mplus User's Guide*; Eighten: Los Angeles, CA, USA, 1998–2017.
27. Hu, L.; Bentler, P.M. Cutoff criteria for fit indexes in covariance structure analysis: Conventional criteria versus new alternatives. *Struct. Equ. Model* **1999**, *6*, 1–55. [CrossRef]
28. Lam, L.W. Impact of competitiveness on salespeople's commitment and performance. *J. Bus. Res.* **2012**, *65*, 1328–1334. [CrossRef]
29. Khatri, J.K.C.; Fitzgerald, G.; Poudyal Chhetri, M.B. Health risks and challenges in earthquake responders in Nepal: A qualitative research. *Prehosp. Disaster Med.* **2019**, *34*, 274–281. [CrossRef] [PubMed]
30. Giorgi, G.; Arcangeli, G.; Ariza-Montes, A.; Rapisarda, V.; Mucci, N. Work-related stress in the Italian banking population and its association with recovery experience. *Int. J. Occup. Med. Environ. Health* **2019**, *32*, 255–265. [CrossRef]
31. Kamijo, T.; Tsukahara, T.; Shimazu, A.; Nomiyama, T. Risk factors for duty-related posttraumatic stress disorder among police officers in the Mt. Ontake eruption disaster-support task force. *Int. J. Environ. Res. Public Health* **2020**, *17*, 3134. [CrossRef]
32. Rodrigues, S.; Paiva, J.S.; Dias, D.; Cunha, J.P.S. Stress among on-duty firefighters: An ambulatory assessment study. *PeerJ* **2018**, *6*, e5967. [CrossRef]
33. Fløvik, L.; Knardahl, S.; Christensen, J.O. How leadership behaviors influence the effects of job predictability and perceived employability on employee mental health—A multilevel, prospective study. *Scand. J. Work. Environ. Health* **2020**, *46*, 392–401. [CrossRef] [PubMed]
34. Heir, T.; Stokke, E.H.; Tvenge, K.P. The role of workplace on work participation and sick leave after a terrorist attack: A qualitative study. *Int. J. Environ. Res. Public Health* **2021**, *18*, 1920. [CrossRef] [PubMed]
35. Grill, M.; Pousette, A.; Nielsen, K.; Grytnes, R.; Törner, M. Safety leadership at construction sites: The importance of rule-oriented and participative leadership. *Scand. J. Work. Environ. Health* **2017**, *43*, 375–384. [CrossRef] [PubMed]
36. Walker, A.; McKune, A.; Ferguson, S.; Pyne, D.B.; Rattray, B. Chronic occupational exposures can influence the rate of PTSD and depressive disorders in first responders and military personnel. *Extrem. Physiol. Med.* **2016**, *5*, 1–12. [CrossRef] [PubMed]

sustainability

Review

Decontamination Methods of N95 Respirators Contaminated with SARS-CoV-2

Thirumaaran Gopalan [1], Rabi'atul 'Adawiyah Mohd Yatim [1], Mohd Ridha Muhamad [1,2,*], Nor Shafina Mohamed Nazari [3], N. Awanis Hashim [4], Jacob John [3] and Victor Chee Wai Hoe [5]

1 Department of Mechanical Engineering, Faculty of Engineering, Universiti Malaya, Kuala Lumpur 50603, Malaysia; thirumaarangopalan@gmail.com (T.G.); rabiatuladawiyahmohdyatim@gmail.com (R.'A.M.Y.)
2 Centre of Advanced Manufacturing and Material Processing (AMMP Centre), Universiti Malaya, Kuala Lumpur 50603, Malaysia
3 Department of Restorative Dentistry, Faculty of Dentistry, Universiti Malaya, Kuala Lumpur 50603, Malaysia; shafina.mnazari@um.edu.my (N.S.M.N.); drjacob@um.edu.my (J.J.)
4 Department of Chemical Engineering, Faculty of Engineering, Universiti Malaya, Kuala Lumpur 50603, Malaysia; awanis@um.edu.my
5 Centre for Epidemiology and Evidence-Based Practice, Department of Social and Preventive Medicine, Faculty of Medicine, Universiti Malaya, Kuala Lumpur 50603, Malaysia; victor@ummc.edu.my
* Correspondence: ridha@um.edu.my; Tel.: +60-3-7967-6806

Abstract: In the preparation and response to the COVID-19 pandemic, a sufficient supply of personal protective equipment (PPE), particularly the face mask, is essential. Shortage of PPE due to growing demand leaves health workers at significant risk as they fight this pandemic on the frontline. As a mitigation measure to overcome potential mask shortages, these masks could be decontaminated and prepared for reuse. This review explored past scientific research on various methods of decontamination of the N95-type respirators and their efficiency against the SARS-CoV-2 virus. Ultraviolet germicidal irradiation (UVGI) and hydrogen peroxide vapor (HPV) show great potential as an effective decontamination system. In addition, UVGI and HPV exhibit excellent effectiveness against the SARS-CoV-2 virus on the N95 respirator surfaces.

Keywords: decontamination; N95 respirators; SARS-CoV-2; COVID-19; ultraviolet germicidal irradiation (UVGI); hydrogen peroxide vapor (HPV); heat; microwave-generated steam (MGS); ethanol

Citation: Gopalan, T.; Mohd Yatim, R.'A.; Muhamad, M.R.; Mohamed Nazari, N.S.; Awanis Hashim, N.; John, J.; Wai Hoe, V.C. Decontamination Methods of N95 Respirators Contaminated with SARS-CoV-2. *Sustainability* **2021**, *13*, 12474. https://doi.org/10.3390/su132212474

Academic Editors: Amir Khorram-Manesh and Krzysztof Goniewicz

Received: 13 September 2021
Accepted: 8 November 2021
Published: 11 November 2021

1. Introduction

According to the WHO, COVID-19 human cases, which are caused by a novel coronavirus named SARS-CoV-2, were first reported in Wuhan City, China, in December 2019 [1]. Due to this unprecedented pandemic, the demand for face mask respirators has surged significantly. The WHO predicted that mask manufacturing industries need to increase manufacturing by 40 percent to meet the demand [2]. Frontline workers rely solely on PPE, especially N95 respirators, to protect themselves from being infected and infecting others. The N95 respirators should be disposed of after a sole patient visit, according to the Centers for Disease Control and Prevention.

Nevertheless, under acute PPE scarcity, it advises prolonged use of N95 respirators (using the same N95 respirator for many patient interactions) with limited reuse (keeping an N95 respirator during interactions for usage across several patients' visits). During the COVID-19 pandemic, due to a shortage of N95 masks, several emergency services have implemented various N95 prolonged use strategies. However, there is insufficient scientific proof that they were successful. In one investigation, researchers examined how often duckbill N95s and dome-shaped N95s masks failed by using fit-tests when they were reused. They concluded that healthcare systems must closely monitor N95 fit throughout extended usage or reuse and avoid using duckbill masks if better options are available [3].

Among the available models of face masks, N95 respirators are designed and intended for healthcare usage [4].

Developing countries whose populations are mostly made up of people living in poverty, such as India, Pakistan, and Sri Lanka, face even greater challenges due to a shortage of masks. The slowed economies in these countries, coupled with a face mask price hike, made people prioritize daily necessities over face masks, promoting the risk of the COVID-19 pandemic still existing in the community [5]. Due to these shortages, health workers were forced to ration their face mask supply to one N95 mask per week with an additional surgical mask on top. In addition, healthcare facilities are restricted to performing some non-COVID-related medical care as these supply limitations are concentrated on COVID-related patients [6].

As a solution, extending the usage of N95 respirators can assist in overcoming the shortage of masks experienced worldwide. Decontamination procedures of face masks that reduce the pathogen burden show great potential to alleviate the shortage of mask issues. According to NIOSH, ultraviolet germicidal irradiation, vaporous hydrogen peroxide, and moist heat have shown the most potential procedures to decontaminate filtering facepiece respirators (FFR) [7].

In essence, the mask shortage problem during the pandemic needs to be addressed immediately. This review aimed to compare the decontamination procedures of the virus on the N95 respirator, particularly highlighting effective but economical methods.

2. Methods

Relevant studies were searched using the PubMed and Preprint platform (medRxiv) electronic databases using a combination of specified MeSH terms that were restricted from 2000 to 2021 (Table 1). Apart from the database searches, several studies were included based on the relevance to this review. In addition, regulatory documents related to the decontamination of N95 respirators were obtained from the official websites of the CDC, the FDA, the WHO, and 3M. Studies were selected for evaluation based on specified inclusion criteria: (a) studies reporting at least one of the selected N95 respirator decontamination procedures for this review (UVGI or HPV or heat or MGS or ethanol); (b) studies reporting at least one of the selected N95 respirator decontamination outcomes (reduction in pathogen load or mask performance or structural integrity of the mask).

Table 1. Studies search strategies and outcomes.

Database	Search Terms	Results (n)	Studies Included (n)
PubMed	((“N95 Respirators”[Mesh]) OR (“Respiratory Protective Devices”[Mesh]) OR (“Personal Protective Equipment”[Mesh])) AND ((“Decontamination”[Mesh]) OR (“Microbial Viability”[Mesh]) OR (“Virus Inactivation”[Mesh]) OR (“Equipment Reuse”[Mesh]) OR (“Sterilization”[Mesh]))	781	35
medRxiv	((N95 respirators) OR (respiratory protective devices)) AND ((decontamination) OR (microbial viability) OR (virus inactivation))	149	12
Other Relevant Studies	Low-cost mask decontamination, N95 decontamination, and SARS-CoV-2 inactivation	-	14

3. SARS-CoV-2

The WHO named the pathogen that causes coronavirus disease (COVID-19) SARS-CoV-2 on 12 February 2020. CoVs is a single-stranded positive-sense RNA (+ssRNA) virus [8]. The schematic structure of the SARS-CoV-2 virus is illustrated in Figure 1. The SARS-CoV-2 virus was reported to possess 80% similarity in the aspect of the genome to previous human coronaviruses. Bats were deduced as the vital host and transmitting medium of the SARS-CoV-2 virus [9]. It was concluded that SARS-CoV-2 is transmitted mainly via respiratory droplets and direct contact [10]. Evaluation of the stability of SARS-CoV-2 on different environmental conditions demonstrated that after seven days, a detectable level of the virus still presents on the outer layer of the surgical mask [11]. The FDA calls for a policy where at least three log reductions must be achieved to sterilize devices intended for skin contact [12].

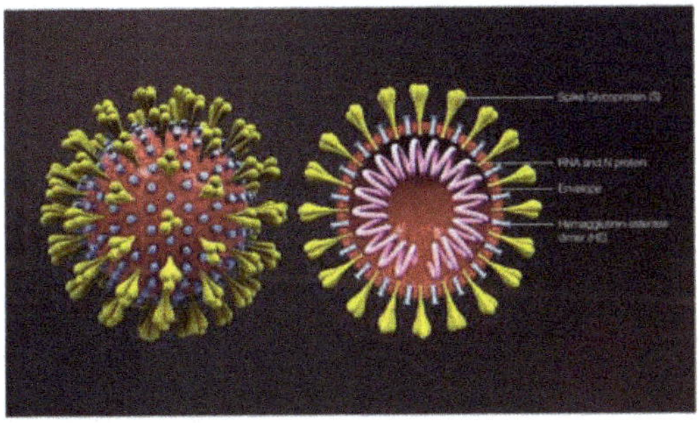

Figure 1. Schematic structure of SARS-CoV-2 [13].

4. The N95 Respirator

The N95 respirator is a type of respiratory protective equipment with a specific design to tightly fit its user. This type of respirator undergoes a testing and evaluation process by NIOSH [14]. In comparison to other FFRs, the N95 respirator offers a minimum of 95% filtration efficiency against particulate aerosols [15]. Quantitative fit testing of FFRs proves the superior protection that the N95 respirator offers [16].

The N95 respirator is made up of four layers, namely, a coverweb, a shell, filter 1, and filter 2 as illustrated in Figure 2. The coverweb and the shell layers are made up of polyester; meanwhile, filter layers are made from polypropylene [4]. The filtration efficiency of the respirator is determined by the internal filtration layer, which is a high-efficiency melt-blown non-woven material [17].

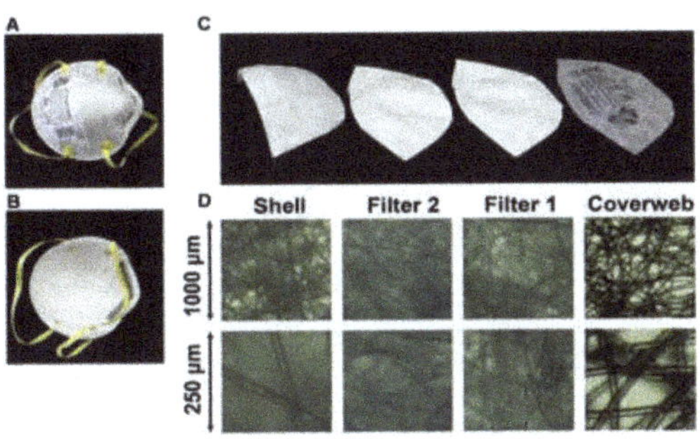

Figure 2. Multilayer sandwich anatomy of N95 mask. (**A**) Environmental interface; (**B**) user interface; (**C**) from left to right: inner layer (shell), middle layers (filter 2 and filter 1), and outer layer (coverweb); (**D**) light microscope images of the four layers, with a lower row at four-fold higher magnification (3M model 8210). Adapted from [18] with permission.

5. Decontamination Treatment for N95 Respirators

5.1. Ultraviolet Germicidal Irradiation (UVGI)

UVGI is a scientifically proven decontamination method that can destroy the protein coating of the SARS-coronavirus, which possesses similar characteristics as the SARS-CoV-2 virus (COVID-19 virus) [19]. Ozog et al. [20] reported excellent decontamination results of the SARS-CoV-2 virus with a 1.5 J/cm^2 UV dose, which was achieved using a 4 UVC lamp set-up. Vo et al. [21] produced the required decontamination levels up to a three-log reduction with a UV dose of 4.32 J/cm^2 and complete decontamination with a $\geq$7.20 J/cm^2 dosage against the MS2 virus. A relatively longer decontamination time was reported due to the low range of UV irradiation used in the research.

Lindsley et al. [22] tested a UV dose up to 950 J/cm^2 on N95 respirators, which resulted in acceptable degradation on filtration performance and no effect in flow resistance. This study reported a perfect range for UVC-based decontamination treatment cycles. Ozog et al. [23] reported excellent fit testing results using N95 respirators with a total exposure of 60 J/cm^2.

5.2. Hydrogen Peroxide Vapor (HPV)

HPV-based decontamination systems are regarded as some of the best decontamination systems due to their efficacy against various microorganisms and their rapid processing cycles [24]. Saini et al. [25] tested the N95 respirator's decontamination against three biological indicators: Escherichia coli, Mycobacterium smegmatis, and spores of Bacillus stearothermophilus using an HPV machine. Excellent decontamination results were reported where decontamination up to a seven-log reduction was achieved using 11–12% HPV against E.coli. Jatta et al. [26] performed decontamination with a 59% HPV concentration using a VPRO maX low-temperature sterilization system. These research results exhibited no significant effect on the filtration performance and fit of the N95 mask after exposure to 59% HPV up to 10 cycles. The range of treatment time reported in this study provides a solid foundation for an HPV-based decontamination system design.

5.3. Heat

5.3.1. Moist Heat

Lore et al. [27] tested moist heat decontamination against the influenza virus applied on an N95 mask. In this study, a contaminated mask was heated to 65 + 5 °C for 3 h. The results show that the required decontamination level (>four-log reduction) was achieved. However, a relatively slow decontamination time can prove to be an inefficient decontamination procedure for everyday application. Rockey et al. [28] investigated the effect of humidity in virus heat inactivation against two bacteriophages (MS2 and phi6), a mouse coronavirus (murine hepatitis virus), and a recombinant human influenza A virus subtype H3N2 (IAV) using a humidity-controlled oven. Heat treatments illustrated greater decontamination results with increasing humidity, where six-log reductions were reported in humidity exceeding 50%.

Bopp et al. [29] tested multiple cycles of autoclaves on N95 respirators. Four different autoclave cycles (115 °C for one hour, 121.1 °C for 30 min, 130 °C for two minutes, and 130 °C for four minutes) were administered to N95 FFRs. N95 FFRs showed negligible differences in their functionality and integrity even after three cycles. Andregg et al. [30] applied heating decontamination to N95 respirators with moisture (85 °C, 60–85% humidity) in a polypropylene container and a convection oven setup. Post-decontamination N95 FFRs exhibited excellent results in both quantitative fit testing and filtration efficiency.

5.3.2. Dry Heat

Xiang et al. [31] implemented dry heat pasteurization for one hour at 70 °C for the N95 respirator's decontamination. This study showed that this procedure can kill six species of respiratory bacteria and one fungi species and can inactivate the H1N1 indicator virus. In addition, neither the performance nor the integrity of N95 respirators showed significant degradation. This study shows that dry heat is capable of deactivating various pathogens but at a relatively slow rate. Pascoe et al. [32] successfully decontaminated pathogen (*S. aureus*) under dry heat of 70 °C by reducing log 4 in 90 min using a laboratory incubator. Despite strong decontamination results, the slow decontamination rate might prove to be the drawback of this method. Viscusi et al. [33] reported a slight increase in average penetration at N95 respirators when exposed to 80 °C after 60 min. These results can potentially act as a limitation for dry heat exposure to an N95 mask.

5.4. Microwave Generated Steam (MGS)

Fischer et al. [34] have proved up to a four-log reduction in bacteriophage MS2 pathogenic virus using sealed steam bags on a 1100-W-rated microwave for 90 s. In addition, tested N95 respirators also passed the minimum required filtration efficiency requirements of 95%. Zulauf et al. [35] reported a reduction greater than four logs measured in PFU on the N95 respirator. They tested MS2-phage-contaminated N95 respirators to microwave-generated steam for 3 min. Moreover, the respirators exhibited the required filtration performance and integrity even after 20 cycles of 3 min.

5.5. Ethanol

By using ethanol, decontamination of pathogens happens by protein denaturation. At a concentration of 60%–80%, ethanol proves to be effective against lipophilic viruses and many hydrophilic viruses [36]. Liao et al. [37] tested N95 respirators using a 75% ethanol treatment, which was immersed and dried. The filtration efficiency of the N95 respirators were affected considerably with treatment, which indicates that ethanol treatment could not retain the mask's reusability properties.

5.6. Other Methods

N95 respirator decontamination procedures other than the methods selected for this review (UVGI or HPV or heat or MGS or ethanol) are highlighted based on their potential as a low-cost and accessible method. Lendvay et al. [38] tested SARS-CoV-2-inoculated N95 masks under methylene blue (MB) photochemical action for decontamination. They showed that MB activated by red or white light significantly inactivates SARS-CoV-2 on N95 mask surfaces without compromising the specimen's integrity. Excellent virucidal activity of 99.8%–>99% was reported, and preservation of mask integrity proved up to five treatment cycles. Their findings suggested a strategy for decontaminating PPE and masks for reuse that is accessible and inexpensive and that can be used in high-resource and low-resource situations amid supply disruptions. This is due to the worldwide availability of MB light at an affordable cost without using specialized instruments. In addition, the New York City Department of Health and Mental Hygiene has released passive decontamination guidance to health workers to use a paper bag or other clean, breathable containers to store used N95 respirators to prolong their efficiency over multiple usages. The method is as follows. Each day, the healthcare workers would use one N95 respirator with a tagged name and the number of the day used and would place it in a paper bag or a ventilated container at the end of the shift. The mask should be disposed of after the seventh day of use. Healthcare workers must be aware that the N95 respirator could be contaminated albeit at a substantially lower rate. Limited storage periods may be considered, although they may raise the chance of contamination. As the more rigorous disinfecting techniques become accessible, this strategy could be integrated for higher efficiency [39]. Heimbuch et al. [40] evaluated the ability of wipe products available commercially to clean filtering facepiece respirators (FFRs) contaminated with pathogenic or non-pathogenic aerosols. They examined the decontamination effect of benzalkonium chloride, hypochlorite, and nonantimicrobial wipes on the N95 FFRs. The highest particle penetration capacity was observed in benzalkonium chloride wipes. They reported effective decontamination results of S aureus up to 99.72% (exterior of N95) and 98.60% (interior of N95) using benzalkonium chloride (BAC) wipes. Decontamination using wipes is readily available for public usage, but penetration of respirator due to wipe decontamination must be approached with caution.

5.7. Comparison of Decontamination Treatments for N95 Respirators

The reusability of a disinfected N95 respirator depends on several factors such as inactivation of the targeted organism, the safety of the user, and consistent filtration function and fit of the respirator. UVGI and HPV have demonstrated excellent results as an efficient decontamination method with effective elimination of SARS-CoV-2 virus while preserving the performance of the respirator. However, extensive studies are needed to incorporate HPV- and UVGI-based decontamination systems into a household-based portable commercial-ready product for commercial use. On the other hand, the MGS-based decontamination method exhibits great potential with rapid disinfection for household applications. Currently, there are still few studies about this method for decontamination application. Its rapid method enables a huge potential of applications. However, use in materials that are sensitive to steam could be a concern for material degradation. The other method includes the heat-based decontamination method, which has a major drawback for its time-consuming process and filtration performance degradation in extensive dosages. The conventional method of using ethanol has shown unavoidable degradation of the respirator by using this procedure. Table 2 demonstrates the effects of using a specified N95 decontamination treatment.

Table 2. Advantages and disadvantages of decontamination treatments for N95 respirators.

Decontamination Treatment	Advantages	Disadvantages
Ultraviolet germicidal irradiation (UVGI)	- Proven efficiency against SARS-CoV-2 - Fast disinfection - Easy parameter control (dosage) - No residue	- Not readily available - Basic expertise in handling needed - Mask performance affected at high doses
Hydrogen peroxide vapor (HPV)	- Proven efficiency against SARS-CoV-2 - Excellent virucidal activity against a variety of viruses. - Integrity of mask preserved - Multiple mask decontamination in one cycle	- Not readily available - Expensive - Basic expertise in handling needed - Complete cycle includes multiple stages of decontamination - Require enclosed air circulation set up
Moist heat	- Readily available - Good virucidal activity - No residue - Better decontamination results compared to dry heat decontamination	- Slow disinfection - Integrity of mask affected at high temperatures
Dry heat	- Readily available - Good virucidal activity - No residue	- Slow disinfection - Integrity of mask affected at high temperatures
Microwave-generated steam (MGS)	- Readily available - Good germicidal activity - No residue - Rapid disinfection	- Limited to one mask decontamination per cycle
Ethanol	- No residue	- Not readily available - Significant degradation to respirator integrity and performance

6. Decontamination System Design for N95 Respirators

6.1. Ultraviolet Germicidal Irradiation

Several factors must be taken into account when designing a UVGI-based decontamination system, namely, the wavelength of the ultraviolet rays, the irradiance, and the exposure time. The effectiveness of a UVGI-based decontamination system depends on the dosage of UVC administered to the N95 mask. A safe dosage range must be estimated beforehand because excessive dosage can affect the integrity of the mask. On the other hand, an insufficient dosage can lead to incomplete deactivation of the virus. The UV dose for a specific system can be calculated using Equation (1) [41]. The system specifications and outcomes of studies related to UVGI-based N95 decontamination are listed in Table 3.

$$\text{UV dose}\left(\frac{\text{J}}{\text{cm}^2}\right) = \text{Irradiance}\left(\frac{\text{W}}{\text{cm}^2}\right) \times \text{Time (s)} \quad (1)$$

Table 3. UVGI-based decontamination system specifications and outcomes.

Study	Wavelength (nm)	Irradiance (W/m^2)	Exposure Time (s)	Dosage (J/cm^2)	Distance (cm)	Outcomes
			Reduction in Pathogen Load (Various Pathogens)			
[20]	254	165	60–70	3	11.5	- Log reduction of >3 in viable SARS-CoV-2 virus - Mask model: 3M 1860
[42]	253.7	NA	0–300	NA	100	- Log reduction of >4.79 in viable SARS-CoV-2 virus - Mask model: 3M 1860
[43]	254	54.3	2–420	0.01086–2.2806	10	- Log reduction of up to 3.5 in viable SARS-CoV-2 virus - Mask model: 3M 8211
[44]	254	10	300	0.3	NA	- Average log reduction of 3.74 in viable SARS-CoV-2 virus at 0.6 J/cm^2 dosage (3M 1860) - Average log reduction of 1.68 in viable SARS-CoV-2 virus at 0.6 J/cm^2 dosage (3M 8210) - Mask model: 3M 1860 and 3M 8210
			600	0.6		
[45]	254	3.18	1980	0.63	NA	- No significant log reduction in viable SARS-CoV-2 RNA - Mask model: 3M 1860
[46]	260–285	5.5	600–3600	0.33–1.98	50	- Log reduction of $\geq$3 in viable SARS-CoV-2 virus - Mask model: AOSafety N9504C
[47]	254	64	NA	0.05–1.5	3.4	- Log reduction of >3 in viable SARS-CoV-2 virus at 0.05–0.5 J/cm^2 dosage - Log reduction of >5 in viable SARS-CoV-2 virus at 0.5–1.5 J/cm^2 dosage - Mask model: 3M 1860
[48]	254	2.32	0–3600	0–0.8352	60.96	- Log reduction of >3 (5 min of exposure) and complete decontamination (15 min of exposure) in viable NL63 coronavirus - Mask model: 3M 1860
[49]	NA	NA	120	2.6	NA	- No virus detection after 2 or 5 cycles (porcine coronavirus and murine norovirus) - Mask model: KN95 FFR (Guangzhou Sunjoy Auto Supplies)
[41]	254	3900	60	1	100	- Log reduction of 3 in viable H1N1 influenza virus - Mask model: 3M 1860
[27]	254	16–22	900	1.8	25	- Log reduction of $\geq$4.65 in viable H5N1 influenza virus - Mask model: 3M 1860

Table 3. *Cont.*

Study	Wavelength (nm)	Irradiance (W/m^2)	Exposure Time (s)	Dosage (J/cm^2)	Distance (cm)	Outcomes
[21]	253.7	4	3600–18,000	1.44–7.2	42	- Log reduction of ≥3 in viable MS2 at 4.32 J/cm^2 - No virus detection at ≥7.20 J/cm^2 - Mask model: Honeywell N1105
[50]	254	≥300	60	≥2	NA	- Log reduction of ≥3 in viable MS2 - Mask model: 3M 1860
[51]	254	25	120–15,960	0.0038–0.4707	NA	- Log reduction of >3 in viable MS2 at 0.1 J/cm^2 - Mask model: 3M 1860
[52]	254	NA	300	0.126	NA	- Complete inactivation of *E. coli* and *B. subtilis* after 300 s of exposure - Mask model: UVEX FFP2
			600	0.256		
			900	0.378		
[53]	200–315	0.069–0.1072	300	NA	180	- Log reduction of 0.5–1.3 in MS2 - Log reduction of 0.0–2.0 in phi6 - Log reduction of 0.8–1.7 in IAV - Log reduction of 1.3–1.7 in MHV - Mask model: 3M 1860
[54]	254	189	60–1200	1.134–22.68	10	- UVA could not decontaminate as effectively as UVC - No bacteria recovered after 5 min of UVC exposure - Mask model: 3M 8210
	365	312		1.872–37.44		
Performance or Structural Integrity						
[22]	254	NA	NA	0–950	6.2	- Filtration performance slightly affected - No effect on flow resistance - Mask model: 3M 1860
[27]	254	16–22	900	1.8	25	- Mean penetration: 0.99% at 300nm - Mask model: 3M 1860s
[37]	254	NA	1800	NA	NA	- Efficiency of meltblown layer: (≥96% at 10 cycles) and (≥93% at 20 cycles) - Mask model: 3M 8210
[45]	254	3.18	57,600 (Exterior)	18.4	NA	- Mask integrity was significantly impaired - Average fit score: ≥ 100 - Mask model: 3M 1860
			14,400 (Interior)	4.6		
[49]	NA	NA	120	2.6	NA	- Remained physically unaffected up to 5 cycles - Filtration efficiency of >95% up to 5 cycles - Breathability well within allowed range after 5 cycles - Mask model: KN95 FFR (Guangzhou Sunjoy Auto Supplies)
[52]	254	NA	300	0.126	NA	- Filtration efficiency maintained up to dosage of 0.378 J/cm^2 - Mask model: UVEX FFP2
			600	0.256		
			900	0.378		
[55]	254	≥24.31	NA	≥1	30.48	- Expected penetration: 1.121% (0.3µm, 5 cycles, 3M 1860) and 0.258% (0.3µm, 5 cycles, 3M 8210) - Mask model: 3M 1860 and 3M 8210
[56]	NA	NA	300	>1	100	- Filtration performance preserved up to 10 cycles - Mask model: 3M 8210
[57]	254	55.56	180	1	36.8	- No visual abnormalities on mask integrity - Mean breaking force of 34.8 ± 5.23 N - Average filtration efficiency = >95% - Fit factor = >100% - Mask model: 3M 8110S

6.2. *Hydrogen Peroxide Vapor (HPV)*

Most of the studies reviewed here used commercially available HPV-based decontamination machines. The efficiency of HPV-based decontamination systems depends on the concentration of the HPV used coupled with the time of exposure to the N95 respirator.

HPV traces on mask surfaces might induce health hazards. Therefore, each HPV-based decontamination system must be able to produce residue-free N95 respirators upon the decontamination cycle. The system specifications and outcomes of studies related to HPV-based N95 decontamination are listed in Table 4.

Table 4. HPV-based decontamination system specifications and outcomes.

Study	Method	Concentration of HPV Used/Achieved	Exposure Time (min)	Outcome
		Reduction in Pathogen Load (Various Pathogens)		
[45]	Bioquell Z vaporizer	30% (Peak 500 ppm)	Gassing: 20 Dwell: 60 Aeration: 210	- Log reduction of ≈5 in viable SARS-CoV-2 RNA - Mask model: 3M 1860
[46]	Panasonic MCO-19AIC-PT	≈ 1000 ppm	Gas: 7	- Log reduction of ≥ 3 viable SARS-CoV-2 virus - Mask model: AOSafety N9504C
[58]	VHP® ARD system	35% (Peak 750 ppm)	Conditioning: 3 Decontamination: 30 Aeration: 20	- Log reduction of 5.2–6.3 in viable SARS-CoV-2 virus - Mask model: 3M 1860 and 3M 8210
[59]	V-PRO maX low-temperature sterilization system by Steris	NA	Non-lumen cycle: 28	- Log reduction of 4 in viable SARS-CoV-2 titer and 5 in HCoV-229E - Mask model: 3M 8210
[60]	Steris ARD1000®	410 ± 83 ppm	Gas: 180	- Log reduction of >4 in viable SARS-CoV-2 - Mask model: 3M 1860
[49]	V-PRO maX low-temperature sterilization system by Steris	59%	Non-lumen cycle: 28	- No virus detection after 2 or 5 cycles (porcine coronavirus and murine norovirus) - Mask model: KN95 FFR (Guangzhou Sunjoy Auto Supplies)
[61]	A novel HPV-based system was constructed	3%	Gassing: 3–5 Dwell: 60 Aeration: 15	- Log reduction of >6 in P22 bacteriophage - Mask model: 3M 1860
[62]	Bioquell® BQ-50	35%	NA	- No growth of 6-log Geobacillus stearothermophilus spores post decontamination - Mask model: 3M 1860
[63]	VHP® VICTORY unit	35% (400–800 ppm)	Conditioning and Gassing: 90 Dwell: 180 Aeration: 900–1080	- No growth of 6-log Geobacillus stearothermophilus spores post decontamination (1st, 7th day) - Mask model: 3M 1860s
		Performance or Structural Integrity		
[26]	V-PRO maX low-temperature sterilization system by Steris	59%	Inject: 18 Aeration: 8	- Mask fit and filtration efficiency preserved up to 10 cycles - Mask model: 3M 8211
[45]	Bioquell Z vaporizer	30% (Peak 500 ppm)	Gassing: 20 Dwell: 60 Aeration: 210	- Mask integrity minimally affected - Average fit score: ≥ 100 - Mask model: 3M 1860
[46]	Panasonic MCO-19AIC-PT	≈ 1000 ppm	Gas: 7	- Filtration performance preserved after 1 treatment - Mask model: AOSafety N9504C

Table 4. *Cont.*

Study	Method	Concentration of HPV Used/Achieved	Exposure Time (min)	Outcome
[49]	V-PRO maX low-temperature sterilization system by Steris	59%	Non-lumen cycle: 28	- Remained physically unaffected up to 5 cycles - Filtration efficiency of >95% up to 5 cycles - Breathability well within allowed range after 5 cycles -Mask model: KN95 FFR (Guangzhou Sunjoy Auto Supplies)
[55]	V-PRO maX low-temperature ster-ilization system by Steris (Masks were enclosed within Vis-U-AllTM low-temperature sterilization pouches)	59%	Full cycle: 28	- Expected penetration: 0.277% (0.3µm, 5 cycles, 3M 1860) and 0.424% (0.3µm, 5 cycles, 3M 8210) - Mask model: 3M 1860 and 3M 8210
[58]	VHP® ARD system	35% (Peak 750 ppm)	Conditioning: 3 Decontamination: 30 Aeration: 20	- Structural and functional integrity preserved - Mask model: 3M 1860 and 3M 8210
[59]	V-PRO maX low-temperature sterilization system by Steris	NA	Non-lumen cycle: 28	- Filtration efficiency retained - Mask model: 3M 8210
[60]	Steris ARD1000®	410 ± 83 ppm	Gas: 180	- Mask fit and filtration efficiency preserved after 1 cycle - Mask model: 3M 1860
[61]	A novel HPV-based system was constructed	3%	Gassing: 3–5 Dwell: 60 Aeration: 15	- Minimum required filtration efficiency value of 95% preserved up to 20 cycles - Mask model: 3M 1860
[62]	Bioquell® BQ-50	35%	NA	- All processed masks passed fit testing - Mask model: 3M 1860
[64]	V-PRO maX low-temperature sterilization system by Steris	NA	Non-lumen cycle: 28	- Filtration efficiency significantly affected (80.4–91.8%), particularly at a lower particle diameter - Mask model: 3M 8210
[65]	VHP® VICTORY unit	35% (400–800 ppm)	Conditioning and Gassing: NA Dwell: 180 Aeration: overnight	- Integrity (mask fit) of the mask preserved up to 8 decontamination cycles - Mask model: 3M 1860s
[66]	V-PRO maX low-temperature ster-ilization system by Steris (masks were enclosed within Tyvek pouches)	NA	Non-lumen cycle: 28	- 66% of the respirators failed fit testing after one decontamination cycle - Mask model: 3M 1860s
[67]	Bioquell Clarus C	35% (±480 ppm)	Gassing: 25 Dwell: 20	- All the tested masks passed fit testing up to 10 cycles - Mask model: 3M 1870 +

6.3. Heat

Heat treatments can sterilize microbes by altering their membranes and denaturing proteins [68]. Heat-related decontaminations can be divided into two main classifications, namely, moist-heat and dry-heat decontamination. The efficiency of a heat-based decontamination system depends on the working temperature, the presence of humidity, and the exposure time. The existence of moisture in the heating procedure is proven to promote better decontamination results. The system specifications and outcomes of studies related to moist heat and dry heat-based N95 decontamination are listed in Tables 5 and 6 respectively.

Table 5. Moist-heat-based decontamination system specifications and outcomes.

Study	Method	Temperature (°C)	Exposure Time (min)	Relative Humidity (%)	Outcome
Reduction in Pathogen Load (Various Pathogens)					
[69]	- 57 L model BD 56 standard incubator - Humidity induced by placing 400 mL of water-filled pan below the incubator	70	180–360	≈<5–32	- Complete decontamination of SARS-CoV-2 at 5 hrs of exposure - Mask model: 3M 1860, 3M 8210, and Moldex 1510
[70]	- Multicookers with the sous vide function - Humidity induced by placing 500 mL of water in the multicooker pot	65	30	94 ± 0.5 (measured inside the paper bag)	- Inactivation of SARS-CoV-2 virus beyond detection limit within 10 min of exposure - Stacked mask does not hinder decontamination - Mask model: 3M 1860 and 3M 8210
[27]	- Mask loaded to a sealed container placed inside a heated oven - Container filled with 1 L tap water	65 ± 5	20	NA	- Log reduction of ≥4.62 log in viable H5N1 influenza - Mask model: 3M 1860
[71]	- Circulating water bath	60 ± 2	30	80 ± 5	- Log reduction of ≥4.35 in influenza A virus (InfA) - Log reduction of >5.32 in *S. aureus* - Mask model: 3M 1860s
[28]	- Conducted using TestEquity 123H temperature/humidity chamber	72, 82	30	1–89	- Increase in treatment temperature and humidity results in an increased log reduction of pathogen - Mask model: 3M 1860
[52]	- Samples were steamed above boiling water	NA	30, 60, 90	70–85	- Log reduction of >4 in *E. coli* and *B. subtilis* at 30 and 90 min of exposure - Mask model: UVEX FFP2

Table 5. *Cont.*

Study	Method	Temperature (°C)	Exposure Time (min)	Relative Humidity (%)	Outcome
[53]	- Ziploc container	80	30	≈70	- Log reduction of >6.9 in MS2 - Log reduction of >7.2 in phi6 - Log reduction of >3.4 in IAV - Log reduction of >0.4 in MHV - Mask model: 3M 1860
	- Humidity-controlled oven	82	30	≈50	- Log reduction of >6.6 in MS2 - Log reduction of >6.7 in phi6 - Log reduction of >3.9 in IAV - Log reduction of >2.7 in MHV - Mask model: 3M 1860
[72]	- BevLes heated holding cabinet with humidity (masks were enclosed within steril-peel pouches)	70, 90	60	0, 25, 40, 50, 70	- Inactivation of E. coli beyond detection limit at (70 °C, 50%RH) and (90 °C, 70%RH) - Mask model: 3M 1860s
		Performance or Structural Integrity			
[27]	- Mask loaded to a sealed container placed inside a heated oven - Container filled with 1 L tap water	65 ± 5	20	NA	- Mean penetration of 1.04% at 300-nm particle size - Mask model: 3M 1860
[29]	- Moist-heat autoclave	115–130	2–60	NA	- Molded N95 respirators failed all tested fit testing - Slight degradation to filtration efficiency was notable - Mask model: 3M 1860
[30]	- Conducted using a convection oven (Despatch LAC1-38-8, 3.7 cu. Ft.)	70–85	30	60–85	- Passed fit testing - Filtration efficiency not affected - Mask model: 3M 1860
[52]	- Samples were steamed above boiling water	NA	30, 60, 90	70–85	- Slight decrease in filtration efficiency from 98.86% and 99.51% to 97.58% and 98.79% for 50 and 100 nm particles, respectively - Mask model: UVEX FFP2
[55]	- Masks were enclosed in STERIL-PEEL® sterilization pouches and loaded into the convection heating system with controlled humidity.	75	60	75	- Expected penetration: 1.195% (0.3 μm, 5 cycles, 3M 1860) and 1.924% (0.3 μm, 5 cycles, 3M 8210) - Mask model: 3M 1860, 3M 8210, and Moldex 1510
[69]	- 57 L model BD 56 standard incubator - Humidity induced by placing 400 mL of water-filled pan below the incubator	70	180–360	≈<5–32	- Structural and functional integrity of the respirators preserved up to five cycles - Mask model: 3M 1860, 3M 8210 and Moldex 1510

Table 5. *Cont.*

Study	Method	Temperature (°C)	Exposure Time (min)	Relative Humidity (%)	Outcome
[70]	- Multicookers with the sous vide function - Humidity induced by placing 500 mL of water in the multicooker pot	65	30	94 ± 0.5 (measured inside the paper bag)	- Collection efficiency and inhalation resistance was above the required value of >95% and <35 mmH2O, respectively, for all tested masks upon 5 treatment cycles - A slight change (<10%) in strap elasticity was noted for mask model 3M 1860 - Mask model: 3M 1860 and 3M 8210
[72]	- BevLes heated holding cabinet with humidity (masks were enclosed within steril-peel pouches)	70, 90	60	0, 50	- All processed masks passed fit testing up to 15 cycles - Excellent filtration efficiency of >95%. - Breathing resistance was well within the tolerable resistant standard - Mask model: 3M 1860s and 3M 8210
[73]	- Cylindrical chamber tabletop autoclave (Kronus S18)	121	17	NA	- No visible damage to the mask after treatment - Slight degradation to filtration capacity of 94.4 ± 1.6% after three cycles - Number of reuse does not affect the flow resistance of the mask - Mask model: 3M Aura 1862+
[74]	- Steris Amsco 400 Series prevacuum steam sterilizer model 20	121	30	NA	- 100% (1 cycle) and 86% (2 cycles) of the samples passed fit testing - Mask model: AO Safety 1054S Pleats Plus
[75]	NA	121	20	NA	- Decrease of 20 Pa in respiratory resistance after 4 cycles - Mask model: Duckbill FPP2
[76]	- Sealed respirator container placed inside boiled water	>65	30	50	- Filtration efficiency was recorded above 97% up to 5 cycles - Mask model: Kimberly Clark

Table 6. Dry-heat-based decontamination system specifications and outcomes.

Study	Method/Equipment	Temperature (°C)	Exposure Time (min)	Outcome
		Reduction in Pathogen Load (Various Pathogens)		
[72]	BevLes heated holding cabinet with humidity (masks were enclosed within steril-peel pouches)	70	60	- Inactivation of SARS-CoV-2 virus beyond the detection limit - Mask model: 3M 1860s and 3M 8210
[77]	Laboratory dry oven (Fisher Scientific Isotemp 500 series)	60–75	30, 60	- N95 coupons placed in tissue culture plate wells yielded better decontamination results compared to the one placed in parchment paper - No required SARS-CoV-2 virus inactivation achieved in suspended intact N95 respirators - Mask model: 3M 1860, 3M 1860s, and 3M 8200
	Open drying (room conditions)	22–23	7200	- 5/9 coupons contained live SARS-CoV-2 virus - Mask model: 3M 1860s
[49]	FFRs hung horizontally on a metal frame were inserted into an electrically heated vessel	102 ± 4	60 ± 15	- No virus detection after 2 or 5 cycles (porcine coronavirus and murine norovirus) - Mask model: KN95 FFR (Guangzhou Sunjoy Auto Supplies)
[31]	Electric oven	60, 70	60–180	- 1 h of exposure could successfully kill 7 types of bacteria as well as inactivate the H1N1 virus - Mask model: 3M 1860
		Performance or Structural Integrity		
[31]	Electric oven	60, 70	60–180	- No significant effect on the shape and filtration efficiency after exposure up to 3 h - Mask model: 3M 1860
[49]	FFRs hung horizontally on a metal frame were inserted into an electrically heated vessel	102 ± 4	60 ± 15	- Signs of degradation or burning visible after 5 cycles - Filtration efficiency dropped to 94.16% after 3 cycles - Breathability well within allowed range after 5 cycles - Mask model: KN95 FFR (Guangzhou Sunjoy Auto Supplies)
[55]	VWR® forced air oven	100	30	- Expected penetration: 0.562% (0.3 µm, 5 cycles, 3M 1860) and 8.107% (0.3 µm, 5 cycles, 3M 8210) - Mask model: 3M 1860 and 3M 8210
[78]	5-sided heating vacuum oven	75	30	-No effect on the fit factor of the mask up to 5 cycles - Mask model: 3M 8210
[79]	Oven (masks were enclosed within nylon heat-resistant bags)	65, 86	34–56	- All processed masks passed fit testing - Mask model: 3M 8810, 3M 8833, and 3M 8835

6.4. Microwave-Generated Steam (MGS)

MGS-based decontamination has enormous potential for wide application as it can be done with household items. It offers a rapid disinfection rate with minimal expertise needed to perform this treatment. The efficiency of MGS-based decontamination is affected by exposure time and is specific to the design of the selected face mask model for the treatment. However, many protocols use commercial steam bags or special materials that are available in laboratories. The system specifications and outcomes of studies related to MGS-based N95 decontamination are listed in Table 7.

Table 7. Microwave-generated steam (MGS)-based decontamination system specifications and outcomes.

Study	Method/Equipment	Exposure Time (s)	Outcome
	Reduction in Pathogen Load (Various Pathogens), Performance or Structural Integrity		
[34]	- N95 respirators placed inside Medela Quick CleanTM MICRO-STEAMTM BAGS - Steam bags were placed inside Sharp Model R-305KS (2450 MHz, 1100 W) microwave oven	90	- Log reduction of ≥3 in viable MS2 - Filtration efficiency preserved after 1 cycle - Mask model: 3M 1860 and 3M 8210
[35]	- 1150 W and 1100 W microwave oven used - 1st set up: N95 respirator placed on mesh over mug containing water - 2nd set up: N95 respirator placed on mesh over glass container containing water	180	- Log reduction of ≥4 in viable MS2 with one cycle - Fit, seal, and filtration preserved up to 20 cycles - Mask model: 3M 1860
[52]	- Household microwave oven (Wave 300, 400 W) was used - FFR circular samples were placed on a plastic Petri dish	4–6 (Multiple specified cycles)	- Log reduction of >4 in *E. coli* and *B. subtilis* at 10 and 20 min of exposure - Filtration efficiency maintained - Mask model: UVEX FFP2

6.5. Ethanol

Ethanol-based disinfection is used widely around the world as an effective decontamination method. However, ethanol-based treatment does not produce an efficient result in the decontamination of N95 respirators. Ethanol is known to degrade the structure of the mask's filtration and thus affects the integrity and performance of treated N95 respirators. The system specifications and outcomes of studies related to ethanol-based N95 decontamination are listed in Table 8.

Table 8. Ethanol-based decontamination system specifications and outcomes.

Study	Concentration Used	Exposure Time (h)	Outcome
	Reduction in Pathogen Load (Various Pathogens)		
[45]	- 70% ethanol was sprayed 10 times on the mask exterior and 5 times on the interior - Placed in a sealed plastic bag overnight	Air drying: ~8	- No detection of viable SARS-CoV-2 RNA - Mask model: 3M 1860
[52]	- Samples were immersed in 75% ethanol for 2 min	Depends on air drying time	- Complete inactivation of *E. coli* and *B. subtilis* - Mask model: UVEX FFP2
	Performance or Structural Integrity		
[37]	- Samples were immersed in 75% ethanol	Depends on air drying time	- Significant decrease in filtration efficiency (56.33 ± 3.03%) - Mask model: 3M 8210
[45]	-70% ethanol was sprayed 10 times on the mask exterior and 5 times on the interior - Placed in a sealed plastic bag overnight	Air drying: ~8	- Mask integrity was significantly impaired - Average fit score: ≥100 - Mask model: 3M 1860
[52]	- Samples were immersed in 75% ethanol for 2 min	Depends on air drying time	- Significant decrease in filtration efficiency - Mask model: UVEX FFP2
[80]	- Approximately 50 mL of 70% ethanol solution was poured over each mask	Air drying: 2–3	- Filtration efficiency of the mask dropped by 20–30% - It was also noted that 99% of their initial filtration efficiency was restored after vacuum drying - Mask model: 3M 8200, 3M 8210, and 3M 8511

7. Effectiveness of Decontamination Systems against SARS-CoV-2

The effectiveness of a specific decontamination system depends on critical parameters such as the exposure time. UVGI and HPV were investigated further in this review on their effectiveness against SARS-CoV-2, specifically from the surfaces of N95 respirators. The relationship between parameter control and effectiveness against the SARS-CoV-2 virus is illustrated in Figures 3 and 4.

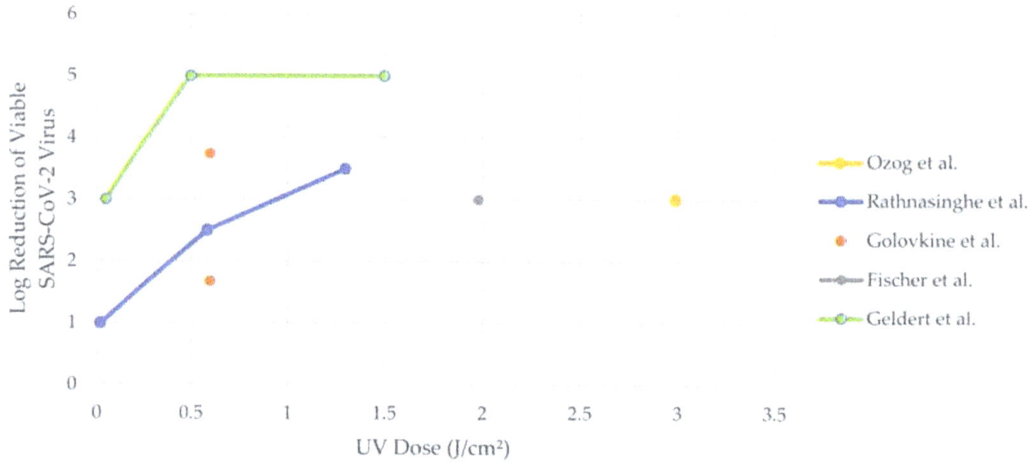

Figure 3. Log reduction of viable SARS-CoV-2 virus with increasing UV dose (data represented in Figure 3 exhibit minimum log reduction achieved by specific dosage as upon reaching the limit of detection (LOD)—real data are not quantifiable).

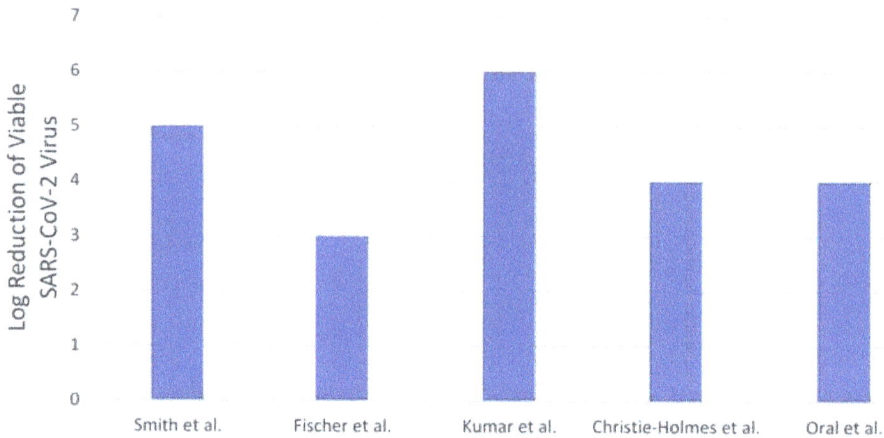

Figure 4. Log reduction of viable SARS-CoV-2 virus with various HPV-based decontamination settings (data represented in Figure 4 exhibit minimum log reduction achieved by specific dosage as upon reaching the limit of detection (LOD)—real data are not quantifiable).

7.1. *Ultraviolet Germicidal Irradiation*

In a study, Ozog et al. [20] had demonstrated successful decontamination when an N95 mask was irradiated with 1.5 J/cm^2 of UVC (254nm). It was concluded that the dose applied was sufficient. However, a concern on the disinfection of the strap arises due to its coverage by UVC on the strap surface. Rathnasinghe et al. [43] presented a simple UVC decontamination device without the mask's strap decontamination. Golovkine et al. [44],

Smith et al. [45], Fischer et al. [46], and Geldert et al. [47] investigated and compared the efficiency of UVC-based decontamination systems for N95 respirators with other decontamination methods such as ethanol, heat, UVA, ethylene oxide, hydrogen peroxide plasma and vapor, MGS, bleach, and liquid hydrogen peroxide. Comparing across the studies, a UVC-based N95 disinfection treatment with a dosage of greater than 0.5 J/cm^2 can achieve the minimum pathogen load reduction required of three-log reduction against the SARS-CoV-2 virus. As Figure 3 illustrates, Geldert et al. [47] demonstrated notable disinfection of five-log reduction at a relatively low dosage of 0.5 J/cm^2. Nevertheless, the reported sharp decline in the log reduction of SARS-CoV-2 [47] at lower UVC doses (0–0.5 J/cm^2) must be addressed with caution.

7.2. Hydrogen Peroxide Vapor (HPV)

Smith et al. [45], Fischer et al. [46], Kumar et al. [58], Christie-Holmes et al. [59], and Oral et al. [60] have investigated the efficiency of HPV-based decontamination systems for N95 respirators against the SARS-CoV-2 virus. All the studies that reported HPV-based decontamination against the SARS-CoV-2 virus were designed using commercially available HPV generating machines. The comparison of the HPV-based N95 decontamination system efficiency across the studies is presented in Figure 4. The concentration of hydrogen peroxide exposed and the treatment time of a complete cycle comprised of four different processes are the variables that play a significant part in HPV-based decontamination systems to deliver the required decontamination efficiency. Notably, Kumar et al. [58] demonstrated a significant reduction in SARS-CoV-2 of six-log reduction while preserving the functional integrity of the N95 respirator post-treatment.

8. Conclusions

The COVID-19 pandemic shows the severity of the needed supply of PPE for healthcare workers to stay protected at all times. Decontamination of PPE could be an essential measure to mitigate the immediate risk of running out of PPE supply. UVGI- and HPV-based decontamination systems exhibit great potential as a good choice for N95 respirator decontamination. The study indicated that the UVGI and HPV methods could be used to deactivate the SARS-CoV-2 virus without affecting the integrity of the respirator. The excellent virucidal activity of UVGI- and HPV-based decontamination systems suggested that they are good candidates for N95 respirator decontamination.

Author Contributions: Conceptualization, M.R.M., N.S.M.N., N.A.H., J.J., and V.C.W.H.; methodology, M.R.M., T.G., and R.'A.M.Y.; software, R.'A.M.Y.; validation, M.R.M., N.S.M.N., N.A.H., J.J., and V.C.W.H.; formal analysis, T.G.; investigation, T.G.; resources, M.R.M., T.G., and R.'A.M.Y.; data curation, T.G.; writing—original draft preparation, T.G.; writing—review and editing, T.G. and R.'A.M.Y.; visualization, M.R.M. and T.G.; supervision, M.R.M.; project administration, M.R.M.; funding acquisition, M.R.M. All authors have read and agreed to the published version of the manuscript.

Funding: This research was funded by AUN/SEED-Net, grant number UMSPRAC 2101.

Institutional Review Board Statement: Not applicable.

Informed Consent Statement: Not applicable.

Data Availability Statement: Data are contained within this article.

Acknowledgments: The authors would like to thank Mohd Fauzi Bakri Hashim for his assistance in this research project.

Conflicts of Interest: The authors declare no conflict of interest.

References

1. World Health Organization. *Coronavirus Disease 2019 (COVID-19): Situation Report, 94*; World Health Organization: Geneva, Switzerland, 2020.
2. World Health Organization. Shortage of Personal Protective Equipment Endangering Health Workers Worldwide. Available online: https://www.who.int/news/item/03-03-2020-shortage-of-personal-protective-equipment-endangering-health-workers-worldwide (accessed on 16 July 2021).
3. Degesys, N.F.; Wang, R.C.; Kwan, E.; Fahimi, J.; Noble, J.A.; Raven, M.C. Correlation Between N95 Extended Use and Reuse and Fit Failure in an Emergency Department. *JAMA* **2020**, *324*, 94–96. [CrossRef] [PubMed]
4. 3M. 3M™ Particulate Respirator, 8210, N95 Technical Specifications. Available online: https://multimedia.3m.com/mws/media/1425070O/3m-particulate-respirator-8210-n95-technical-specifications.pdf (accessed on 16 July 2021).
5. Gray, A. Exploring the Shortage of Affordable Masks in Developing Countries. Available online: https://www.borgenmagazine.com/affordable-masks/ (accessed on 6 September 2021).
6. Parshley, L. The Mask Shortage Is Forcing Health Workers to Disregard Basic Coronavirus Infection Control. Available online: https://www.vox.com/2020/4/3/21206726/coronavirus-masks-n95-hospitals-health-care-doctors-ppe-shortage (accessed on 6 September 2021).
7. Centers for Disease Control and Prevention. Implementing Filtering Facepiece Respirator (FFR) Reuse, Including Reuse after Decontamination, When There Are Known Shortages of N95 Respirators. Available online: https://www.cdc.gov/coronavirus/2019-ncov/hcp/ppe-strategy/decontamination-reuse-respirators.html (accessed on 16 July 2021).
8. Chen, Y.; Liu, Q.; Guo, D. Emerging coronaviruses: Genome structure, replication, and pathogenesis. *J. Med. Virol.* **2020**, *92*, 418–423. [CrossRef] [PubMed]
9. Shereen, M.A.; Khan, S.; Kazmi, A.; Bashir, N.; Siddique, R. COVID-19 infection: Emergence, transmission, and characteristics of human coronaviruses. *J. Adv. Res.* **2020**, *24*, 91–98. [CrossRef] [PubMed]
10. Zhang, Y.; Geng, X.; Tan, Y.; Li, Q.; Xu, C.; Xu, J.; Hao, L.; Zeng, Z.; Luo, X.; Liu, F.; et al. New understanding of the damage of SARS-CoV-2 infection outside the respiratory system. *Biomed. Pharmacother.* **2020**, *127*, 110195. [CrossRef]
11. Chin, A.W.H.; Chu, J.T.S.; Perera, M.R.A.; Hui, K.P.Y.; Yen, H.L.; Chan, M.C.W.; Peiris, M.; Poon, L.L.M. Stability of SARS-CoV-2 in different environmental conditions. *Lancet Microbe* **2020**, *1*, e10. [CrossRef]
12. Turtil, S. Sterility Review of 510(k) Submissions: Common Microbiology Issues Found in 510(k) Submissions. Available online: https://www.fda.gov/media/141277/download (accessed on 16 July 2021).
13. Scientific Animations Inc. 3D Medical Animation Corona Virus. Available online: https://commons.wikimedia.org/wiki/File:3D_medical_animation_corona_virus.jpg (accessed on 16 July 2021).
14. Centers for Disease Control and Prevention (CDC); National Institute for Occupational Safety and Health. Understanding the Diffrence. Available online: https://www.cdc.gov/niosh/npptl/pdfs/understanddifferenceinfographic-508.pdf (accessed on 16 July 2021).
15. Ji, D.; Fan, L.; Li, X.; Ramakrishna, S. Addressing the worldwide shortages of face masks. *BMC Mater.* **2020**, *2*, 9. [CrossRef]
16. O'Kelly, E.; Arora, A.; Pirog, S.; Ward, J.; Clarkson, P.J. Comparing the fit of N95, KN95, surgical, and cloth face masks and assessing the accuracy of fit checking. *PLoS ONE* **2021**, *16*, e0245688. [CrossRef]
17. Henneberry, B. How to Make N95 Masks. Available online: https://www.thomasnet.com/articles/plant-facility-equipment/how-to-make-n95-masks/#_How_are_N95 (accessed on 16 July 2021).
18. Huber, T.; Goldman, O.; Epstein, A.; Stella, G.; Sakmar, T. Principles and practice of SARS-CoV-2 decontamination of N95 masks with UV-C. *Biophys. J.* **2020**, *120*, 2927–2942. [CrossRef]
19. U.S. Food Drug Administration. UV Lights and Lamps: Ultraviolet-C Radiation, Disinfection, and Coronavirus. Available online: https://www.fda.gov/medical-devices/coronavirus-covid-19-and-medical-devices/uv-lights-and-lamps-ultraviolet-c-radiation-disinfection-and-coronavirus (accessed on 16 July 2021).
20. Ozog, D.M.; Sexton, J.Z.; Narla, S.; Pretto-Kernahan, C.D.; Mirabelli, C.; Lim, H.W.; Hamzavi, I.H.; Tibbetts, R.J.; Mi, Q.S. The effect of ultraviolet C radiation against different N95 respirators inoculated with SARS-CoV-2. *Int. J. Infect. Dis.* **2020**, *100*, 224–229. [CrossRef]
21. Vo, E.; Rengasamy, S.; Shaffer, R. Development of a test system to evaluate procedures for decontamination of respirators containing viral droplets. *Appl. Environ. Microbiol.* **2009**, *75*, 7303–7309. [CrossRef]
22. Lindsley, W.G.; Martin, S.B., Jr.; Thewlis, R.E.; Sarkisian, K.; Nwoko, J.O.; Mead, K.R.; Noti, J.D. Effects of Ultraviolet Germicidal Irradiation (UVGI) on N95 Respirator Filtration Performance and Structural Integrity. *J. Occup. Environ. Hyg.* **2015**, *12*, 509–517. [CrossRef] [PubMed]
23. Ozog, D.; Parks-Miller, A.; Kohli, I.; Lyons, A.B.; Narla, S.; Torres, A.E.; Levesque, M.; Lim, H.W.; Hamzavi, I.H. The importance of fit testing in decontamination of N95 respirators: A cautionary note. *J. Am. Acad. Dermatol.* **2020**, *83*, 672–674. [CrossRef] [PubMed]
24. Sciences, S.L. The Advantages of Decontaminating with Vapor Phase Hydrogen Peroxide. Available online: https://www.sterislifesciences.com/resources/documents/technical-tips/the-advantages-of-decontaminating-with-vapor-phase-hydrogen-peroxide (accessed on 16 July 2021).

25. Saini, V.; Sikri, K.; Batra, S.D.; Kalra, P.; Gautam, K. Development of a highly effective low-cost vaporized hydrogen peroxide-based method for disinfection of personal protective equipment for their selective reuse during pandemics. *Gut Pathog.* **2020**, *12*, 29. [CrossRef] [PubMed]
26. Jatta, M.; Kiefer, C.; Patolia, H.; Pan, J.; Harb, C.; Marr, L.C.; Baffoe-Bonnie, A. N95 reprocessing by low temperature sterilization with 59% vaporized hydrogen peroxide during the 2020 COVID-19 pandemic. *Am. J. Infect. Control* **2021**, *49*, 8–14. [CrossRef]
27. Lore, M.B.; Heimbuch, B.K.; Brown, T.L.; Wander, J.D.; Hinrichs, S.H. Effectiveness of three decontamination treatments against influenza virus applied to filtering facepiece respirators. *Ann. Occup. Hyg.* **2012**, *56*, 92–101. [CrossRef]
28. Rockey, N.; Arts, P.J.; Li, L.; Harrison, K.R.; Langenfeld, K.; Fitzsimmons, W.J.; Lauring, A.S.; Love, N.G.; Kaye, K.S.; Raskin, L.; et al. Humidity and Deposition Solution Play a Critical Role in Virus Inactivation by Heat Treatment of N95 Respirators. *mSphere* **2020**, *5*. [CrossRef]
29. Bopp, N.; Bouyer, D.; Gibbs, C.; Nichols, J.; Ntiforo, C.; Grimaldo, M. Multicycle Autoclave Decontamination of N95 Filtering Facepiece Respirators. *Appl. Biosaf.* **2020**, *25*, 150–156. [CrossRef]
30. Anderegg, L.; Meisenhelder, C.; Ngooi, C.O.; Liao, L.; Xiao, W.; Chu, S.; Cui, Y.; Doyle, J.M. A scalable method of applying heat and humidity for decontamination of N95 respirators during the COVID-19 crisis. *PLoS ONE* **2020**, *15*, e0234851. [CrossRef]
31. Xiang, Y.; Song, Q.; Gu, W. Decontamination of surgical face masks and N95 respirators by dry heat pasteurization for one hour at 70 °C. *Am. J. Infect. Control* **2020**, *48*, 880–882. [CrossRef]
32. Pascoe, M.J.; Robertson, A.; Crayford, A.; Durand, E.; Steer, J.; Castelli, A.; Wesgate, R.; Evans, S.L.; Porch, A.; Maillard, J.Y. Dry heat and microwave-generated steam protocols for the rapid decontamination of respiratory personal protective equipment in response to COVID-19-related shortages. *J. Hosp. Infect.* **2020**, *106*, 10–19. [CrossRef]
33. Viscusi, D.; King, W.P.; Shaffer, R. Effect of Decontamination on the Filtration Efficiency of Two Filtering Facepiece Respirator Models. *J. Int. Soc. Respir. Prot.* **2007**, *24*, 93.
34. Fisher, E.M.; Williams, J.L.; Shaffer, R.E. Evaluation of microwave steam bags for the decontamination of filtering facepiece respirators. *PLoS ONE* **2011**, *6*, e18585. [CrossRef] [PubMed]
35. Zulauf, K.E.; Green, A.B.; Nguyen Ba, A.N.; Jagdish, T.; Reif, D.; Seeley, R.; Dale, A.; Kirby, J.E. Microwave-Generated Steam Decontamination of N95 Respirators Utilizing Universally Accessible Materials. *mBio* **2020**, *11*. [CrossRef] [PubMed]
36. Centers for Disease Control and Prevention. Chemical Disinfectants. Available online: https://www.cdc.gov/infectioncontrol/guidelines/disinfection/disinfection-methods/chemical.html (accessed on 16 July 2021).
37. Liao, L.; Xiao, W.; Zhao, M.; Yu, X.; Wang, H.; Wang, Q.; Chu, S.; Cui, Y. Can N95 Respirators Be Reused after Disinfection? How Many Times? *ACS Nano* **2020**, *14*, 6348–6356. [CrossRef] [PubMed]
38. Lendvay, T.S.; Chen, J.; Harcourt, B.H.; Scholte, F.E.M.; Lin, Y.L.; Kilinc-Balci, F.S.; Lamb, M.M.; Homdayjanakul, K.; Cui, Y.; Price, A.; et al. Addressing personal protective equipment (PPE) decontamination: Methylene blue and light inactivates severe acute respiratory coronavirus virus 2 (SARS-CoV-2) on N95 respirators and medical masks with maintenance of integrity and fit. *Infect. Control. Hosp. Epidemiol.* **2021**, 1–10. [CrossRef]
39. The NYC Health Department. COVID-19: Potential Decontamination Strategies for N95 Respirators. Available online: https://www1.nyc.gov/assets/doh/downloads/pdf/imm/n95-decontamination-strategies.pdf (accessed on 12 October 2021).
40. Heimbuch, B.K.; Kinney, K.; Lumley, A.E.; Harnish, D.A.; Bergman, M.; Wander, J.D. Cleaning of filtering facepiece respirators contaminated with mucin and Staphylococcus aureus. *Am. J. Infect. Control* **2014**, *42*, 265–270. [CrossRef]
41. Mills, D.; Harnish, D.A.; Lawrence, C.; Sandoval-Powers, M.; Heimbuch, B.K. Ultraviolet germicidal irradiation of influenza-contaminated N95 filtering facepiece respirators. *Am. J. Infect. Control* **2018**, *46*, e49–e55. [CrossRef]
42. Simmons, S.E.; Carrion, R.; Alfson, K.J.; Staples, H.M.; Jinadatha, C.; Jarvis, W.R.; Sampathkumar, P.; Chemaly, R.F.; Khawaja, F.; Povroznik, M.; et al. Deactivation of SARS-CoV-2 with pulsed-xenon ultraviolet light: Implications for environmental COVID-19 control. *Infect. Control. Hosp. Epidemiol.* **2021**, *42*, 127–130. [CrossRef]
43. Rathnasinghe, R.; Karlicek, R.F.; Schotsaert, M.; Koffas, M.A.; Arduini, B.; Jangra, S.; Wang, B.; Davis, J.L.; Alnaggar, M.; Costa, A.; et al. Scalable, effective, and rapid decontamination of SARS-CoV-2 contaminated N95 respirators using germicidal ultra-violet C (UVC) irradiation device. *medRxiv* **2020**. [CrossRef]
44. Golovkine, G.R.; Roberts, A.W.; Cooper, C.; Riano, S.; DiCiccio, A.M.; Worthington, D.L.; Clarkson, J.P.; Krames, M.; Zhang, J.; Gao, Y.; et al. Practical considerations for Ultraviolet-C radiation mediated decontamination of N95 respirator against SARS-CoV-2 virus. *PLoS ONE* **2021**, *16*, e0258336. [CrossRef]
45. Smith, J.S.; Hanseler, H.; Welle, J.; Rattray, R.; Campbell, M.; Brotherton, T.; Moudgil, T.; Pack, T.F.; Wegmann, K.; Jensen, S.; et al. Effect of various decontamination procedures on disposable N95 mask integrity and SARS-CoV-2 infectivity. *J. Clin. Transl. Sci.* **2020**, *5*, e10. [CrossRef] [PubMed]
46. Fischer, R.J.; Morris, D.H.; van Doremalen, N.; Sarchette, S.; Matson, M.J.; Bushmaker, T.; Yinda, C.K.; Seifert, S.N.; Gamble, A.; Williamson, B.N.; et al. Assessment of N95 respirator decontamination and re-use for SARS-CoV-2. *medRxiv* **2020**. [CrossRef]
47. Geldert, A.; Su, A.; Roberts, A.W.; Golovkine, G.; Grist, S.M.; Stanley, S.A.; Herr, A.E. Nonuniform UV-C dose across N95 facepieces can cause 2.9-log variation in SARS-CoV-2 inactivation. *medRxiv* **2021**. [CrossRef]
48. Weaver, D.T.; McElvany, B.D.; Gopalakrishnan, V.; Card, K.J.; Crozier, D.; Dhawan, A.; Dinh, M.N.; Dolson, E.; Farrokhian, N.; Hitomi, M.; et al. UV decontamination of personal protective equipment with idle laboratory biosafety cabinets during the COVID-19 pandemic. *PLoS ONE* **2021**, *16*, e0241734. [CrossRef]

49. Ludwig-Begall, L.F.; Wielick, C.; Jolois, O.; Dams, L.; Razafimahefa, R.M.; Nauwynck, H.; Demeuldre, P.-F.; Napp, A.; Laperre, J.; Thiry, E.; et al. "Don, doff, discard" to "don, doff, decontaminate"—FFR and mask integrity and inactivation of a SARS-CoV-2 surrogate and a norovirus following multiple vaporised hydrogen peroxide-, ultraviolet germicidal irradiation-, and dry heat decontaminations. *PLoS ONE* **2021**, *16*, e0251872. [CrossRef]
50. Kayani, B.J.; Weaver, D.T.; Gopalakrishnan, V.; King, E.S.; Dolson, E.; Krishnan, N.; Pelesko, J.; Scott, M.J.; Hitomi, M.; Cadnum, J.L.; et al. UV-C tower for point-of-care decontamination of filtering facepiece respirators. *Am. J. Infect. Control* **2021**, *49*, 424–429. [CrossRef]
51. Fisher, E.M.; Shaffer, R.E. A method to determine the available UV-C dose for the decontamination of filtering facepiece respirators. *J. Appl. Microbiol.* **2011**, *110*, 287–295. [CrossRef]
52. He, W.; Guo, Y.; Gao, H.; Liu, J.; Yue, Y.; Wang, J. Evaluation of Regeneration Processes for Filtering Facepiece Respirators in Terms of the Bacteria Inactivation Efficiency and Influences on Filtration Performance. *ACS Nano* **2020**, *14*, 13161–13171. [CrossRef]
53. Wigginton, K.R.; Arts, P.J.; Clack, H.L.; Fitzsimmons, W.J.; Gamba, M.; Harrison, K.R.; LeBar, W.; Lauring, A.S.; Li, L.; Roberts, W.W.; et al. Validation of N95 Filtering Facepiece Respirator Decontamination Methods Available at a Large University Hospital. *Open Forum Infect. Dis.* **2021**, *8*, ofaa610. [CrossRef]
54. Lin, T.H.; Tang, F.C.; Hung, P.C.; Hua, Z.C.; Lai, C.Y. Relative survival of Bacillus subtilis spores loaded on filtering facepiece respirators after five decontamination methods. *Indoor Air* **2018**, *28*, 754–762. [CrossRef]
55. Chen, P.Z.; Ngan, A.; Manson, N.; Maynes, J.T.; Borschel, G.H.; Rotstein, O.D.; Gu, F.X. Transmission of aerosols through pristine and reprocessed N95 respirators. *medRxiv* **2020**. [CrossRef]
56. Ou, Q.; Pei, C.; Chan Kim, S.; Abell, E.; Pui, D.Y.H. Evaluation of decontamination methods for commercial and alternative respirator and mask materials—View from filtration aspect. *J. Aerosol Sci.* **2020**, *150*, 105609. [CrossRef]
57. Ontiveros, C.C.; Sweeney, C.L.; Smith, C.; MacIsaac, S.; Bennett, J.L.; Munoz, S.; Stoddart, A.K.; Gagnon, G.A. Assessing the impact of multiple ultraviolet disinfection cycles on N95 filtering facepiece respirator integrity. *Sci. Rep.* **2021**, *11*, 12279. [CrossRef]
58. Kumar, A.; Kasloff, S.B.; Leung, A.; Cutts, T.; Strong, J.E.; Hills, K.; Vazquez-Grande, G.; Rush, B.; Lother, S.; Zarychanski, R.; et al. N95 Mask Decontamination using Standard Hospital Sterilization Technologies. *medRxiv* **2020**. [CrossRef]
59. Christie-Holmes, N.; Tyli, R.; Budylowski, P.; Guvenc, F.; Weiner, A.; Poon, B.; Speck, M.; Naugler, S.; Rainville, A.; Ghalami, A.; et al. Vapourized hydrogen peroxide decontamination in a hospital setting inactivates SARS-CoV-2 and HCoV-229E without compromising filtration efficiency of unexpired N95 respirators. *Am. J. Infect. Control* **2021**, *49*, 1227–1231. [CrossRef]
60. Oral, E.; Wannomae, K.K.; Connolly, R.; Gardecki, J.; Leung, H.M.; Muratoglu, O.; Griffiths, A.; Honko, A.N.; Avena, L.E.; McKay, L.G.A.; et al. Vapor H2O2 sterilization as a decontamination method for the reuse of N95 respirators in the COVID-19 emergency. *medRxiv* **2020**. [CrossRef]
61. Dave, N.; Pascavis, K.S.; Patterson, J.; Wallace, D.; Chowdhury, A.; Abbaszadegan, M.; Alum, A.; Herckes, P.; Zhang, Z.; Kozicki, M.; et al. Characterization of a novel, low-cost, scalable vaporized hydrogen peroxide system for sterilization of N95 respirators and other COVID-19 related personal protective equipment. *medRxiv* **2020**. [CrossRef]
62. Moschella, P.; Liao, W.; Litwin, A.; Foulk, J.; Anthony, J.; Player, M.; Chang, J.; Cole, C. Repeated vaporised hydrogen peroxide disinfection of 3M 1860 N95 mask respirators does not degrade quantitative fit performance. *Br. J. Anaesth.* **2021**, *126*, e125–e127. [CrossRef] [PubMed]
63. Russo, R.; Levine, C.; Grady, C.; Peixoto, B.; McCormick-Ell, J.; Block, T.; Gresko, A.; Delmas, G.; Chitale, P.; Frees, A.; et al. Decontaminating N95 respirators during the COVID-19 pandemic: Simple and practical approaches to increase decontamination capacity, speed, safety and ease of use. *J. Hosp. Infect.* **2021**, *109*, 52–57. [CrossRef]
64. Al-Hadyan, K.; Alsbeih, G.; Nobah, A.; Lindstrom, J.; Falatah, S.; Faran, N.; Al-Ghamdi, S.; Moftah, B.; Alhmaid, R. In-House Filtration Efficiency Assessment of Vapor Hydrogen Peroxide Decontaminated Filtering Facepiece Respirators (FFRs). *Int. J. Environ. Res. Public Health* **2021**, *18*, 7169. [CrossRef] [PubMed]
65. Levine, C.; Grady, C.; Block, T.; Hurley, H.; Russo, R.; Peixoto, B.; Frees, A.; Ruiz, A.; Alland, D. Use, re-use or discard? Quantitatively defined variance in the functional integrity of N95 respirators following vaporized hydrogen peroxide decontamination during the COVID-19 pandemic. *J. Hosp. Infect.* **2021**, *107*, 50–56. [CrossRef]
66. Lieu, A.; Mah, J.; Zanichelli, V.; Exantus, R.C.; Longtin, Y. Impact of extended use and decontamination with vaporized hydrogen peroxide on N95 respirator fit. *Am. J. Infect. Control* **2020**, *48*, 1457–1461. [CrossRef]
67. Beam, E.; Nesbitt, J.C.; Austin, M.D.; Ramar, K. Effect of vaporized hydrogen peroxide reprocessing on N95 respirators. *Infect. Control. Hosp. Epidemiol.* **2021**, *42*, 907–908. [CrossRef] [PubMed]
68. Veronique Greenwood; Quanta Magazine. Why Does Heat Kill Cells? Available online: https://www.theatlantic.com/science/archive/2017/05/heat-kills-cells/526377/ (accessed on 16 July 2021).
69. Kumar, A.; Kasloff, S.B.; Cutts, T.; Leung, A.; Sharma, N.; Vazquez-Grande, G.; Drew, T.; Laframboise, D.; Orofino, O.; Tanelli, J.; et al. Standard hospital blanket warming cabinets can be utilized for complete moist heat SARS-CoV2 inactivation of contaminated N95 masks for re-use. *Sci. Rep.* **2021**, *11*, 18316. [CrossRef] [PubMed]
70. Choi, Y.W.; Richardson, A.W.; Sunderman, M.; Mladineo, M.J.; Keyes, P.H.; Hofacre, K.C.; Middleton, J.K. Decontamination of SARS-CoV-2 contaminated N95 filtering facepiece respirators (FFRs) with moist heat generated by a multicooker. *Lett. Appl. Microbiol.* **2021**, *72*, 366–374. [CrossRef] [PubMed]

71. Oral, E.; Wannomae, K.K.; Gil, D.; Connolly, R.; Gardecki, J.A.; Leung, H.M.; Muratoglu, O.K.; Tsurumi, A.; Rahme, L.; Jaber, T.; et al. Efficacy of moist heat decontamination against various pathogens for the reuse of N95 respirators in the COVID-19 emergency. *medRxiv* **2020**. [CrossRef]
72. Daeschler, S.C.; Manson, N.; Joachim, K.; Chin, A.W.H.; Chan, K.; Chen, P.Z.; Tajdaran, K.; Mirmoeini, K.; Zhang, J.J.; Maynes, J.T.; et al. Effect of moist heat reprocessing of N95 respirators on SARS-CoV-2 inactivation and respirator function. *CMAJ* **2020**, *192*, E1189–E1197. [CrossRef]
73. Harskamp, R.E.; van Straten, B.; Bouman, J.; van Maltha-van Santvoort, B.; van den Dobbelsteen, J.J.; van der Sijp, J.R.; Horeman, T. Reprocessing filtering facepiece respirators in primary care using medical autoclave: Prospective, bench-to-bedside, single-centre study. *BMJ Open* **2020**, *10*, e039454. [CrossRef]
74. Czubryt, M.P.; Stecy, T.; Popke, E.; Aitken, R.; Jabusch, K.; Pound, R.; Lawes, P.; Ramjiawan, B.; Pierce, G.N. N95 mask reuse in a major urban hospital: COVID-19 response process and procedure. *J. Hosp. Infect.* **2020**, *106*, 277–282. [CrossRef]
75. Benboubker, M.; Oumokhtar, B.; Hmami, F.; Mabrouk, K.E.; Alami, L.E.; Arhoune, B.; Belahsen, M.F.; Aboutajeddine, A. Covid-19 respiratory protection: The filtration efficiency assessment of decontaminated FFP2 masks responding to associated shortages. *medRxiv* **2021**. [CrossRef]
76. Doshi, S.; Banavar, S.P.; Flaum, E.; Kulkarni, S.; Kumar, S.; Chen, T.; Bhattacharya, A.; Prakash, M. Applying Heat and Humidity using Stove Boiled Water for Decontamination of N95 Respirators in Low Resource Settings. *medRxiv* **2020**. [CrossRef] [PubMed]
77. Perkins, D.J.; Nofchissey, R.A.; Ye, C.; Donart, N.; Kell, A.; Foo-Hurwitz, I.; Muller, T.; Bradfute, S.B. COVID-19 global pandemic planning: Dry heat incubation and ambient temperature fail to consistently inactivate SARS-CoV-2 on N95 respirators. *Exp. Biol. Med.* **2021**, *246*, 952–959. [CrossRef]
78. Price, A.; Cui, Y.; Liao, L.; Xiao, W.; Yu, X.; Wang, H.; Zhao, M.; Wang, Q.; Chu, S.; Chu, L. Is the fit of N95 facial masks effected by disinfection? A study of heat and UV disinfection methods using the OSHA protocol fit test. *medRxiv* **2020**. [CrossRef]
79. Loh, M.; Clark, R.; Cherrie, J. Heat treatment for reuse of disposable respirators during Covid-19 pandemic: Is filtration and fit adversely affected? *medRxiv* **2020**. [CrossRef]
80. Nazeeri, A.I.; Hilburn, I.A.; Wu, D.-A.; Mohammed, K.A.; Badal, D.Y.; Chan, M.H.W.; Kirschvink, J.L. Ethanol-Drying Regeneration of N95 Respirators. *medRxiv* **2020**. [CrossRef]

sustainability

MDPI

Article

Civilian-Military Collaboration before and during COVID-19 Pandemic—A Systematic Review and a Pilot Survey among Practitioners

Amir Khorram-Manesh [1,2,*], Luc J. Mortelmans [3,4], Yohan Robinson [1,2], Frederick M. Burkle [5] and Krzysztof Goniewicz [6,*]

1 Institute of Clinical Sciences, Sahlgrenska Academy, Gothenburg University, 413 45 Gothenburg, Sweden; yohan.robinson@gu.se
2 Department of Research and Development, Armed Forces Center for Defense Medicine, 426 76 Västra Frölunda, Sweden
3 Center for Research and Education in Emergency Care, University of Leuven, 3000 Leuven, Belgium; luc.mortelmans@zna.be
4 Regedim, VUB, Brussels and Department of Emergency Medicine, ZNA, Stuivenberg, 2060 Antwerp, Belgium
5 Harvard Humanitarian Initiative, T.H. Chan School of Public Health, Harvard University, Boston, MA 02115, USA; skipmd77@aol.com
6 Department of Security, Military University of Aviation, 08-521 Dęblin, Poland
* Correspondence: amir.khorram-manesh@surgery.gu.se (A.K.-M.); k.goniewicz@law.mil.pl (K.G.)

Abstract: Due to the similarity in skills and assets, Civilian-Military collaboration has emerged as one of the most reliable partnerships during the disaster and public health emergency management to address all necessary elements of surge capacity, i.e., staff, stuff, structure (space), and systems. This study aimed to evaluate this collaboration before and during the coronavirus 2019 pandemic. The outcomes of the systematic review revealed several published reports on successful civilian-military collaboration and proposed a need for further improvement. One hundred sixty-six individuals from 19 countries responded to nine questions, included in an online survey with the possibility to leave comments if necessary. The questionnaire referred to elements such as command and control, safety, communication, assessment, triage, treatment, and transport, as the crucial components of emergency management. The comprehensive examination of the survey results together with registered comments revealed a possible improvement in collaboration particularly on the strategic levels, i.e., meetings at the command-and-control level, safety, communication, and networking issues. While logistic collaboration seemed to be unchanged, the practical parts of the collaboration, i.e., clinical and non-clinical operational partnership (Triage and Treatment), mutual education, training, and operational understanding of each organization remained unchanged. In conclusion, although the current pandemic may have facilitated a more intense collaboration between civilian and military healthcare organizations, it lacks practical partnership and operative engagement, representing two crucial elements necessary for harmony and compatibility of both systems. Such collaboration may require a political will and perhaps a mutual civilian-military authority.

Keywords: civilian-military collaboration; interagency partnership; pandemic; public health

Citation: Khorram-Manesh, A.; Mortelmans, L.J.; Robinson, Y.; Burkle, F.M.; Goniewicz, K. Civilian-Military Collaboration before and during COVID-19 Pandemic—A Systematic Review and a Pilot Survey among Practitioners. *Sustainability* **2022**, *14*, 624. https://doi.org/10.3390/su14020624

Academic Editors: John Rennie Short and Marc A. Rosen

Received: 12 November 2021
Accepted: 5 January 2022
Published: 6 January 2022

Publisher's Note: MDPI stays neutral with regard to jurisdictional claims in published maps and institutional affiliations.

1. Introduction

Multiagency collaboration (MC) is universally accepted as an important part of the management of disasters and public health emergencies [1–5]. Among various factors influencing MC, leadership and communication are seemingly the most crucial [3–5]. While experience and transparent leaderships govern the functional relationships and the clarity of the roles between various partners, insufficient leaderships create significant challenges to MC and influence the trust, understanding, and mutual respect between the agencies [6–9]. Moreover, good inter-and intra-organizational communication facilitates a successful collaboration, although requiring adequate resourcing and financial assets to achieve the established goals [2,4,5].

Inter-organizational collaboration is a situation-dependent complex process with diversified scope, and structure, thus yielding different understandings, interpretations, and outcomes. Distinctions may arise when two organizations experience diverse responsibilities, autonomy, legacy, organizational framework, and authority structure [10,11]. Consequently, even well-formulated collaboration may fail to achieve its expected outcomes due to several factors, such as asymmetrical structures, and requires continuous supervision and cultivation [12–14].

1.1. Theoretical Framework

The collaboration aims at bringing two independent organizations together in a new structure, where they share the same commitments to conduct the same planning and mission to achieve the same outcomes, and ultimately produce or create something unique [11,13,14]. According to Vangen and Huxham [15], a successful collaboration consists of five perspectives:

1. Substantive outcomes (e.g., better use of funds and resources, increase in awareness)
2. High productivity
3. Emergent milestones (e.g., mutual and united targets, joint events, and considering each other's interests)
4. Recognizing and valuing their partnership
5. Creating individual and organizational pride to highlight their collaborative success and compatible organizational culture.

These perspectives are necessary for a successful relationship between two organizations and influence their aims, working processes, communication, trust, and accountability [16–18]. Considering these perspectives in civilian-military relations, Shanks Kaurin [19], proposes that the outcome will create five diverse situations when civilian-military populations:

1. Share values but have conflicting understanding.
2. Share values but have different priorities.
3. Share the process without sharing values.
4. Have no shared substantive or procedural values at all.
5. Are indifferent towards the outcomes of their actions.

Within healthcare, one way to measure the outcomes of collaboration is to use the acronym CSCATTT used in MIMMS (Major Incident Medical Management and Support) courses [20]. CSCATTT stands for C: Command and control; S: Safety; C: Communication; A: Assessment; T: Triage; T: Treatment; and T: Transport. These factors illustrate medical and non-medical aspects of disaster and emergency management and should be included in healthcare planning and response and synchronized with other organizations, such as the military healthcare, in collaboration to achieve a fruitful outcome.

Applying the described theoretical framework to the elements of CSCATTT may facilitate a unique opportunity to measure and evaluate changes in disaster and emergency management processes over time.

1.2. Civilian-Military Collaboration in Healthcare

Historically, Civilian-Military Collaboration (CMC) has connected both agencies in various areas, e.g., the pyrotechnics industry and clinical practice, but a formalized collaboration started in educational sectors when military staff established academic carriers in civilian universities [20–24]. Nowadays, an increasing number of public health emergencies, armed conflicts, and disasters, together with the global financial awareness and healthcare-related technological developments, have enforced new constraints on the healthcare sector, necessitating a new round of CMC collaboration in healthcare [5,25–27]. Lessons learned indicate that CMC should become compatible in both medical and non-medical aspects to achieve desired results [3,4,28–32]. Medical factors that influence the outcomes of CMC include differences in triage systems, treatment and intervention alternatives, and logistics for patients' evacuation, while non-medical factors encompass differences in command and control and leadership, security, situation assessment, communication, information-sharing, and reporting systems [3,4,33,34]. These aspects are included in CSCATTT as essential elements of emergency management.

The coronavirus 2019 (COVID-19), as well as several others incidents, has resulted in several societal changes and revealed weaknesses and strengths of the current management system [27,35–37]. Political and economic-based decision-making has been one, affecting major public health decisions, preventing the crucial collaborative efforts in implementing public health strategies, and halting healthcare leaders from making unpopular but necessary public health decisions. The lack of proper communication has equally contributed to the failure in achieving the established goal, the inability of information sharing, and disrespect for medical decisions [36–43]. However, this pandemic has also provided a good opportunity to evaluate and compare the current collaboration with that reported in the past [11,40–47]. An evaluation is particularly crucial since disasters and public health emergencies are increasingly impacted by cross-border factors that place increasing demands on society to initiate a broader dialogue of partnership [27,45–48]. Moreover, it is important to not only review experts' publications but also the opinions of the operational populations to identify potential gaps in outcomes and comprehension.

This article attempts to identify the status of CMC before and after the COVID-19 pandemic, based on the aforementioned theoretical background and using CSCATTT, in two steps:

(1) A systematic review of published literature aims at evaluating the status of CMC, presenting researchers' viewpoints.
(2) A survey among civilian and military staff to investigate the individuals' perception of CMC at the operational level, using CSCATTT.

2. Materials and Method

2.1. The Systematic Literature Review

A systematic literature review was conducted, using the following search engines; Science Direct, Scopus, PubMed, Web of Science, and Gothenburg University's online library, according to the PRISMA (Preferred Reporting Items for Systematic Reviews and Meta-Analyses) guidelines to evaluate the status of CMC (Figure 1) [49]. The quality of each included study was assessed using Health Evidence Quality Assessment Tool (Appendix A) [50].

Inclusion criteria: Original research studies published in English (1995–2021).

Exclusion criteria: Conference papers, abstracts, reports, non-scientific publications.

Search string: Civilian Military Collaboration AND/OR Civilian Military Partnership, separately or in combination. The terms "collaboration" and "partnership" were chosen based on the definition provided by the Oxford dictionary, ensuring the words were synonymous [51].

Two authors assessed all abstracts and titles independently to agree on included and excluded articles. Whenever disagreed, the third author was consulted. After achieving a mutual consensus, the full texts of the studies were reviewed. The reasons for all excluded papers were documented. For included studies, data regarding the name of authors, article title, year of publication, the title of the journal, the used methods, main results, and conclusions were all collected in Appendix B.

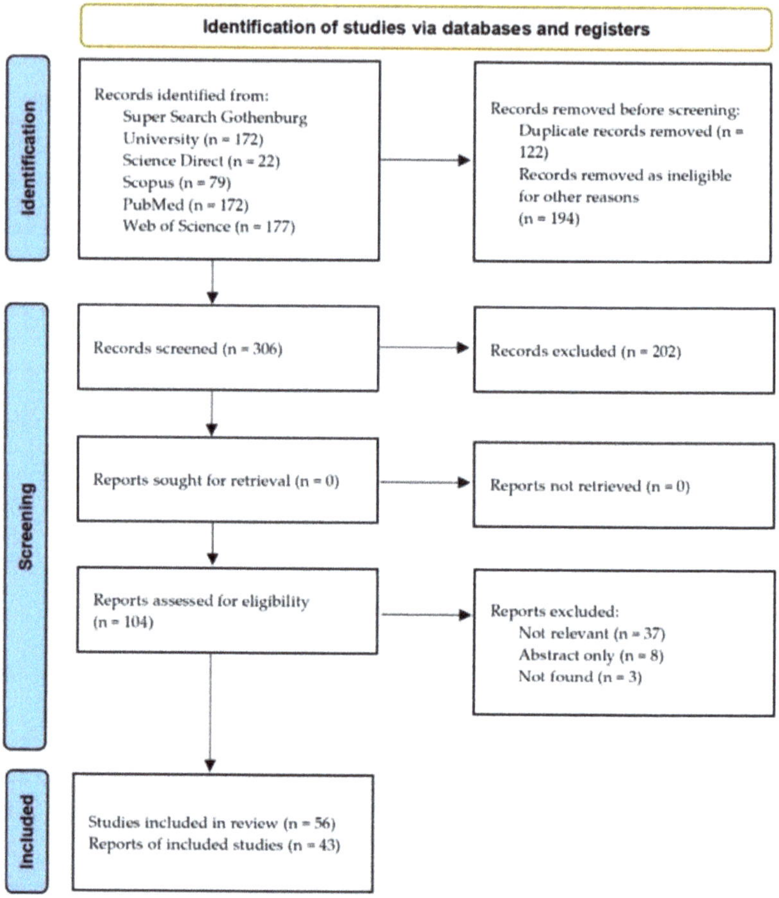

Figure 1. The process of literature selection according to PRISMA flow chart for new systematic reviews [49].

2.2. Questionnaire Preparation

The research group with experience from both civilian and military healthcare systems, formulated a questionnaire, consisting of eight questions, representing eight different dimensions, inspired by CSCATTT, i.e., Command and control, Safety, Communication, Assessment, Triage, Treatment, and Transport [20]. The tool identifies the leading strategic, tactical and operational parts of collaboration during emergencies [2,3,11]. Command and control encompassed three parts: administrative, practical, and mutual activities such as issuing directives and recommendations. The remaining five questions concerned safety and security issues, situational assessment, communication, medical issues, and logistics. The final questionnaire included free space to allow participants to include their comments (question 9). All authors reviewed, evaluated, and approved the questionnaire in consensus and based on a combination of clarity, logic, relevance, eligibility, comprehension, and usability. Each defined question could be answered by using a Likert scale, which was marked as 1 to 5, where 1 was defined as a weak collaboration and 5 a strong collaboration, before and during the COVID-19 pandemic (Appendix C).

2.3. Distribution of the Questionnaire

The research subject was introduced as a discussion topic on ResearchGate (RG), from 1 January to the end of May 2021. RG represents a European social networking site, engaging over 19 million scientists and researchers, being, the largest European academic network in terms of active users. The members of RG actively share papers, ask and answer questions voluntarily. They also find research collaborators [52]. Individuals interested in the topic could, after reading the purpose of the study, click on a link to a google document page and answer questions voluntarily (see "Ethical Considerations"). The use of the RG represents a so-called "virtual snowball sampling," method, which has been used in numerous studies [22,53–55]. The method helps to identify individuals of interest for this research, thus, allowing an increase in the representativeness of the results. It can also, increase the number of responses, is inexpensive, and decreases the sampling time. However, the sample selection is biased toward the characteristics of the online population like gender, age, education level, and socioeconomic belonging [53–55].

2.4. Ethical Considerations

The survey was anonymous, and all respondents agreed to participate voluntarily by clicking on the available link, where information about their participation and the purpose of the study was provided additionally. No name, affiliation, or other searchable information was registered. Confidentiality was strictly respected during data collection and obtained information was stored in a secure and safe area. The study complied with the ethical guidelines stipulated by Swedish law (SFS 2008:192). In Sweden, ethical approval is necessary if the research includes data regarding participants' race, ethnic heritage, political views, religion, sexual habits, or if it uses health or physical interventions or methods that aim to affect the person physically or psychologically (SFS 2003:460). Since this study did not include any of these aspects and all individuals freely contributed with their views on an available scientific site, it was exempt from ethics approval [22,55].

2.5. Statistics

Data were transferred to a spreadsheet, where the scores for each question before and under the COVID-19 pandemic were inserted. The mean and SD for each question before and during the pandemic was calculated, and the means were compared by using a *t*-test for the entire study cohort and each involved nation to obtain statistically significant changes, using a GraphPad Prism *t*-test calculator.

3. Results

3.1. Literature Review

The term, "Civilian-Military Collaboration", returned over 80,000 hits for all search engines. Using "Civilian-Military Collaboration" AND OR "Civilian-Military Partnership" in combination or separately resulted in a manageable number of references. Of the total 602 publications identified, 306 papers remained after removing duplicates and ineligible publications. These papers were sifted by looking at the abstracts, methods, and aims, and the eligible papers (n = 104), were studied in detail (Figure 1). Abstracts and non-relevant papers with no association to the main search key and case studies were removed. The final 43 papers were included and reported in Appendix B.

3.2. The Core Findings of the Review

There was a lack of consistency in defining civilian-military relations. While words such as coordination, cooperation, and collaboration were used interchangeably, the publication did not necessarily deal with collaboration. Furthermore, the majority of papers did not illustrate the view of practitioners, i.e., individuals who are operationally active in the field and were reviewed or presented the views of strategic level, researchers, or experts in the field.

Although several authors reported the importance of CM cooperation in diverse fields like technological area [7], others reported that such cooperation results in a dual capacity building, which can enhance the integration between CM organizations, creating dual capacity and resource availability as a valuable advantage in prolonged disaster and emergency management [31]. However, besides a considerable cost, such integration causes primarily some confusion regarding the role of each organization in a specific event or activity, including pandemics [6,23,30,45]. It is well recognized that CM collaboration has resulted in advances in medical treatment of injuries, reduction of the number of deaths, and improvement of the Emergency Medical Systems. However, there seems to remain a need for new guidelines and directives to guarantee the benefits of such cooperation for both organizations and to eliminate or at least minimize some of the challenges between the two organizations, such as, in leadership, operative, and logistics partnership [3,4,9,24,46]. One way to make these organizations compatible seems to be mutual educational and training initiatives [25,30,56], which not only synchronize their activities but equally help clear the role and responsibility of each organization, joint operating mechanism, and treatment policies and reduce the organizational tensions that may exist between two populations [57].

The lack of trust has been reported as one of the core arguments for an insufficient engagement between two organizations [9,22,28]. Sharing information, planning, and developing a mutual administrative working activity, may however help to increase the trust between two organizations and enhance the development of a valuable partnership in all aspects of integration. Within healthcare, there are several contact points between civilian and military organizations [3,4,22,28]. Following the CSCATTT acronym, there is a need for synchronization between these two populations in leadership, safety, and communication issues to achieve mutual assessment of the situation. Such synchronization enables both organizations to achieve and obtain the advantages of dual capacity in staff, stuff, space, and system, i.e., all crucial elements of surge capacity, and in the outcomes of treatment and survival [3,4,32,35,58,59].

Although educational initiatives and training courses—besides other types of planning programs—are associated with a cost [60], they enable a multiagency collaboration that encompasses all agencies and not only, CM. These initiatives clarify the roles, increase the skills, and pave the way for achieving an established goal, individually and as a team [8,55,61]. Additionally, they may prompt agencies, especially CM, closer to creating one organization with responsibility for the development of all involved entities and in an all-risk scenario pattern [36,48,62], demonstrating practical, financial, and political advantages of such collaboration [44,63].

One significant advantage of CM collaboration is what both organizations can learn from each other. The collaboration aims at generating the same goal and such partnership requires opportunities that enhance learning of each other's limitations and capabilities [64,65], which also eases up and enables better resource and capacity sharing. The ideal collaboration should be developed through time [29,66]. Long-term development of such collaboration promotes and offers opportunities of creating one organization with responsibility for all development, education, and administration. Such an organization might be a necessity at the time of war and armed conflicts [28,55,59,67,68] to address all aspects of collaboration, socially and politically and in several levels: nationally and internationally. Consequently, increasing the trust needed for implementing delicate measures and making crucial decisions [41,42,69,70], without allowing one organization to be superior to the other [43,71].

A mutual organization may additionally provide other important elements of relief operations, considering cultural and linguistic understanding, human rights promotion, community-based needs assessment, besides role identification, team working and communication [28,47,55,59,72].

In summary, most publications emphasized the significance of the civilian-military partnership, prominently in how military support was incorporated in the national response, including support to national health systems, military repatriation and evacuation, and support to wider public systems. Additionally, the majority of studies suggest that collaborative educational initiatives in disaster medicine, public health and complex humanitarian emergencies, and international humanitarian law, along with advanced training in competency-based skill sets, should be included in the undergraduate education of health professionals. Finally, the most common CMC reported in the works of literature were in the fields of logistics and trauma. Other fields for CMC collaboration, e.g., infectious diseases, were poorly investigated [3,4,6–9,20–25,35,36,41–48,51–71,73,74].

3.3. Survey Results

A sum of 166 respondents answered the optimized questionnaires from the following 19 countries: Australia (2), Belgium (32), England (3), France (1), Germany (1), Greece (4), Iran (1), Italy (2), Israel (1), Mexico (1), Netherlands (3), Norway (3), Romania (8), Saudi Arabia (2), Sri Lanka (1), Sweden (11), Poland (80), Thailand (3), and the United Kingdom (3). Four respondents did not contribute their country of origin. All responses were sorted into four different groups for statistical analysis. Besides countries with over 10 participants (i.e., Belgium, Poland, and Sweden), all other nations, including responses with no country name, made up the fourth group called "others." Table 1 shows the age and gender distribution of all respondents. In total 128 respondents were physicians and 38 were other professionals, including nurses, psychologists, trainees, and strict military staff. The majority of participants were between 41–50 years of age, followed by 34 between 41–50 years of age, and 27 respondents with ages between 51–60 years. The number of male participants was twice that of females.

Table 1. Shows the gender and age distribution of respondents in this study.

Respondents	Number	<30	31–40	41–50	51–60	>60	Phys.	Other	Mil
Total	166	19	40	52	32	23	128	38	20
Female	52	7	15	15	8	7	44	8	6
Male	114	12	25	37	24	16	84	30	14

The collected results were analyzed using qualitative research methods. After identifying the thematic contents, they were categorized into core contents. The representative statements were outlined at a point where no novel information was retrieved from the data [75].

3.4. Changes in CSCATTT

For all respondents, there was an increase in the mean number of all CSCATTT dimensions under the COVID-19 pandemic. However, these changes were not statistically significant for any of the dimensions (Figure 2). Looking at the individual countries, none of the countries with more than 10 participants demonstrated any statistically significant increase in collaboration before and after the COVID-19 pandemic. Nevertheless, the results obtained solely from Belgium displayed a possible tendency toward significance in dimensions 2 (practical interface in command and control), 4 (safety and security), and 8 (transport). In Poland, only dimension 5 (communication and information), and in Sweden only dimension 1 (administrative part of command and control) showed a tendency to a significant increase.

Finally, the group called others did not demonstrate any statistically significant increase, although some of them such as the UK showed a very high numeric increase (Figure 2).

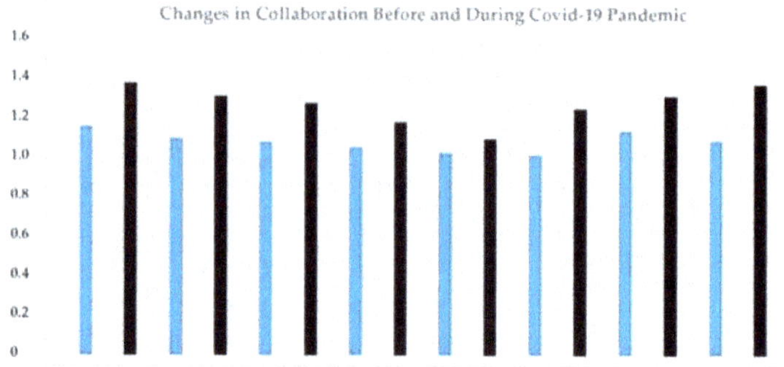

Dimension	1	2	3	4	5	6	7	8
Total	0.64	0.69	0.67	0.53	0.55	0.67	0.71	0.71
Belgium	0.44	0.32	0.53	0.36	0.46	0.46	0.45	0.32
Poland	0.53	0.81	0.75	0.52	0.26	0.57	0.62	0.75
Sweden	0.38	0.65	0.44	0.41	0.44	0.60	0.60	0.55
Others	0.83	0.93	0.50	0.47	0.65	0.76	0.86	0.86

Figure 2. Shows the differences in collaboration before and during COVID-19 for all countries, and some specific countries with a larger number of participants displayed as mean. It also shows the *p*-value for each significant change (CI 95%), where the light bars are the values before and darker (black bars) are values after the COVID-19 pandemic.

3.5. Comments

There were over 50 comments. All comments were grouped into four categories of No Collaboration (29/49 = 59.2%), Some Collaboration (12/49 = 24.5%), Full Collaboration (3/49 = 6%), and others (5/49 = 10.3%). In the latter group, two comments were technical and questionnaire-related (Table 2). Some of the comments were not about the subject but an expression of general dissatisfaction with slow progress in a specific country or the political interference with no results.

Table 2. Comments given by respondents were categorized into four groups.

No Collaboration	► No true collaboration. ► No Changes. ► Was bad, now is worse. no help, no support. ► We only have "so-called collaboration" ► I would say it is not better than it was. Before we could have at least some support (small but some) and now there is no help. Of course not everywhere but in most healthcare facilities. ► I see no big changes. ► It is worse now. ► Cooperation exists only in documents. ► We have plans we have big dreams and nothing has changed. ► CM was never a strong point. I think this is partly because of the intense administration involved with it. ► During the planning, the military role was not yet defined. The military means were on standby for emergencies. ► In my humble opinion, the collaboration between civil and military medical services is severely lacking. A widely recognized and supported permanent collaboration platform would be ideal but, if it even exists, it is lacking the prominent position it would deserve. ► I think the current pandemic was a chance for better collaboration in clinical practice. The military is the first to help in many areas just like in diagnostic or using a laboratory to support us. Did they do this? No.

Table 2. *Cont.*

	► I remember when we were in a communist system and there was integration with the civil sector. I was the first medic in the big division and we always support the local community. Thought the last years the potential of the medical background of the army was limited almost to zero. There are no people (MD) and stuff. The territorial defense force is one component of this system that might be useful during mass casualties and disasters. But, they are not trained. For now, there is no true collaboration and no support from the army. As a retired soldier, I am very disappointed due to this fact. ► CM collaboration is null during the pandemic. Rather strong logistics cooperation was implemented with the Civil Protection (of which I am part). ► No changes. It looked bad before and looks bad now. Maybe one in News they are talking about some great cooperation but there is nothing in reality. ► Cooperation only during major incidents. Or to show on TV. ► There were no CIMIC in XXX. Maybe some little support from TDF (Territorial defense force) is applied during disasters or emergencies but COVID did not bring anything new. ► Nothing has changed. ► It should be improved to get better results. ► Our expectation was verified by COVID. We could do much more but to politicians, the military was forced to do the stuff, which is not necessary. They should use them to help us in the way we need them. Not to be a guard. ► Before COVID, we at least have some meetings (rare) but now there is nothing. ► There is no real collaboration with the military in France, but with civil security. During COVID military offered help in some areas by transferring critical care patients from crowded regions to others less impacted by COVID. ► Lesson not learned. We could do much more but politicians (decisions) fail like always. ► Cooperation does not exist. There is also no longer any military health service. For example in the army, today there are 6 specialists in the field of emergency medicine. What can they do? Nobody wants to be in the army anymore. And the army is doing nothing for the civilian sector. ► Finally, we have guards at every entrance. ► CM Collaboration was disturbed by COVID. Military personnel was isolated to decrease the spread of the virus, through the CMC. ► There is no true CIMIC in XXX. The so-called Territorial defense, which is a more private gov army rather checks if we do our job instead of providing true help in the field we need. ► Failed by government.
Some collaboration	► The northern part of XXXX has many mountains; patient transportations are usually needed through air transport. Therefore, hospitals in that part have very well collaboration. ► There are working protocols for air transportation with the military plane. ► The military was engaged to support the building of emergency surge capacity. This happened quickly and effectively, as per plans agreed beforehand. ► Improved compared to previous crisis (XXX attacks 2016)—implementation of Lessons Learned as soon as COVID crisis began. ► Besides, some small improvements with reporting which we can call communication, I do not see any changes. ► Only Communication has changed. ► Besides communication and some logistics support (if I can name being guard support) no big change. ► Some minor upgrades are applied but there is still a lot to do. ► Communication is improved. But, before COVID we have some annual meetings mostly with TDF. Now there is no coordination. They (military) used to "help" as a guard, which could be done by local guards units. ► Some cooperation during COVID was observed but there were many actions that should never happen, i.e., monitoring hospitals by soldiers to check if we avoid patients. ► Some of these lay outside my field. However, there has since 2018, been an ongoing total-defense reform, and over the last 3–4 of years, while not directly during COVID, there have been examples of increased and well-functioning health CM collaboration during e.g., NATO collaboration exercises. There have also been examples of CM collaboration during COVID, but then more aimed towards border-control assistance. ► The Pandemic has brought a great understanding between military and civilian services, during the event. Logistic skills are always generally strong within the military. ► Before COVID, we haven't had much practical experience of CM collaboration. There wasn´t much during COVID either, but there was a clear ambition and progress. I find that the military part had more understanding for the civilian, compared to the opposite. My own experience and CM collaboration made my collaboration good (importance of network and understanding), but I found that several in my (civilian) organization lacked this.

Table 2. *Cont.*

Full collaboration	► Collaboration between civilians and the military in the medical field is strong before and during the COVID. ► Being engaged in 30 years of civil war, there has been a good CM collaboration as a necessity for wartime military injury burden. However, before COVID, after the war, there was no pressing demand for CM collaboration. During the COVID, the ministry of health used military assets effectively by formulation of joint operational command comprising of both Director General Health Services and Commander to the Army. ► I have a long tradition of CM collaboration.
Others	► Would be an easier answer if little examples were given. ► All questions should have a N/A (non-applicable) option. ► Big differences depending on the incidence of infections in the region of the hospital and the size of the hospital. ► To my knowledge, there are vast differences in both organizational cultures as well as planning and leadership methodology between civilian and military professions. To merge these two organizations to a certain degree, there should first be a framework grounded in political consensus, which is lacking at present time. As long as this first crucial step is not agreed upon, there will be no long-lasting collaborative structures being built. Then and only then agencies of the state may find cooperative areas to endorse. There may be two ways to perform this: either through time-consuming legislation or by the foundation of a new state agency being the major responsible actor in this process. ► The question is whether the learning experiences are written down, followed up afterward, and included in CM educations so that better collaboration as well as improvements and better preparedness overall.

4. Discussion

Although the necessity of CMC in the management of evolving health crises has been reported and discussed in several publications [3,4,6,22–25,30–33,35,36], this study confirms the need and significance of CMC but fails to illustrate any significant improvement during the COVID-19 pandemic. The results from the survey may suggest possible improvements in some strategic areas, while the practical collaboration (e.g., training and operative engagement) remains missing or unchanged (e.g., logistics).

Theoretically, a successful CMC should encompass several perspectives, which are not completely visible during the current COVID-19 pandemic, globally, indicating that some nations may have a long way ahead to achieve an improved collaboration [16–18]. Although substantive outcomes and the more proficient use of resources represent a mutual target and may raise some awareness, there is still separate funding for both organizations and financial advantages might be a possible cause of collaboration. The current CMC may thus lack a political consensus and framework as cited by one of the participants;

> *Participants 1: To my knowledge, there are vast differences in both organizational culture as well as planning and leadership methodology between civilian and military professions. To merge these two organizations to a certain degree, there should first be a framework grounded in political consensus, which is lacking at present time. As long as this first crucial step is not agreed upon, there will be no long-lasting collaborative structures being built. Then and only then agencies of the state may find cooperative areas to endorse. There may be two ways to perform this: either through time-consuming legislation or by the foundation of a new state agency being the major responsible actor in this process.*

There are different definitions of high productivity, probably due to diverse definitions of what collaboration is. The Oxford Dictionary [51] offers the following definitions: Collaboration is the act of working with another person or group of people to create or produce something. Cooperation is the fact of doing something together or of working together towards a shared aim. Finally, coordination is the act of making parts of something, groups of people, etc. work together in an efficient and organized way. While the literature seems to deal with reports of successful cooperation, few publications describe a unique production of CMC.

Emergent milestones are partly lacking. There are some joint events but practical collaboration with a mutual target, when both organizations may share a benefit barely exist. In most cases, military healthcare assists the civilian partner; there might be a different outcome if civilian healthcare is asked to assist the military partner in an armed conflict while confronting a constrained system with overloaded emergency departments [59,72–74]. Several participants in the pilot survey expressed their views;

Participants 2: Communication has improved, but before COVID-19, we have some annual meetings. Now there is no coordination. They (military) used to "help" as a guard, which could be done by local guards' units.

There has been broad recognition of CMC during the current pandemic, mainly from strategic sources, while a few operational participants, in this study, declared their sincere pride to highlight their successful collaboration in a compatible organizational culture. Thus, affecting communication, trust, accountability, and consequently the outcomes of collaboration. As mentioned by Shanks Kaurin [19], civilian-military populations may share the same values but have a conflicting understanding of a situation, and different priorities while sharing the process, as cited below;

Participants 3: We have plans we have big dreams and nothing has changed.

Participants 4: In my humble opinion, the collaboration between civil and military medical services is severely lacking. A widely recognized and supported permanent collaboration platform would be ideal but, if it even exists, it is lacking the prominent position it would deserve.

The differences between participating countries in survey data may indicate a lack of unified definition, diverse social and historical background, and nation's involvement in earlier conflicts [22,47,50,58,66,68]. The prominent changes in this study were chiefly within the administration of the command-and-control section, while the logistics cooperation was unchanged. These coordinating and cooperative activities aim at achieving collaboration but may not necessarily target similar goals and outcomes [19].

Participants 5: Before COVID-19, we did not have much practical experience with CM collaboration. There wasn´t much during COVID-19 either, but there was a clear ambition and progress. I find that the military part had more understanding for the civilian, compared to the opposite. My own experience and CM collaboration made my collaboration good (importance of the network and understanding), but I found that several in my (civilian) organization lacked this.

In some countries, e.g., Belgium, a mutual production of guidelines and instructions, safety and security considerations, communication and situational assessment, might indicate the first steps for a collaboration, however, defined by the Oxford Dictionary [51], achieving a collaboration, shared outcomes and goals, and establishing a control mechanism to ensure the operational outcome, are mandatory. Some countries with a few participants claimed a higher civilian-military collaboration level. The UK appears to be enjoying a fruitful and continuous interagency collaboration. Sri Lanka and Morocco also report prevailing collaboration between civilian and military healthcare systems. These successful collaborations may depend on previous involvement in international or national armed conflicts, which may necessitate such partnership or an apparent and continuous interest from the government. On the opposite, in countries such as Poland, there seems to be no trustful relationship between government and involved organizations, indicating the negative impacts of political interference in medical decision-making [27–29]. Nevertheless, there are not enough respondents from these countries to achieve a statistically significant result.

Participants 6: Being engaged in 30 years of civil war, there has been a good CM collaboration as a necessity for wartime military injury burden. However, before COVID-19, after the war, there was no pressing demand for CM collaboration. During the COVID, the ministry of health used military assets effectively by formulation of joint operational command comprising of both Director General Health Services and Commander to the Army.

There are several essential factors for a successful partnership in disaster and emergency management. Factors such as relation-building focus on mutual learning and information sharing, bilateral and multilateral agreements, comprehending the concept of CMC, trust, and mutual practical exercises, were all crucial elements of such partnership [8,9,30,31,56–58,62]. These conditions seem to be met in countries, such as the UK, while lacking in other European countries, such as Poland. A recent literature review, targeting six European countries reported that the most prominent partnership in these countries during COVID-19 consisted of incorporation of military support into the national COVID-19 response, e.g., support to national health and broader public systems, and military repatriation and evacuation [71], confirming the supportive role of the military in CMC, but no real collaboration.

A fruitful CMC depends on organizations' mutual values, situational interpretations, priorities, processes and moral principles [2,22,63,74,76,77]. Since a fruitful and strong collaboration relies on a homogenous and synchronized relationship as well as compatible ethics, the goal in a collaboration should be having shared values and interpretation towards the same goal. The diverse responses from respondents included in this study regarding CMC dimensions indicate a difference between their perceptions compared to that of authorities, which also calls for the evaluation of ethical views in CMC. Firm leadership, collaboration, coordination, and decision-making are all crucial for planning, executing, and harmonizing all efforts needed for successful crisis management [3,4,64,77]. In opposition to previous studies, the current study may indicate that COVID-19 has offered new opportunities for a fruitful collaboration in command and control between military and civilian authorities [78–81]. Increasing administrative measures demand good communication to improve and enable situational awareness and assessment, resource distribution, technological development, practicing decision-making, and information sharing and provides new incentives for educational initiatives, and training [78,80,82]. An improved administrative meeting for mutual planning during the current pandemic inevitably has resulted in improved understanding of each other's abilities and shortcomings, issuing mutual documents and recommendations, and consequently an increase in partnership for smooth distribution of resources and logistics in some countries. While factors, such as a political will and unity, a trustful political-military-public relationship, transparency, and evidence-based approaches are necessary elements of any collaboration, collaboration should be practiced to allow all involved parties to realize their limitations and capabilities, practicing the crucial decision-making step in an environment where mistakes can be made with no harm [1,2,4,22,29,41,83].

5. Limitations

One limitation to this study is the small number of respondents in the survey, necessitating a larger population study to achieve greater statistically significant results. The overwhelming majority of respondents came from two specific countries and given the uniqueness of civil-military relations in each country; the generalizability of such results is very limited. Diversities and peculiarities in cultures, national health systems, and CMC attitudes and experiences should be deeply inquired, and taken into strong account when testing and explaining CMC in different countries with diverse institutions.

Another limitation of the study was the use of English in the questionnaire and the search of the literature, which may have created some misunderstandings among participants and limited our search results, respectively.

Furthermore, there might be some doubts about using snowball sampling. However, the method has been used in several studies and is scientifically accepted. CMC may have a greater impact in larger nations with large militaries or in countries, which have built-in CMC into their medical infrastructures. However, even small countries such as Sweden without independent military healthcare seem to have a good collaboration, while larger countries such as Italy with different systems seem to have lost their routine partnership.

Finally, the use of coordination, cooperation, and collaboration in the literature to define the success and failure of CMC may have limited the results of the search. The use of a defined and united terminology is necessary for future publications.

6. Recommendation

- Define collaboration for future research and development.
- Create a trustful relationship between politic-public and profession (3P).
- Plan interaction through meetings, discussion, training, and practical work.
- Increase mutual research and teaching activities to increase the interest in CMC.
- Share information and educate the public to understand CMC.
- Create a mutual administrative activity or organization with similar goals and planning.

7. Conclusions

The COVID-19 pandemic has been associated with several changes and has revealed weaknesses and strengths in the current disaster and public health emergency management system, highlighting the importance of multiagency collaboration, particularly CMC. Although COVID-19 seems to have resulted in some progress in communication, coordination, resource distribution, and information sharing, there is still a need for stronger leadership, organizational closeness, and educational and training initiatives to guarantee a synchronized and well-functioning CMC. These steps are necessary to safeguard the practical partnership, operative management, harmony, and compatibility of CMC and require a political will and perhaps a mutual civilian-military authority.

Author Contributions: A.K.-M. provided the main framework, identified primary materials, and collaborated on the writing of the paper. K.G. organized research materials, identified appropriate references, and collaborated on the writing of the paper. A.K.-M., L.J.M., Y.R., F.M.B., and K.G. collaborated on the writing and editing of the paper. F.M.B. edited the final version. All authors have read and agreed to the published version of the manuscript.

Funding: This research received no external funding.

Institutional Review Board Statement: Not applicable.

Informed Consent Statement: Not applicable.

Data Availability Statement: Not applicable.

Conflicts of Interest: The authors declare no conflict of interest.

Appendix A

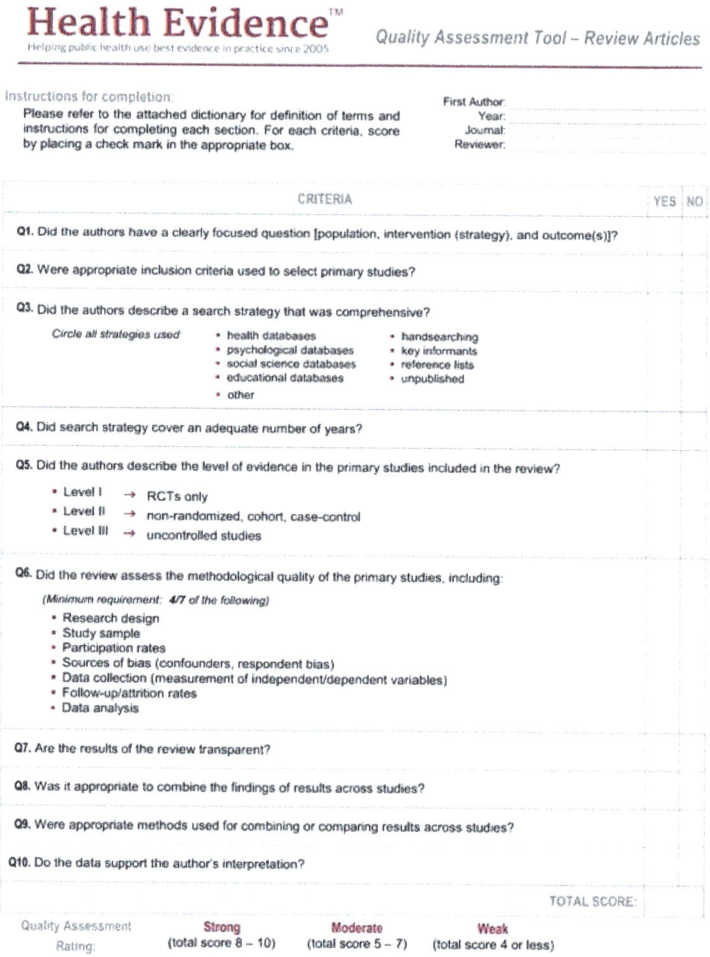

Health Evidence™
Helping public health use best evidence in practice since 2005

Quality Assessment Tool – Review Articles

Instructions for completion:
Please refer to the attached dictionary for definition of terms and instructions for completing each section. For each criteria, score by placing a check mark in the appropriate box.

First Author:
Year:
Journal:
Reviewer:

CRITERIA	YES	NO
Q1. Did the authors have a clearly focused question [population, intervention (strategy), and outcome(s)]?		
Q2. Were appropriate inclusion criteria used to select primary studies?		
Q3. Did the authors describe a search strategy that was comprehensive? *Circle all strategies used:* • health databases • psychological databases • social science databases • educational databases • other • handsearching • key informants • reference lists • unpublished		
Q4. Did search strategy cover an adequate number of years?		
Q5. Did the authors describe the level of evidence in the primary studies included in the review? • Level I → RCTs only • Level II → non-randomized, cohort, case-control • Level III → uncontrolled studies		
Q6. Did the review assess the methodological quality of the primary studies, including: *(Minimum requirement: **4/7** of the following)* • Research design • Study sample • Participation rates • Sources of bias (confounders, respondent bias) • Data collection (measurement of independent/dependent variables) • Follow-up/attrition rates • Data analysis		
Q7. Are the results of the review transparent?		
Q8. Was it appropriate to combine the findings of results across studies?		
Q9. Were appropriate methods used for combining or comparing results across studies?		
Q10. Do the data support the author's interpretation?		
TOTAL SCORE:		

Quality Assessment Rating: **Strong** (total score 8 – 10) **Moderate** (total score 5 – 7) **Weak** (total score 4 or less)

Figure A1. The protocol used for quality assessment of the included papers according to healthevidence.org, accessed on 14 June 2021.

Appendix B

Table A1. Included and Evaluated studies; Title, Author, Year, Journal, Summary, Topic, Evidence.

No	Title	Author (Ref No.)	Year	Journal	Summary	Topic	Evidence
1	Civilian military cooperation strategies in developing new technologies	Kulve, et al. [7]	2003	Research Pol	This paper focuses on the cooperation between civilian and military actors in developing new technology, suggesting the establishment of dual capacity networks, as part of a possible strategy towards an integrated civilian-military technology and industrial base.	Co-operation, strategic, tactical	M
2	A novel civilian-military partnership in emergency medical services during a prolonged disaster: patient characteristics, resources utilization, and future recommendations.	Avegno, et al. [31]	2006	Ann Emerg Med	This study describes a civilian-military partnership in the delivery of emergency medical services (EMS) in a disaster area, including medical needs, and resource utilization of patients presenting to an EMS unit in a prolonged disaster event and the benefits of such a partnership for the staff involved and the community at large.	Co-operation at all levels	S
3	Civilian-military coordination in emergency response in Indonesia	Joyce, et al. [6]	2006	Mil Med	Specific events and activities illustrate the comparative roles of civilian and military organizations and the importance of recognition of each organization's abilities and limitations.	Coordination	M
4	A Review of Nurses in Disaster Preparedness and Response: Military & Civilian Collaboration.	Rivers, et al. [23]	2010	JHSEM	This review of the literature provides an overview and reveals some of the difficulties and lessons learned from civilian-military coordination over time.	Cooperation, strategic, tactical levels, and research	S
5	Pandemic Influenza preparedness and response in Israel: A unique model of civilian-military collaboration	Kohn, et al. [45]	2010	JPHP	Discussing pandemics and pandemic preparedness protocols as a collaboration tool in medical decision-making within the defense sector. Although not generalizable, it offers a unique forum for all agencies to evaluate this interface within the context of pandemic influenza.	Strategic collaboration	M

Table A1. *Cont.*

No	Title	Author (Ref No.)	Year	Journal	Summary	Topic	Evidence
6	Collaboration between civilian and military healthcare professionals: a better way for planning, preparing, and responding to all-hazard domestic events	Marklund, et al. [30]	2010	Prehosp Disaster Med	This review summarizes the long and rich history of collaboration between civilians and the military in various countries and provides support for the continuation and improvement of collaborative efforts.	Collaboration	M
7	Civilian Military Cooperation in crisis management in Africa: American and European union's policy compared.	Olsen, et al. [24]	2011	J Int Rel Dev	This paper discusses the need for widespread consensus among various actors, necessary to combine civilian and military instruments in crisis management.	Strategic and Cooperative models	M
8	Using the military in disaster relief: systemizing challenges and opportunities	Heaslip, et al. [46]	2014	J Human Log Supply Chain Manag	Discusses the challenges of civil- military logistical cooperation, coordination, and collaboration in humanitarian relief logistics.	Coordination, cooperation, collaboration at operational level, Research	S
9	Role clarity, swift trust, and multi-agency coordination.	Curnin, et al. [9]	2015	J Conting Crisis Manag	Discuss the importance of swift trust and role clarity in temporary organizations during emergency management coordination.	Coordination Research	M
10	The Best of Both Worlds: Psychiatry Training at Combined Civilian-Military Programs.	Welton, et al. [25]	2015	Acad Psych	Discuss the role of collaboration in creating hybrid-training programs in Psychiatry.	Educational Strategic tactical Cooperation and coordination	M
11	Military-civilian cooperative emergency response to infectious disease prevention and control in China	Ma, et al. [57]	2016	Mil Med Res	The Chinese CMC in management of infectious disease prevention and control, focusing on mechanisms in several levels and stages like the military-cooperative emergency response to infectious diseases -the joint working mechanism, the information-sharing mechanism, the research collaboration mechanism, and the joint disposal mechanism-and presents a sorted summary of the practices and experiences of cooperative emergency responses to infectious diseases.	All level Cooperation	M

Table A1. *Cont.*

No	Title	Author (Ref No.)	Year	Journal	Summary	Topic	Evidence
12	Military and Civilian Collaboration: The Power of Numbers	Stinner, et al. [32]	2017	Mil Med	Compare the number and types of extremity injuries treated at civilian trauma centers vs. military treatment facilities and investigate the potential benefits of a clinical research network that includes both civilian trauma centers and military trauma facilities.	Coordination Cooperation	M
13	Military-Civilian Collaborations for mTBI Rehabilitation Research in an Active Duty Population: Lessons Learned From the Assessment of Military Multitasking Performance Project	McCulloch, et al. [33]	2017	J Head Trauma Rehab	This article describes lessons learned in the planning, development, and administration of a collaborative military-civilian research project, the Assessment of Military Multitasking Performance.	Strategic, Tactical Collaboration Research	M
14	Non-Medical aspects of civilian-military collaboration in the management of major incidents.	Khorram-Manesh, et al. [3]	2017	Eur J Trauma Emerg Surg	The paper builds up a discussion about civilian-military collaboration by presenting the result of simulation training.	Simulation and Education all level Collaboration	S
15	Obstacles to civil-military collaboration in conflict zones when organizations go to war	Leprince, C. [58]	2017	Etudes Internationales	Discussed the reasons for organizational tensions The results shed new light on the study of civil-military cooperation and yield policy lessons for optimizing Canada's international interventions.	Research, Strategic-Tactical Cooperation	M
16	The military partnerships	Brandt. [59]	2017	J Trauma Acute Care Surg	Expanding the mission of all of the Military Treatment Facilities (MTF) in the United States to include the medical care of the poor and disadvantaged patients in those communities. To expand the civilian/military collaboration beyond trauma care to maintain competency and readiness of all military medical personnel in war and peace. In war and disaster relief, in addition to the care of service members, the military medical professionals often care for the local population.	Operative collaboration Strategic planning	w

Table A1. *Cont.*

No	Title	Author (Ref No.)	Year	Journal	Summary	Topic	Evidence
17	Civilian-military pooling of health care resources in Haiti: a theory of complementarities perspective: The Swedish perspectives.	Naor [35]	2018	Int J Product Res	This study investigates opportunities and barriers for relief organizations to pool complementary resources originating from multiple countries, by examining five case studies that represent the breadth of organizational types, including charter (civilian, military, university-affiliated. and public/private), facility type (primary, secondary, and tertiary care), and duration of stay.	Research and Education, Strategic planning	M
18	Facilitators and constrainers of civilian-military collaboration.	Khorram-Manesh, et al. [4]	2018	Eur J Trauma Emerg Surg	The paper discusses how the current global and domestic security threats and challenges make CMC critical and inevitable. However, there is a need for careful analysis of its consequences, impact, possibilities, and limitations to differentiate between our expectations and the current reality.	Operative Collaboration Strategic Planning	M
19	Military-Civilian Partnerships in Training, Sustaining, Recruitment, Retention, and Readiness: Proceedings from an Exploratory First-Steps Meeting	Knudson, et al. [61]	2018	J Am Coll Surg	Discusses longer-term goals, and several shorter-term tasks that describe best practices for both military-based and civilian-based training and sustainment platforms.	Educational, Training Strategic Planning Collaboration	M
20	Characterizing the importance of clarity of roles and responsibilities in government inter-organizational collaboration and information sharing initiatives.	Gil-Garcia, et al. [8]	2019	Gov Info Quarter	Further discussion about three significant determinants of Clarity of Roles and Responsibility in Cross-Boundary Information Sharing, namely (1) the extent participants use boundary objects, (2) participant skills in terms of collaboration, coordination, and communication, and (3) the diversity of the participating organizations and their goals.	Coordination Cooperation Collaboration Research	M

Table A1. *Cont.*

No	Title	Author (Ref No.)	Year	Journal	Summary	Topic	Evidence
21	Immediate response to major incidents: defining an immediate responder!	Khorram-Manesh, et al. [56]	2019	Eur J Trauma Emerg Surg	This paper discusses the use of civilians and immediate responders in MCI and concludes that the use of immediate responders is a life-saving approach in MCIs and situations when every minute counts and every human resource is an invaluable asset.	Strategic, operative planning for civilian preparedness.	M
22	Implementation and Evaluation of a Military-Civilian Partnership to Train Mental Health Specialists	Simpson, et al. [62]	2019	Mil Med	The study describes a novel military-civilian collaboration in training.	Training, Educational, strategic planning for collaboration	M
23	The Territorial Defence Force in Disaster Response in Poland: Civil-Military Collaboration during the State of Emergency	Goniewicz, et al. [48]	2019	Sustainability	The recreation of the existing Polish Territorial Defense Force in disaster-related missions, limited to the territory of the country and largely focused on cooperation with the civilian sector.	Strategic, tactical, and operative cooperation	M
24	A short report on an interprofessional mobilizer team: innovation and impact during the COVID-19 pandemic.	Stifter, et al. [36]	2020	J Int Prof Care	Inter-professional collaboration is an integral component when implementing a robust and comprehensive response to crises.	Strategic, tactical, and operational collaboration	M
25	Rapid Response: Civilian-military medical collaboration-an everyday medical implementation?	Mitchel, [44]	2020	BMJ	Short comments about various practical, financial, and political pros and cons to integrating civilian-military collaboration into everyday medical practice, but following the eventual passing of this pandemic, isn't it worth considering its medical role in more than simply major incident response?	Strategic, Planning	W
26	Developing a blueprint for a civilian-military collaborative program in trauma training for Northern European countries: A South African experience	van der Wal, et al. [64]	2020	Injury	To describe and create a collaborative program between a major South African trauma service and a NATO country military medical service, with a synergistic effect on both partners.	Training, education, strategic planning for collaboration	M

Table A1. *Cont.*

No	Title	Author (Ref No.)	Year	Journal	Summary	Topic	Evidence
27	Flexible surge capacity—Public health, public education, and disaster management.	Khorram-Manesh, [60]	2020	Health Pro Pers	This study evaluates the concept of surge capacity, which intends to achieve a balance between the needs and resources in affected areas by providing staff, stuff, structure, and system and enhancing multiagency cooperation, coordination, and collaboration.	Coordination, cooperation, and collaboration	M
28	Pilot study of a longitudinal integrated disaster and military medicine education program for undergraduate medical students	Tsai, et al. [65]	2020	Medicine	The need for understanding disaster medicine and the health care system during massive casualty incidents is an integral part of the medical curriculum.	Educational, strategic, and tactical planning	M
29	Military Planning. What the NHS is learning from the British army in the COVID-19 crisis.	Watts, et al. [66]	2020	BMJ	Short discussion regarding how the civilian part can learn from the military side by considering some factors; Planning not plans, Speed and scale, and Chain of commands.	Strategic, Planning	W
30	Swedish Emergency Hospitals surgical surge capacity to mass casualty incidents.	Blimark, et al. [29]	2020	SJTREM	This paper discusses the preparedness in Swedish hospitals and their capacity during MCI and concludes that the MCI preparedness of Swedish emergency care hospitals needs further attention. To improve Swedish surgical MCI preparedness a national strategy for trauma care in disaster management is necessary.	Strategic, tactical, and operational planning	W
31	The History of Swedish Military Healthcare System and Its Path Toward Civilian-Military Collaboration from a Total Defense Perspective.	Khorram-Manesh, et al. [67]	2020	MilMed	This paper discusses the historical development of military medicine and the need for civilian-military collaboration from a Swedish perspective and concludes that the Swedish concept of total defense's healthcare system integration and collaboration may be a more fruitful approach. The collaboration within the total defense healthcare system will result in technical achievements, innovations, and medical advancements for the benefit of the whole nation.	Strategic, tactical, and operational planning	M

Table A1. *Cont.*

No	Title	Author (Ref No.)	Year	Journal	Summary	Topic	Evidence
32	Use of military forces in the COVID-19 emergency.	Cancian. [63]	2020	Web CSIS	This analysis addresses the distinctive roles of U.S. federal military forces and state National Guard units, the ways U.S. forces could be most helpful, the limitations on military forces, and the potential cost of employing the military to help fight the coronavirus.	Strategic planning for Cooperation	W
33	Total Defence Resilience: Viable or Not During COVID-19? A Comparative Study of Norway and the UK. Risk Hazards Crisis Public Policy.	Pollock et al. [68]	2020	Risk Haz Crisis Public Policy	Studying the application of total defense (TD) during the COVID-19 crisis and exploring what makes the TD a viable system with resilience capabilities in the face of the crisis by comparing British and Norwegian TD systems.	Strategic and research-based description for Collaborative actions	M
34	How do we fight COVID-19? Military medical actions in the war against the COVID-19 pandemic in France.	Pasquier, et al. [69]	2020	BMJ	Presenting multiagency collaboration in France as well as overseas.	Strategic, tactical Collaboration	M
35	Pandemics meet democracy: Experimental evidence from the COVID-19 crisis in Spain.	Amat, et al. [41]	2020	arXiv	The results of a set of survey experiments in Spain together with longitudinal evidence from a panel survey fielded right before and after the virus outbreak.	Experts, Opinion, Civilian, Collaboration	S
36	The effect of COVID-19 lockdowns on political support: Some good news for democracy?	Bol, et al. [42]	2020	Eur J Politic Res	A web-based survey in Western Europe to compare the political support of those who took the survey right before and right after the start of the lockdown in their country.	Opinion, Civilian, Collaborative, Strategic planning	M
37	Civilian perception of the role in Nigeria's 2014 Ebola outbreak and health-related responses in the North East region	Kwaja, et al. [47]	2021	BMJ Mil Health	Robust civilian-military relations require an appropriately defined role of the military and clear communication. Some important considerations include military cultural-linguistic understanding, human rights promotion, and community-based needs assessments; such foci can facilitate the military's understanding of community norms and civilian cooperation with military aims.	Opinion, Strategic, tactical all level Collaboration	M

Table A1. *Cont.*

No	Title	Author (Ref No.)	Year	Journal	Summary	Topic	Evidence
38	Delivering resilience training to pre-registration student nurses in partnership with a reservist military organization: A qualitative study	Corlett, et al. [74]	2021	Nurse Ed Today	In collaboration with a military reservist organization, the teams aimed at fostering resilience by promoting teamwork and leadership skills in student nurses.	Educational, Research	M
39	Severe pediatric war trauma: A military-civilian collaboration from retrieval to repatriation	Samuel, et al. [70]	2021	J Trauma Acute Care Surg	This paper describes a unique model of a coordinated military-civilian response for the stabilization, transport, and in-hospital management of severe pediatric warzone trauma.	Operational Coordination	M
40	The Development of Swedish Military Healthcare System: Part II-Re-evaluating the Military and Civilian Healthcare Systems in Crises Through a Dialogue and Study Among Practitioners.	Khorram-Manesh, et al. [22]	2021	Mil Med	This study investigated the challenges and views of practitioners regarding the benefits of CMC and it would be initiated.	All level collaboration, educational	S
41	Military crisis responses to COVID-19.	Kalkman, et al. [43]	2021	J Contingen Crisis Manag	Describes how current contributions of armed forces due to an urgent need for additional personnel and resources, facilitated by a framing of the crisis in terms of war were in the interest of armed forces and enabled them to improve their operational readiness, boost their societal standing and support societies with their expertise.	Opinion, civilian, operational, cooperation	M
42	Civilian-Military coordination in disaster preparedness and response.	Puckett, et al. [71]	2021	Nat Hazard Rev	This paper identifies common civil-military coordination challenges in disaster preparedness and the response among actors who operate at the regional, national, and international levels.	Coordination, opinion, experts, and strategic level	M

Table A1. *Cont.*

No	Title	Author (Ref No.)	Year	Journal	Summary	Topic	Evidence
43	Civil–military cooperation in the early response to the COVID-19 pandemic in six European countries.	Gad, et al. [72]	2021	BMJ Mil Health	This qualitative literature review targeted six European countries and found 19 distinct descriptive categories of civil–military cooperation extending across seven analytical themes of which the most prominent included how military support was incorporated in the national COVID-19 response, e.g., support to national health systems, military repatriation, and evacuation, and support to wider public systems.	Cooperation, support, repatriation, public system support	M

Appendix C The Questionnaire

Introduction

Civilian-Military Collaboration (CMC) is desired for the successful management of emergencies, disasters, and pandemics. This short survey aims to identify differences between two periods, BEFORE and DURING COVID-19 pandemic.

By conducting this survey, you agree to participate voluntarily. No name, affiliation, or other searchable information, but your profession and civilian/military status are registered. The data is handled in strict confidentiality and secure data storage and the study complies with the ethical principles stipulated by Swedish law, SFS 2008:192 and SFS 2003:460.

Please choose one of the options below, as indicated on the Likert Scale, for each question before and during the current COVID-19 pandemic in the table.

1: Weak 2: Fair 3: Undecided 4: Good 5: Strong

You may provide an example if needed. Comments are welcomed.

General information

A. Country: B. Gender: C. Profession: D. Civilian/Military E. Age: under 30 31–40 41–50 51–60 >60

No.	Questions/Dimensions	before	during	CSCATTT
1	CMC, defined as the overall assessment of meetings and planning regarding healthcare issues.			Command and control (administrative)
2	CMC, defined as the overall assessment of practical interferences regarding healthcare issues.			Command and control (practical)
3	The practical implementation of CM mutual decisions, defined as the overall assessment of mutual directives, recommendations, and plans.			Command and control (Mutual guidelines)
4	CMC and coordination of safety issues, defined as an overall assessment of sharing information, knowledge, and items such as protective equipment.			Safety, Security
5	CMC, defined as the overall assessment of contacts, meetings, and sharing communication systems.			Communication, Information
6	The mutual assessment of the incident/situation, defined as CM situational awareness through overall assessment and mutual analysis of the incident.			Assessment
7	Planning and practical clinical collaboration, defined as the overall assessment and contribution of medical staff and resources.			Triage, Treatment
8	Planning and performance of medical support logistics, defined as overall assessment and contribution of medical logistics resources.			Transport
9	Comments/Examples			Free text

References

1. Atkinson, M.; Jones, M.; Lamont, E. Multi-Agency Working and Its Implications for Practice. A Review of the Literature. 2007. Available online: https://www.nfer.ac.uk/nfer/publications/mad01/mad01.pdf (accessed on 14 June 2021).
2. Khorram-Manesh, A.; Berner, A.; Carlström, E. Facilitating Multiagency Collaboration Before Mass Gatherings—The Development of MAGRAT (Mass Gathering Risk Assessment Tool). *Biomed. J. Sci. Tech. Res.* **2020**, *24*, 18607–18616. [CrossRef]
3. Khorram-Manesh, A.; Lönroth, H.; Rotter, P.; Wilhelmsson, M.; Aremyr, J.; Berner, A.; Andersson, A.N.; Carlström, E. Non-medical aspects of civilian-military collaboration in the management of major incidents. *Eur. J. Trauma Emerg. Surg.* **2017**, *43*, 595–603. [CrossRef] [PubMed]
4. Khorram-Manesh, A. Facilitators and constrainers of civilian-military collaboration: The Swedish perspectives. *Eur. J. Trauma Emerg. Surg.* **2020**, *46*, 649–656. [CrossRef] [PubMed]
5. Kapucu, N. Interagency communication networks during emergencies: Boundary spanners in multiagency coordination. *Am. Rev. Public Adm.* **2006**, *36*, 207–225. [CrossRef]
6. Joyce, N. Civilian-Military Coordination in the Emergency Response in Indonesia. *Mil. Med.* **2006**, *171*, 66–70. [CrossRef]
7. Kulve, H.T.; Smit, W.A. Civilian–military co-operation strategies in developing new technologies. *Res. Policy* **2003**, *32*, 955–970. [CrossRef]
8. Gil-Garcia, J.R.; Guler, A.; Pardo, T.A.; Burke, B. Characterizing the importance of clarity of roles and responsibilities in government inter-organizational collaboration and information sharing initiatives. *Gov. Inf. Quart.* **2019**, *36*, 101393. [CrossRef]

9. Curnin, S.; Owen, C.; Paton, U.; Trist, C.; Parsons, D. Role clarity, swift trust, and multi-agency coordination. *J. Conting Crisis Manag.* **2015**, *23*, 29–35. [CrossRef]
10. Kaiser, F.M. Interagency Collaborative Arrangements and Activities: Types, Rationales, Considerations. Congressional Research Service 7-5700, R41803. 2011. Available online: https://www.fas.org/sgp/crs/misc/R41803.pdf (accessed on 12 December 2021).
11. Perrault, E.; McClelland, R.; Austin, C.; Sieppert, J. Working Together in Collaborations: Successful Process Factors for Community Collaboration. *Adm. Soc. Work.* **2011**, *35*, 282–298. [CrossRef]
12. Sienkiewicz-Małyjurek, K. Strategic Approach and Initiatives Streamlining Emergency Operations in Poland. *Acad. J. Interdiscip. Stud.* **2014**, *3*, 385–392. [CrossRef]
13. Leung, Z.C.S. Boundary Spanning in Interorganizational Collaboration. *Adm. Soc. Work.* **2013**, *37*, 447–457. [CrossRef]
14. Kożuch, B.; Sienkiewicz-Małyjurek, K. Factors of effective inter-organizational collaboration: A framework for public management. *Transylv. Rev. Adm. Sci.* **2016**, *47*, 97–115.
15. Vangen Huxham Vangen, S.; Huxham, C. Introducing the Theory of Collaborative Advantage. In *The New Public Governance? Emerging Perspectives on the Theory and Practice of Public Governance*; Osborne, S.P., Ed.; Routledge: London, UK; New York, NY, USA, 2010; pp. 163–184.
16. Arya, B.; Lin, Z. Understanding Collaboration Outcomes from an Extended Resource-Based View Perspective: The Roles of Organizational Characteristics, Partner Attributes, and Network Structures. *J. Manag.* **2007**, *33*, 697–723. [CrossRef]
17. Hansen, M.T.; Nohria, N. How to Build Collaborative Advantage. *MIT Sloan Manag. Rev.* **2004**, *46*, 20–30.
18. Hardy, C.; Phillips, N.; Lawrence, T.B. Resources, Knowledge and Influence: The Organizational Effects of Interorganizational Collaboration. *J. Manag. Stud.* **2003**, *40*, 321–347. [CrossRef]
19. Kaurin, P.S. An "Unprincipled Principal": Implications for Civil-Military Relations. *Strateg. Stud. Q.-Perspect.* **2021**, *15*, 50–68. Available online: https://www.jstor.org/stable/27032896 (accessed on 1 November 2021).
20. Hodgetts, T.J. Major Incident Medical Training: A Systematic International Approach. *Int. J. Disaster Med.* **2003**, *1*, 13–20. [CrossRef]
21. Ellern, H. Military and Civilian Pyrotechnics. Chemical Publishing Company. 1968. Available online: http://www.getanewgun.com/Pyrotechnic/Pyrotechnic_Books/Fireworks_Ellernh_M_Cp.pdf (accessed on 1 November 2021).
22. Khorram-Manesh, A.; Burkle, F.M., Jr.; Phattharapornjaroen, P.; Marzaleh, M.A.; Al Sultan, M.; Mäntysaari, M.; Carlström, E.; Goniewicz, K.; Santamaria, E.; Comandante, J.D.; et al. The Development of Swedish Military Healthcare System: Part II—Re-evaluating the Military and Civilian Healthcare Systems in Crises Through a Dialogue and Study Among Practitioners. *Mil. Med.* **2021**, *186*, e442–e450. [CrossRef]
23. Rivers, F.; Speraw, S.; Phillips, K.D.; Lee, J. A review of nurses in disaster preparedness and response: Military and Civilian Collaboration. *J. Homel. Secur. Emerg. Manag.* **2010**, *7*. [CrossRef]
24. Olsen, G.R. Civil-military cooperation in crisis management in Africa: American and European Union policies compared. *J. Int. Relat. Dev.* **2011**, *14*, 333–353. [CrossRef]
25. Welton, R.S.; Hamaoka, D.A.; Broderick, P.J.; Schillerstrom, J.E. The Best of Both Worlds: Psychiatry Training at Combined Civilian-Military Programs. *Acad. Psychiatry* **2015**, *39*, 360–364. [CrossRef]
26. Wennman, I.; Wittholt, M.; Carlström, E.; Carlsson, T.; Khorram-Manesh, A. Urgent care centre in Sweden—The integration of teams and perceived effects. *Int. J. Health Plan. Manag.* **2019**, *34*, 1205–1216. [CrossRef]
27. Pollock, A.M.; Dunnigan, M.G.; Gaffney, D.; Price, D.; Shaoul, J. The private finance initiative: Planning the "new" NHS: Downsizing for the 21st century. *BMJ* **1999**, *319*, 179–184. [CrossRef]
28. Khorram-Manesh, A.; Burkle, F.M., Jr. Disasters and Public Health Emergencies—Current Perspectives in Preparedness and Response. *Sustainability* **2020**, *12*, 8561. [CrossRef]
29. Blimark, M.; Örtenwall, P.; Lönroth, H.; Mattsson, P.; Boffard, K.; Robinson, Y. Swedish emergency hospital surgical surge capacity to mass casualty incidents. *Scand. J. Trauma Resusc. Emerg. Med.* **2020**, *28*, 12. [CrossRef]
30. Marklund, L.A.; Graham, A.M.; Morton, P.G.; Hurst, C.G.; Motola, I.; Robinson, D.W.; Kelley, V.A.; Elenberg, K.J.; Russler, M.F.; Boehm, D.E.; et al. Collaboration between civilian and military healthcare professionals: A better way for planning, preparing, and responding to all hazard domestic events. *Prehosp. Disaster Med.* **2010**, *25*, 399–412. [CrossRef]
31. Avegno, J.; Moises, J.; Tatford, S.; Herbert, K.; Zickerman, E. A novel civilian-military partnership in emergency medical services during a prolonged disaster: Patient characteristics, resource utilization, and future recommendations. *Ann. Emerg. Med.* **2006**, *48*, 52. [CrossRef]
32. Stinner, M.D.J.; Wenke, J.C.; Ficke, C.J.R.; Gordon, L.C.W.; Toledano, C.J.; Carlini, A.R.; Scharfstein, D.O.; Hsu, J.R.; the Major Extremity Trauma Research Consortium (METRC); MacKenzie, E.J.; et al. Military and Civilian Collaboration: The Power of Numbers. *Mil. Med.* **2017**, *182*, 10–17. [CrossRef]
33. McCulloch, K.L.; Cecchini, A.S.; Radomski, M.V.; Scherer, M.R.; Smith, L.; Cleveland, C.; McMillan, H.P.; Davidson, L.F.; Weightman, M.M. Military-Civilian Collaborations for mTBI Rehabilitation Research in an Active Duty Population: Lessons Learned From the Assessment of Military Multitasking Performance Project. *J. Head Trauma Rehabil.* **2017**, *32*, 70–78. [CrossRef]
34. Khorram-Manesh, A.; Nordling, J.; Carlström, E.; Goniewicz, K.; Faccincani, R.; Burkle, F.M. A translational triage research development tool: Standardizing prehospital triage decision-making systems in mass casualty incidents. *Scand. J. Trauma Resusc. Emerg. Med.* **2021**, *29*, 119. [CrossRef]

35. Naor, M. Civilian-military pooling of health care resources in Haiti: A theory of complementarities perspective. *Int. J. Prod. Res.* **2018**, *56*, 6741–6757. [CrossRef]
36. Stifter, J.; Terry, A.; Phillips, J.; Heitschmidt, M. A short report on an interprofessional mobilizer team: Innovation and impact during the COVID-19 pandemic. *J. Interprof. Care* **2020**, *34*, 716–718. [CrossRef] [PubMed]
37. Khorram-Manesh, A.; Dulebenets, M.A.; Goniewicz, K. Implementing Public Health Strategies—The Need for Educational Initiatives: A Systematic Review. *Int. J. Environ. Res. Public Health* **2021**, *18*, 5888. [CrossRef] [PubMed]
38. Burkle, F.M. Political Intrusions into the International Health Regulations Treaty and Its Impact on Management of Rapidly Emerging Zoonotic Pandemics: What History Tells Us. *Prehosp. Disaster Med.* **2020**, *35*, 426–430. [CrossRef]
39. Kettl, D.F. States divided: The implications of American federalism for COVID-19. *Public Adm. Rev.* **2020**, *80*, 595–602. [CrossRef]
40. Khorram-Manesh, A.; Carlström, E.; Hertelendy, A.J.; Goniewicz, K.; Casady, C.B.; Burkle, F.M. Does the Prosperity of a Country Play a Role in COVID-19 Outcomes? *Disaster Med. Public Health Prep.* **2020**, 1–10. [CrossRef]
41. Amat, F.; Arenas, A.; Faló-Gimeno, A.; Muñoz, J. Pandemics meet democracy: Experimental evidence from the COVID-19 crisis in Spain. *arXiv* **2020**. Available online: https://osf.io/preprints/socarxiv/dkusw/ (accessed on 14 June 2021).
42. Bol, D.; Giani, M.; Blais, A.; Loewen, P.J. The effect of COVID-19 lockdowns on political support: Some good news for democracy. *Eur. J. Politic Res.* **2021**. [CrossRef]
43. Kalkman, J.P. Military crisis responses to COVID-19. *J. Conting Crisis Manag.* **2021**, *29*, 99–103. [CrossRef]
44. Mitchell, R.M.W. Rapid Response: Civilian-Military Medical Collaboration—An Everyday Medical Implementation? Available online: https://www.bmj.com/content/369/bmj.m2055/rr-0 (accessed on 11 November 2021).
45. Kohn, S.; Barnett, D.J.; Leventhal, A.; Reznikovich, S.; Oren, M.; Laor, D.; Grotto, I.; Balicer, R.D. Pandemic influenza preparedness and response in Israel: A unique model of civilian-defense collaboration. *J. Public Health Policy* **2010**, *31*, 256–269. [CrossRef]
46. Heaslip, G.; Barber, E. Using the military in disaster relief: Systemizing challenges and opportunities. *J. Hum. Logist. Supply Chain. Manag.* **2014**, *4*, 60–81. [CrossRef]
47. Kwaja, C.M.A.; Olivieri, D.J.; Boland, S.; Henwood, P.C.; Card, B.; Polatty, D.P.; Levine, A.C. Civilian perception of the role of the military in Nigeria's 2014 Ebola outbreak and health-related responses in the North East region. *BMJ Mil. Health* **2021**, e001696. [CrossRef]
48. Goniewicz, K.; Goniewicz, M.; Burkle, F.M., Jr. The Territorial Defence Force in Disaster Response in Poland: Civil-Military Collaboration during a State of Emergency. *Sustainability* **2019**, *11*, 487. [CrossRef]
49. Page, M.J.; McKenzie, J.E.; Bossuyt, P.M.; Boutron, I.; Hoffmann, T.C.; Mulrow, C.D.; Shamseer, L.; Tetzlaff, J.M.; Akl, E.A.; Brennan, S.E.; et al. The PRISMA 2020 statement: An updated guideline for reporting systematic reviews. *BMJ* **2021**, *372*, n71. [CrossRef]
50. Health Evidence Quality Assessment Tool (HEQAT). Available online: https://www.healthevidence.org/documents/our-appraisal-tools/QA_Tool&Dictionary_10Nov16.pdf (accessed on 14 June 2021).
51. Oxford Dictionary Online. Available online: https://www.oxfordlearnersdictionaries.com/ (accessed on 14 June 2021).
52. Nicholas, D.; Clark, D.; Herman, E. ResearchGate: Reputation uncovered. *Learn. Publ.* **2016**, *29*, 173–182. [CrossRef]
53. Kirchherr, J.; Charles, K. Enhancing the sample diversity of snowball samples: Recommendations from a research project on anti-dam movements in Southeast Asia. *PLoS ONE* **2018**, *13*, e0201710. [CrossRef]
54. Baltar, F.; Brunet, I. Social research 2.0: Virtual snowball sampling method using Facebook. *Internet Res.* **2018**, *22*, 55–74. [CrossRef]
55. Khorram-Manesh, A.; Plegas, P.; Högstedt, Å.; Peyravi, M.; Carlström, E. Immediate response to major incidents: Defining an immediate responder! *Eur. J. Trauma Emerg. Surg.* **2020**, *46*, 1309–1320. [CrossRef]
56. Ma, H.; Dong, J.P.; Zhou, N.; Pu, W. Military-civilian cooperative emergency response to infectious disease prevention and control in China. *Mil. Med. Res.* **2016**, *30*, 39. [CrossRef]
57. Leprince, C. Obstacles to civil-military collaboration in conflict zones when organizations go to war. *Etudes Int.* **2017**, *48*, 37–61. [CrossRef]
58. Brandt, M.M. Civilian-military partnerships. *J. Trauma Acute Care Surg.* **2017**, *82*, 977–978. [CrossRef]
59. Khorram-Manesh, A. Flexible Surge capacity—Public health, public education, and disaster management. *Health Promot. Perspect.* **2020**, *10*, 175–179. [CrossRef]
60. Knudson, M.M.; Elster, E.; Bailey, J.A.; Johannigman, J.A.; Bailey, P.V.; Schwab, C.W.; Kirk, G.G.; Woodson, J.A. Military–Civilian Partnerships in Training, Sustaining, Recruitment, Retention, and Readiness: Proceedings from an Exploratory First-Steps Meeting. *J. Am. Coll. Surg.* **2018**, *227*, 284–292. [CrossRef]
61. Simpson, S.A.; Goodwin, M.; Thurstone, C. Implementation and Evaluation of a Military-Civilian Partnership to Train Mental Health Specialists. *Mil. Med.* **2019**, *184*, e184–e190. [CrossRef]
62. Cancian, M.E. Use of Military Forces in the COVID-19 Emergency. Center for Strategic & International Studies. (CSIS). Available online: https://www.csis.org/analysis/use-military-forces-covid-19-emergency (accessed on 14 June 2021).
63. van der Wal, H.; van Dongen, T.T.; Vermeulen, C.F.; Bruce, J.L.; Bekker, W.; Manchev, V.; Kong, V.; van Waes, O.; Clarke, D.L.; Hoencamp, R. Developing a blueprint for a civilian-military collaborative program in trauma training for Northern European countries: A South African experience. *Injury* **2020**, *51*, 70–75. [CrossRef]
64. Tsai, Y.-D.; Tsai, S.-H.; Chen, S.-J.; Chen, Y.-C.; Wang, J.-C.; Hsu, C.-C.; Chen, Y.-H.; Yang, T.-C.; Li, C.-W.; Cheng, C.-Y. Pilot study of a longitudinal integrated disaster and military medicine education program for undergraduate medical students. *Medicine* **2020**, *99*, e20230. [CrossRef]

65. Watts, G.; Wilkinson, E. Military Planning. What the NHS is learning from the British army in the COVID-19 crisis. *BMJ* **2020**, *369*, m2055. [CrossRef]
66. Khorram-Manesh, A.; Robinson, Y.; Boffard, K.; Örtenwall, P. The History of Swedish Military Healthcare System and Its Path Toward Civilian-Military Collaboration From a Total Defense Perspective. *Mil. Med.* **2020**, *185*, e1492–e1498. [CrossRef] [PubMed]
67. Pollock, K.; Steen, R. Total Defence Resilience: Viable or Not During COVID-19? A Comparative Study of Norway and the UK. *Risk Hazards Crisis Public Policy* **2020**, *12*, 73–109. [CrossRef] [PubMed]
68. Pasquier, P.; Luft, A.; Gillard, J.; Boutonnet, M.; Vallet, C.; Pontier, J.-M.; Duron-Martinaud, S.; Dia, A.; Puyeo, L.; Debrus, F.; et al. How do we fight COVID-19? Military medical actions in the war against the COVID-19 pandemic in France. *BMJ Mil. Health* **2020**. [CrossRef] [PubMed]
69. Samuel, N.; Epstein, D.; Oren, A.; Shapira, S.; Hoffmann, Y.; Friedman, N.; Shavit, I. Severe pediatric war trauma: A military-civilian collaboration from retrieval to repatriation. *J. Trauma Acute Care Surg.* **2021**, *90*, e1–e6. [CrossRef]
70. Puckett, L.M. Civilian-Military coordination in disaster preparedness and response. *Nat. Hazard Rev.* **2021**, *22*, 04021005. [CrossRef]
71. Gad, M.; Kazibwe, J.; Quirk, E.; Gheorghe, A.; Homan, Z.; Bricknell, M. Civil–military cooperation in the early response to the COVID-19 pandemic in six European countries. *BMJ Mil. Health* **2021**. [CrossRef]
72. Khorram-Manesh, A.; Burkle, F.M.; Goniewicz, K.; Robinson, Y. Estimating the Number of Civilian Casualties in Modern Armed Conflicts-A Systematic Review. *Front. Public Health* **2021**, *9*, 765261. [CrossRef]
73. Corlett, J.; McConnachie, T. Delivering resilience training to pre-registration student nurses in partnership with a reservist military organization: A qualitative study. *Nurse Educ. Today* **2021**, *97*, 104730. [CrossRef]
74. Sultan, M.A.S.; Khorram-Manesh, A.; Carlström, E.; Berli, J.; Sörensen, J. Impact of Virtual Disaster Collaboration Exercises on Disaster Leadership at Hospitals in Saudi Arabia. *Int. J. Disaster Risk. Sci.* **2021**, *12*, 879–889. [CrossRef]
75. Graneheim, U.H.; Lundman, B. Qualitative content analysis in nursing research: Concepts, procedures and measures to achieve trustworthiness. *Nurse Educ. Today* **2004**, *24*, 105–112. [CrossRef]
76. Khorram-Manesh, A.; Angthong, C.; Pangma, A.; Sulannakarn, S.; Burivong, R.; Jarayabhand, R.; Örtenwall, P. Hospital Evacuation; Learning from the Past? Flooding of Bangkok 2011. *J. Adv. Med. Med. Res.* **2013**, *4*, 395–415. [CrossRef]
77. Angthong, C.; Kumjornkijjakarn, P.; Pangma, A.; Khorram-Manesh, A. Disaster Medicine in Thailand: A Current Update. Are We Prepared? *J. Med. Assoc. Thai* **2012**, *95*, 42–50.
78. Phattharapornjaroen, P.; Glantz, V.; Carlström, E.; Dahlén Holmqvist, L.; Khorram-Manesh, A. Alternative Leadership in Flexible Surge Capacity—The Perceived Impact of Tabletop Simulation Exercises on Thai Emergency Physicians Capability to Manage a Major Incident. *Sustainability* **2020**, *12*, 6216. [CrossRef]
79. Shah, S.; Diwan, S.; Kohan, L.; Rosenblum, D.; Gharibo, C.; Soin, A.; Sulindro, A.; Nguyen, Q.; Provenzano, D.A. The technological impact of COVID-19 on the future of education and health care delivery. *Pain Physician* **2020**, *23*, S367–S380. [CrossRef] [PubMed]
80. Moreno, C.; Wykes, T.; Galderisi, S.; Nordentoft, M.; Crossley, N.; Jones, N.; Cannon, M.; Correll, C.U.; Byrne, L.; Carr, S.; et al. How mental health care should change as a consequence of the COVID-19 pandemic. *Lancet Psychiatry* **2020**, *7*, 813–824. [CrossRef]
81. Dwivedi, Y.K.; Hughes, D.L.; Coombs, C.; Constantiou, I.; Duan, Y.; Edwards, J.S.; Gupta, B.; Lal, B.; Misra, S.; Prashant, P.; et al. Impact of COVID-19 pandemic on information management research and practice: Transforming education, work and life. *Int. J. Inf. Manag.* **2020**, *55*, 102211. [CrossRef]
82. Kramer, A.; Kramer, K.Z. The potential impact of the COVID-19 pandemic on occupational status, work from home, and occupational mobility. *J. Vocat. Behav.* **2020**, *119*, 103442. [CrossRef] [PubMed]
83. Khorram-Manesh, A.; Berlin, J.; Carlström, E. Two Validated Ways of Improving the Ability of Decision-Making in Emergencies; Results from a Literature Review. *Bull. Emerg. Trauma* **2016**, *4*, 186–196. [PubMed]

International Journal of
Environmental Research and Public Health

MDPI

Article

A Critical Analysis of the COVID-19 Hospitalization Network in Countries with Limited Resources

Marcio L. V. Araujo [1,2,3,*,†], José G. V. Miranda [4,†], Rodrigo N. Vasconcelos [5,†], Elaine C. B. Cambui [6,†], Raphael S. Rosário [4,†], Márcio C. F. Macedo [4,†], Antonio C. Bandeira [7,†], Márcia S. P. L. Souza [7,†], Ana C. F. N. Silva [7,†], Aloisio S. Nascimento Filho [3,8,†], Thiago B. Murari [3,8,†], Eduardo M. F. Jorge [3,9,†] and Hugo Saba [1,3,9,†]

1 Modelagem Computacional e Tecnologia Industrial (PPG MCTI), Centro Universitário SENAI CIMATEC, Av. Orlando Gomes, 1845—Piatã, Salvador 41650-010, Brazil; hugosaba@gmail.com
2 Department of Computer Science, Federal Institute of Bahia, Rua São Cristóvão, s/n—Novo Horizonte, Lauro de Freitas 42700-000, Brazil
3 Núcleo de Pesquisa Aplicada e Inovação (NPAI), Universidade do Estado da Bahia—UNEB/Centro Universitário SENAI CIMATEC, Salvador 41650-010, Brazil; aloisio.nascimento@gmail.com (A.S.N.F.); mura.learning@gmail.com (T.B.M.); emjorge1974@gmail.com (E.M.F.J.)
4 Department of Physics, Federal University of Bahia, Campus Universitário de Ondina—Ondina, Salvador 40210-340, Brazil; vivasm@gmail.com (J.G.V.M.); phaoso@gmail.com (R.S.R.); marciocfmacedo@gmail.com (M.C.F.M.)
5 Department of Earth and Environmental Sciences, State University of Feira de Santana, Av. Transnordestina, s/n—Feira de Santana, Novo Horizonte 44036-900, Brazil; rnvuefsppgm@gmail.com
6 Department of Ecology, Federal University of Bahia, Campus Universitário de Ondina—Ondina, Salvador 40210-340, Brazil; elainecambui@gmail.com
7 Health Secretary of the State of Bahia, 4ª Avenida Centro Administrativo da Bahia, 400—Centro Administrativo da Bahia, Salvador 40301-110, Brazil; antoniobandeira@gmail.com (A.C.B.); marcia.saopedro@saude.ba.gov.br (M.S.P.L.S.); anaclaudianunes@hotmail.com (A.C.F.N.S.)
8 Gestão e Tecnologia Industrial (PPG GETEC), Centro Universitário SENAI CIMATEC, Av. Orlando Gomes, 1845—Piatã, Salvador 41650-010, Brazil
9 Department of Exact and Earth Sciences, University of the State of Bahia, R. Silveira Martins, 2555—Cabula, Salvador 41180-045, Brazil
* Correspondence: marcioaraujo@ifba.edu.br; Tel.: +55-719-8889-6527
† These authors contributed equally to this work.

Citation: Araujo, M.L.V.; Miranda, J.G.V.; Vasconcelos, R.N.; Cambui, E.C.B.; Rosário, R.S.; Macedo, M.C.F.; Bandeira, A.C.; Souza, M.S.P.L.; Silva, A.C.F.N.; Nascimento Filho, A.S.; et al. A Critical Analysis of the COVID-19 Hospitalization Network in Countries with Limited Resources. *IJERPH* **2022**, *19*, 3872. https://doi.org/10.3390 ijerph19073872

Academic Editors: Amir Khorram-Manesh and Krzysztof Goniewicz

Received: 8 February 2022
Accepted: 21 March 2022
Published: 24 March 2022

Abstract: To effectively combat the COVID-19 pandemic, countries with limited resources could only allocate intensive and non-intensive care units to a low number of regions. In this work, we evaluated the actual displacement of infected patients in search of care, aiming to understand how the networks of planned and actual hospitalizations take place. To assess the flow of hospitalizations outside the place of residence, we used the concepts of complex networks. Our findings indicate that the current distribution of health facilities in Bahia, Brazil, is not sufficient to effectively reduce the distances traveled by patients with COVID-19 who require hospitalization. We believe that unnecessary trips to distant hospitals can put both the sick and the healthy involved in the transport process at risk, further delaying the stabilization of the COVID-19 pandemic in each region of the state of Bahia. From the results found, we concluded that, to mitigate this situation, the implementation of health units in countries with limited resources should be based on scientific methods, and international collaborations should be established.

Keywords: government; hospitalization; pandemics; public policy; transportation

1. Introduction

The state of Bahia, Brazil, has a total area of approximately 565,000 square kilometers and, by the end of 2020, had an estimated population of about 15 million people, which is superior to the estimated population of European countries, such as Belgium, Greece, Sweden, and Portugal [1]. The human development index (HDI) of the state of Bahia is 0.660, similar to other countries with limited resources such as Guatemala, Honduras, India, Bangladesh, and Morocco. In this sense, while in normal conditions it is already difficult to provide free, high-quality health care services to the population that live in Bahia, on 11 March 2020, with the World Health Organization (WHO) announcement of the coronavirus disease 2019 (COVID-19) outbreak, caused by the new severe acute respiratory syndrome coronavirus 2 (SARS-CoV-2), as a pandemic, the provision of high-quality health care services has become even more challenging, since the high transmissibility of SARS-CoV-2 may quickly overload the health care services of a state or a country [2].

Possibly inspired by the National Health Service of the United Kingdom [3], the Brazilian National Health System (Sistema Único de Saúde—SUS) is a public health system created by the Constitution of the Federative Republic of Brazil [4]. The SUS is a universal access system, which allows any Brazilian to use low-, medium-, and high-complexity health services. In addition, management is divided between federal, state, and municipal sectors. States and municipalities have autonomy in defining policies in favor of health [5]. Previous studies in Brazil have found that, although there was a favorable expansion in Universal Health Coverage (UHC), structural problems remained in the SUS, from gaps in organization and governance to a scarcity of public resources. Thus, it is evident that there are regional disparities in terms of health services [6]. However, the geographic and economic differences do not allow for a comparison between these countries in terms of the flow of hospitalization. Previous works deal with the use of resources in health services [7,8]. This work aims to analyze the flow of hospitalizations in a country with limited resources. The displacement of patients receiving hospital treatment during the COVID-19 pandemic has proved to be a problem for some countries [9,10].

In the state of Bahia, Brazil, the management of SUS is done by the state government of Bahia, which must provide financial resources and stimulate the municipalities of Bahia to achieve the responsible management of their health care services, and must also assume that responsibility in the case some of those municipalities are not able to achieve that goal [5]. As resources are limited and the territorial space of Bahia is large, the creation of health units, in a few areas, is presented as a single alternative, so large displacements of infected patients are inevitable.

By the end of October 2020, following the State Contingency Plan for Confrontation of the New Coronavirus SARS-CoV-2 [11], the state government of Bahia distributed 2286 intensive and non-intensive care units in 61 out of the 417 municipalities of Bahia, in order to provide better assistance to the COVID-19 patients that live in Bahia [12], 41% higher than the previous healthcare network. In Bahia, the room availability follows a protocol based on clinical severity, risk potential, health problems or degree of suffering [13]. Many of these health rooms were created to serve COVID-19 patients, as part of a municipal, state, and federal effort. Therefore, COVID-19 patients that reside in municipalities not capable of providing appropriate treatment or hospitalization for such a disease must travel to another municipality to be better assisted by SUS. In order to reduce the distance and duration of those travels, the state government of Bahia has distributed health care units into municipalities located into nine regions (i.e., North, Northeast, North-Central, East-Central, East, West, Southwest, South, and Extreme-South) that geographically divide the state of Bahia, such that COVID-19 patients could be ideally treated or hospitalized in health care units available at the regions where they reside, promoting a region-based control of the COVID-19 pandemic inside the state of Bahia.

Related work has already shown that we need to analyze transportation networks between the municipalities and states of a country [14–17] to be able to study the dynamics of dissemination of infectious diseases, such as COVID-19 [18–24], as well as to evaluate how we can guarantee a safe transportation for COVID-19 patients to be hospitalized in the health care units [25–27] of Bahia.

In this paper, we aim to evaluate whether the distribution of intensive and non-intensive care units among 61 out of the 417 municipalities in Bahia is sufficient to assist COVID-19 patients inside each one of the nine distinct regions that divide the state of Bahia. On the basis of a dataset provided by the Health Secretary of the State of Bahia (Secretária de Saúde do Estado da Bahia—SESAB) and by the Brazilian Ministry of Health (Ministério da Saúde do Brasil), from open health systems data, we have built a hospitalization network for COVID-19 patients in Bahia, Brazil, based on the concepts of complex networks and using geoprocessing. We have also analyzed whether COVID-19 patients are indeed being hospitalized in health care units located in the same region where they live, and if that is not the case, we determined the relation of importation and exportation of hospitalized COVID-19 patients between distinct regions in Bahia. The specificity of the study and the absence of an index that could be used to compare the level of care and hospitalization provided by a given region led to the development of the Degree of External Search for Hospitalization (DESH) index, used to estimate the saturation level of the municipalities that offer in-hospital assistance for COVID-19 patients that come from other regions of the state of Bahia.

The network approach allowed us to evaluate the relationship between the external demand for COVID-19 care units and the supply of these units in the region. The DESH measure does not represent a new topological index of the network, but rather a simple evaluation of the external pressure for care units in the municipality relativized with respect to the total number of care units available in it. We believe that the discussions presented in this paper may be helpful to the state government of Bahia, which may improve its decision-making process to effectively control the COVID-19 pandemic in Bahia, and we also believe that this kind of study may be replicated for other states and countries around the world to verify whether the hospitalization networks previously estimated by governments match the real ones obtained in practice.

2. Materials and Methods

2.1. Data Collection

In this study, we considered the COVID-19 patients that were hospitalized in intensive or non-intensive care units provided by SUS in the state of Bahia, Brazil, between 1 March 2020 and 30 July 2020, and that have been reported in the hospital systems. To build the hospitalization networks, the data represent all hospitalizations of patients affected by COVID-19 (4387) who were removed from their city of residence to another city. The objective was to measure the displacement of these patients due to the unavailability of health units in their municipality of residence.

2.2. Hospitalization Network

On the basis of the graph theory, we represent the hospitalization networks for COVID-19 patients in Bahia as a directed graph, where each node is assigned to a municipality in Bahia, each node's size is directly proportional to its DESH index to be presented in the next subsection, each directed edge represents a travel going from an origin (i.e., municipality of residence) to a destination (i.e., municipality of hospitalization), and each directed edge is weighted by the number of patients that traveled between the corresponding pair of origin–destination municipalities. Hence, the hospitalization networks provides a visual representation of the patients that needed to be hospitalized because of the severity of COVID-19, but could not be hospitalized in their municipality of residence due to the unavailability of a health care unit at that location and at that moment.

2.3. Simulation of the Expected Network

In order to evaluate whether the strategy of the state government of Bahia to distribute health care units among the nine regions in Bahia was successful, we simulated the expected hospitalization networks idealized by the state government. To do so, we redirected each edge of the observed hospitalization networks to connect the node representing the municipality of residence of the patient to another node representing the closest municipality with an available health care unit, such that each redirected edge could represent the expected path traveled by a patient when searching for hospitalization by COVID-19 in Bahia.

2.4. DESH (Degree of External Search for Hospitalization) Index

To favor a comparison between the level of assistance and hospitalization provided by each region of the state of Bahia, we have developed the DESH index. With such an index, we can measure the saturation level of the 61 municipalities able to hospitalize COVID-19 patients. While each one of those 61 municipalities must provide assistance to the internal demand for hospitalization, by providing support to the patients that live inside the corresponding municipality, the DESH index only takes into account the external demand for hospitalization. In other words, this index measures how much each municipality is involved in the importation of COVID-19 patients provided by other municipalities that could be located inside or outside of the corresponding region of the state of Bahia.

The DESH index of a municipality i, or node i, with at least one intensive or non-intensive care unit available can be described in terms of Equation (1):

$$DESH_i = \frac{\sum_{j=1}^{N-1} w_{ij}}{\gamma_i} \quad (1)$$

where w_{ij} is the weight of a directed edge that connects node i to node j (i.e., the number of patients that traveled from municipality j to municipality i), i is the total number of intensive and non-intensive care units available at that municipality i, N is the total number of municipalities being evaluated, and γ_i represents the municipalities.

Each one of the nine regions of Bahia is represented by a specific color. Each node (red circle) of the directed graph represents a municipality of Bahia. Each node size is directly proportional to its DESH index. The weight of each directed edge (black line) is directly proportional to the number of patients that have been transported to the corresponding municipality for hospitalization.

3. Results

As we can see in Figure 1a, according to the original planning of the state government of Bahia, even if not every one of the 417 municipalities of Bahia has a reference hospital or health care unit able to treat COVID-19 patients, the expected hospitalization networks for COVID-19 patients would be the one in which each patient would be hospitalized in the nearest reference unit available in the region where the patient is residing, such that COVID-19 patients would travel as minimum a distance as possible to be hospitalized, consequently allowing for a faster and more efficient treatment of those patients, as well as for a lower exposition to COVID-19 of the professionals involved in the transportation process. Hence, as can be seen by the weights of the directed edges shown in Figure 1a, once the health care units of each region would concentrate the hospitalization cases of the patients that live in the corresponding municipalities, the hospitalization networks would be more distributed all over the state, and the COVID-19 pandemic could be handled locally, per region of the state of Bahia. However, on the basis of the anonymized data collected from SESAB, we could estimate that the observed hospitalization networks for hospitalized patients are more similar to the one illustrated in Figure 1b. In this case, we can see that several COVID-19 patients need to travel from one region to another to be properly hospitalized, which suggests that some regions of the state of Bahia are not able to handle the high demands of hospitalization that may be happening due to COVID-19. In the ideal, expected scenario depicted in Figure 1a, each region would hospitalize only resident patients diagnosed with COVID-19. However, Table 1 shows that, while the North, East, and Southwest regions exported a few patients to the other regions of the state of Bahia, the North-Central, East-Central, and Northwest regions exported more than three times the number of patients that they could hospitalize. We also observed that both the East and Southwest regions concentrate the highest percentage of imported hospitalizations. In this case, it is worth noting that almost 50% of the hospitalizations done in the East region, which includes the capital of the state of Bahia, Salvador, are imported from other regions, while only 0.5% of the hospitalized cases are exported to other regions.

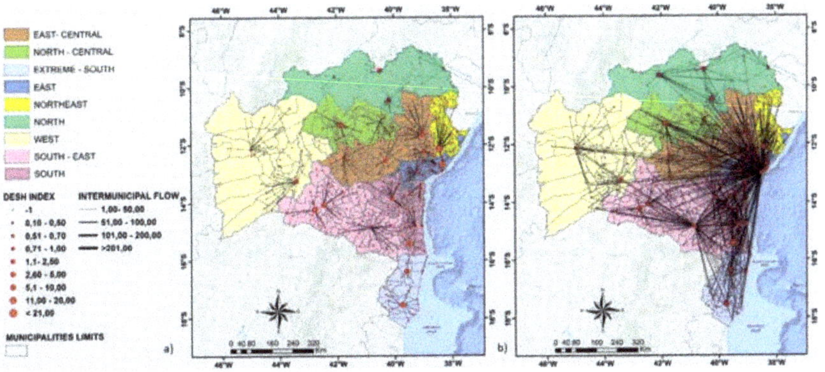

Figure 1. A visual comparison between the expected (**a**) and observed (**b**) hospitalization networks for COVID-19 patients in Bahia, Brazil. Source: Author.

Table 1. A numerical overview of the observed hospitalization networks for COVID-19 patients with respect to the nine regions of the state of Bahia.

Region	Patients That Live in That Region	Patients Imported from Other Regions	Patients Exported to Other Regions
North	158 (81.9%)	0 (0.0%)	35 (18.1%)
Northeast	11 (3.7%)	0 (0.0%)	290 (96.3%)
North-Central	12 (12.9%)	2 (2.2%)	79 (84.9%)
East-Central	77 (10.7%)	70 (9.7%)	571 (79.5%)
East	1686 (54.9%)	1369 (44.6%)	14 (0.5%)
West	62 (67.4%)	0 (0.0%)	30 (32.6%)
Southwest	263 (54.3%)	140 (28.9%)	81 (16.7%)
South	401 (47.3%)	61 (7.2%)	385 (45.5%)
Extreme-South	74 (31.8%)	1 (0.4%)	158 (67.8%)

4. Discussion

One of the main problems caused by such an unbalanced observed hospitalization networks is illustrated in Figure 2, which shows that, while in the expected hospitalization networks, some travel would be required to transport patients between the municipalities of the same region, in the observed scenario, more patients needed to travel longer distances to be hospitalized outside of their region of residence.

In our point of view, this unnecessary transportation of patients may affect the state of Bahia in two ways: First, this scenario may reduce the effectiveness in the reduction of the number of new cases of COVID-19 per region of the state of Bahia, since new patients diagnosed with COVID-19 might end up being hospitalized in another region that has already stabilized the COVID-19 pandemic, exposing the healthcare professionals of such a region to the coronavirus, which, once they are infected by COVID-19, could further disseminate the infectious disease to other people, contributing to a new rise in the number of new cases of COVID-19 per day. Second, this unnecessary transportation may result in additional costs for the state and the municipalities of Bahia, since they both are financially responsible for the management of the healthcare professionals and the infrastructure used to transport the patients to be hospitalized, and for the maintenance of the intensive and non-intensive care units that otherwise would be empty or at least less occupied, assuming a scenario in which a region is exporting new COVID-19 patients to be hospitalized to another region that has achieved stabilization with few new cases of COVID-19.

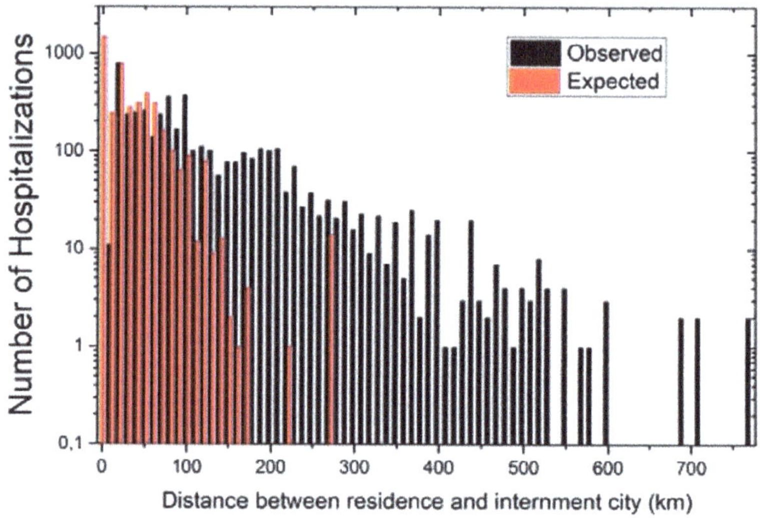

Figure 2. A histogram with the frequencies of expected (red) and observed (black) distances traveled by COVID-19 patients. Source: Author.

In Figures 3, 4, 5a, and 6, we show a more detailed visualization of the observed hospitalization networks previously shown in Figure 1b. These figures detail the transportation network for hospitalized COVID-19 patients with a focus on the relation between distinct regions of the state of Bahia and the East region, which contains the capital of the state of Bahia and the highest number of intensive and non-intensive care units, and concentrates the highest number of imported patients from other regions.

Many patients of the regions that are neighbours of the East region, such as the East-Central (Figure 3a), Northeast (Figure 5a), and South (Figure 6b) regions, are hospitalized in the East region, which may indicate that there is an unbalanced distribution of health care units in those neighbouring regions. Moreover, Figures 3, 4, 5a, and 6 show that the regions that are more distant to the East one, such as the North-Central (Figure 3b) and Extreme-South (Figure 4a) regions, also contribute to the exportation of patients to the East region. On the other hand, both the West (Figure 6a) and North (Figure 5b) regions are able to handle the demand for the hospitalization of their patients, even through the West region exported some patients for hospitalization to the East and Southwest regions, and the North region also exported some cases for hospitalization to the East region.

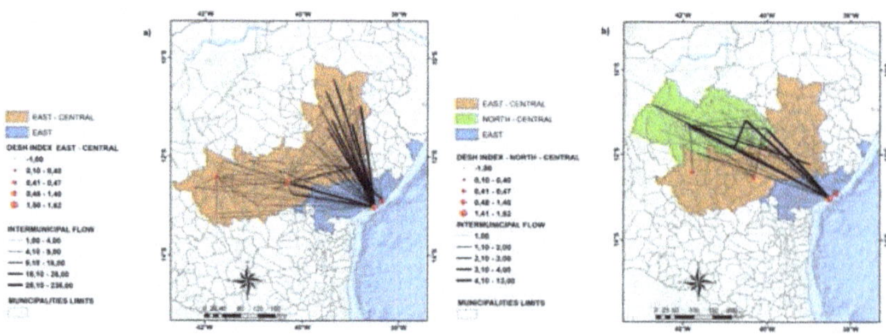

Figure 3. (**a**) A visualization of the East and East-Central regions. (**b**) A visualization of the East, East-Central, and North-Central regions. Source: Author.

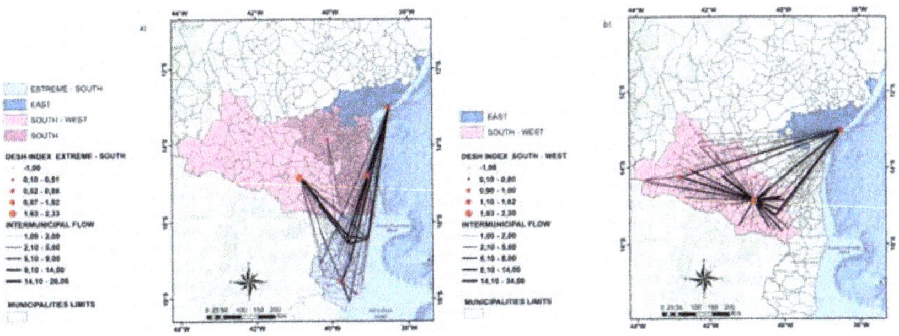

Figure 4. (**a**) A visualization of the Extreme-South, East, South-West, and South regions. (**b**) A visualization of the East and South-West regions. Source: Author.

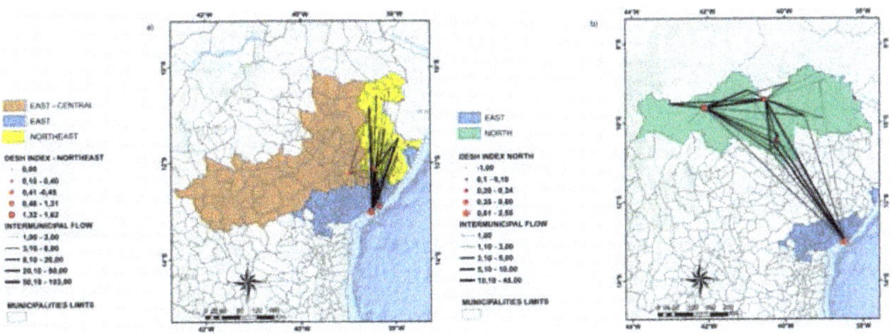

Figure 5. (**a**) A visualization of the East-Central, East, Northeast regions. (**b**) A visualization of the East and North regions. Source: Author.

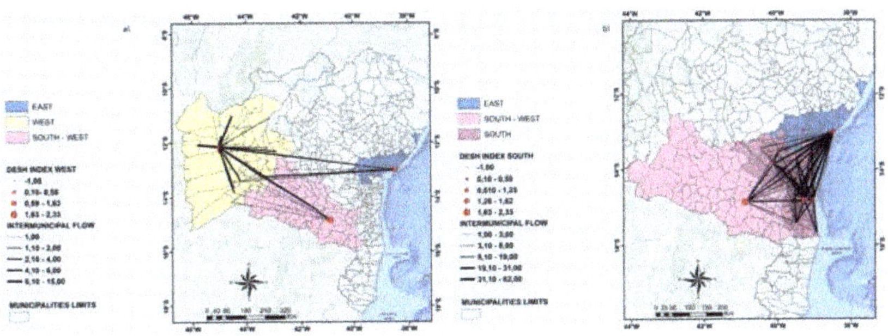

Figure 6. (**a**) A visualization of the East, West, South-West regions. (**b**) A visualization of the East, South-West and South regions. Source: Author.

It is known that the state of Bahia has a health care regulation system, and it can be seen from the results of this research that the logistics included in the process of control and the distribution of care needs to be reviewed. This is not only based on the number of inhabitants per square meter in a health region or city, but also on the need for certain medical specialties and the growth in demand for care, suggesting that this may be the reality in other countries with limited resources.

5. Conclusions

As we have shown in this paper, the distribution of intensive and non-intensive care units in the state of Bahia, Brazil, is limited, since many patients had to travel more than 300 km to be hospitalized, as shown in Figure 2. Hence, a redistribution of the available health care units, or alternatively a selective, adaptive expansion of the health care infrastructure in the regions that are exporting most of their patients to be hospitalized in other regions, may contribute to a more successful reduction in the length of these travels.

COVID-19 is a dangerous infectious disease that requires new policies of the governments in order to effectively combat the further prolongation of this pandemic. Such policies could be based on scientific research that considers the local realities of the population and other variables that can provide optimized health facility distribution arrangements. In this sense, the provision and distribution of new hospitals and health care units based on scientific criteria that are capable of caring for and admitting patients with COVID-19 would allow for the faster and more effective treatment of these patients.

Finally, we hope that the publication of this manuscript will be an encouraging factor for the state government of Bahia, and other governments around the world, to reproduce the methodology presented in this paper, so as to better evaluate their care unit distribution policies. This approach allows for a clear visualization of demand pressure and migration between different regions, which can help to determine whether the expected strategies previously planned are being observed in practice and thus reducing the social and economic impact and, most importantly, saving lives.

Author Contributions: Conceptualization: M.L.V.A., J.G.V.M., R.N.V., E.C.B.C., M.S.P.L.S. and H.S.; methodology: all authors; software: M.L.V.A., J.G.V.M., R.N.V., E.C.B.C., R.S.R., E.M.F.J. and H.S.; validation: all authors; formal analysis: all authors; investigation: all authors; resources: M.L.V.A., A.C.B., M.S.P.L.S., A.C.F.N.S., A.S.N.F., T.B.M., E.M.F.J. and H.S.; data curation: M.L.V.A., J.G.V.M., M.S.P.L.S., A.C.F.N.S. and H.S.; writing—original draft preparation: all authors; writing—review and editing: all authors; visualization: all authors; supervision: M.L.V.A. and H.S.; project administration: M.L.V.A. and H.S.; funding acquisition: M.L.V.A., M.S.P.L.S., A.C.F.N.S. and H.S. All authors have read and agreed to the published version of the manuscript.

Funding: This research was funded by PPSUS FAPESB: TO SUS0013/2021, grant number: 4370/2020. Received financial support from the National Council for Scientific and Technological Development—CNPq (http://cnpq.br/, accessed on 20 November 2021), grant numbers 306306/2021-2 (M.L.V.A.), 431990/2018-2 (H.S.) and 313423/2019-9 (H.S.).

Institutional Review Board Statement: Not applicable. The data used in this research were anonymous, without any personal data of the patients.

Informed Consent Statement: Not applicable.

Data Availability Statement: The original database used is public and available at https://bi.saude.ba.gov.br/transparencia/ (accessed on 22 October 2021), https://opendatasus.saude.gov.br/dataset/srag-2020 (accessed on 22 October 2021), and https://opendatasus.saude.gov.br/dataset/srag-2021-e-2022 (accessed on 22 October 2021). Summarized data from hospitalizations used in the analysis can be found at https://github.com/dataNPAI/UTIdata.git (accessed on 5 January 2022).

Acknowledgments: This work was supported by The Foundation for Research Support of the State of Bahia—FAPESB and the National Council for Scientific and Technological Development—CNPq.

Conflicts of Interest: The authors declare that there is no conflict of interest. The funders had no role in the design of the study; in the collection, analyses, or interpretation of data; in the writing of the manuscript; or in the decision to publish the results.

Abbreviations

The following abbreviations are used in this manuscript:

CNPq	National Council for Scientific and Technological Development
COVID-19	Coronavirus Disease 2019
DESH	Degree of External Search for Hospitalization
FAPESB	The Foundation for Research Support of the State of Bahia
HDI	Human Development Index
SESAB	Health Secretary of the State of Bahia
SUS	Brazilian National Health System
WHO	World Health Organization

References

1. Brazilian Institute of Geography and Statistics. Estimated population in Bahia, Brazil. Available online: https://cidades.ibge.gov.br/brasil/ba/panorama (accessed on 20 November 2021).
2. World Health Organization. *Considerations for Quarantine of Individuals in the Context of Containment for Coronavirus Disease (COVID-19): Interim Guidance*; No. WHO/2019-nCov/IHR_Quarantine/2020.1; World Health Organization: Geneva, Switzerland, 2020.
3. Tanaka, O.Y.; Oliveira, V.E. Reforms and organization of the British National Health System: Lessons to the Brazilian National Health System. *Saúde Soc.* **2007**, *16*, 7–17. [CrossRef]
4. Constitution of the Federative Republic of Brazil Available online: http://www.planalto.gov.br/ccivil_03/constituicao/constituicao.htm (accessed on 20 November 2021).
5. Lei Orgânica de Saúde. Lei nº 8.080. 1990. Available online: http://www.planalto.gov.br/ccivil_03/leis/l8080.htm (accessed on 20 November 2021).
6. Massuda, A.; Hone, T.; Leles, F.A.G.; De Castro, M.C.; Atun, R.The Brazilian health system at crossroads: progress, crisis and resilience. *BMJ Global Health* **2018**, *3*, e000829. [PubMed]
7. Punnakitikashem, P.; Hallinger, P. Bibliometric review of the knowledge base on healthcare management for sustainability, 1994–2018. *Sustainability* **2019**, *12*, 205. [CrossRef]
8. Nuti, S.; Vainieri, M.; Bonini, A. Disinvestment for re-allocation: a process to identify priorities in healthcare. *Health Policy* **2010**, *95*, 137–143. [CrossRef] [PubMed]
9. Park, H.A.; Kim, S.; Ha, S.O.; Han, S.; Lee, C. Effect of Designating Emergency Medical Centers for Critical Care on Emergency Medical Service Systems during the COVID-19 Pandemic: A Retrospective Observational Study. *J. Clin. Med.* **2022**, *11*, 906. [CrossRef] [PubMed]
10. Katayama, Y.; Tanaka, K.; Kitamura, T.; Takeuchi, T.; Nakao, S.; Nitta, M.; Iwami, T.; Fujimi, S.; Uejima, T.; Miyamoto, Y.; et al. Incidence and Mortality of Emergency Patients Transported by Emergency Medical Service Personnel during the Novel Corona Virus Pandemic in Osaka Prefecture, Japan: A Population-Based Study. *J. Clin. Med* **2021**, *10*, 5662. [CrossRef] [PubMed]
11. Health Secretary of the State of Bahia. Plano Estadual de Contingências para Enfrentamento do Novo Coronavírus—SARS—CoV—2. Available online: http://www.saude.ba.gov.br/wp-content/uploads/2020/06/Plano-de-Continge%CC%82ncia-Coronav%C3%ADrus-Bahia-2020-2606.pdf (accessed on 20 November 2021).
12. Health Secretary of the State of Bahia. Central Integrada de Comando e Controle de Saúde—COVID-19. Available online: https://bi.saude.ba.gov.br/transparencia/ (accessed on 20 January 2022).
13. Health Secretary of the State of Bahia. Regulation System. Available online: http://www.saude.ba.gov.br/atencao-a-saude/comofuncionaosus/sistema-de-regulacao/ (accessed on 5 February 2022).
14. Saba, H.; Vale, V.C.; Moret, M.A.; Miranda, J.C.V. Spatio-temporal correlation networks of dengue in the state of Bahia. *BMC Public Health* **2014**, *14*, 1085. [CrossRef]
15. Saba, H.; Moret, M.A.; Barreto, F.R.; Araujo, M.L.V.; Jorge, E.M.F.; Filho, A.S.N.F.; Miranda, J.G.V. Relevance of transportation to correlations among criticality, physical means of propagation, and distribution of dengue fever cases in the state of Bahia. *Sci. Total Environ.* **2018**, *618*, 971–976. [CrossRef] [PubMed]
16. Tiracini, A.; Cats, O. COVID-19 and public transportation: Current assessment, prospects, and research needs. *J. Public Trans.* **2020**, *22*, 1. [CrossRef]
17. Zheng, R.; Xu, Y.; Wang, W.; Ning, G.; Bi, Y. Spatial transmission of COVID-19 via public and private transportation in China. *Travel. Med. Infect. Dis.* **2020**, *34*, 101626. [CrossRef] [PubMed]
18. Du, Z.; Wang, L.; Cauchemez, S.; Xu, X.; Wang, X.; Cowling, B.J.; Meyers, L.A. Risk for Transportation of Coronavirus Disease from Wuhan to Other Cities in China. *Emerg. Infect. Dis.* **2020**, *26*, 1049. Available online: https://wwwnc.cdc.gov/eid/article/26/5/20-0146_article (accessed on 20 November 2021). [PubMed]
19. Wei, J.T.; Liu, Y.X.; Zhu, Y.C.; Qian, J.; Ye, R.Z.; Li, C.Y.; Ji, X.K.; Li, H.K.; Qi, C.; Wang, Y.; et al. Impacts of transportation and meteorological factors on the transmission of COVID-19. *Int. J. Hyg. Environ. Health* **2020**, *230*, 113610. [CrossRef] [PubMed]
20. Lee, H.; Park, S.J.; Lee, G.R.; Kim, J.E.; Lee, J.H.; Jung, Y.; Nam, E.W. The relationship between trends in COVID-19 prevalence and traffic levels in South Korea. *Int. J. Infect. Dis.* **2020**, *96*, 399–407. [CrossRef] [PubMed]

21. Carmo, R.F.; Nunes, B.E.B.R.; Machado, M.F.; Armstrong, A.C.; Souza, C.D.F. Expansion of COVID-19 within Brazil: the importance of highways. *J. Travel. Med.* **2020**, *27*, taaa106. [CrossRef] [PubMed]
22. Zhong, P.; Guo, S.; Chen, T. Correlation between travellers departing from Wuhan before the Spring Festival and subsequent spread of COVID-19 to all provinces in China. *J. Travel. Med.* **2020**, *27*, taaa036. [CrossRef] [PubMed]
23. Hu, M.; Lin, H.; Wang, J.; Xu, C.; Tatem, A.J.; Meng, B.; Zhang, X.; Liu, Y.; Wang, P.; Wu, G.; et al. The risk of COVID-19 transmission in train passengers: An epidemiological and modelling study. *Clin. Infect. Dis.* **2020**, *72*, 604–610. [CrossRef]
24. Bajardi, P.; Poletto, C.; Ramasco, J.J.; Tizzoni, M.; Colizza, V.; Vespignani, A. Human Mobility Networks, Travel Restrictions, and the Global Spread of 2009 H1N1 Pandemic. *PLoS ONE* **2011**, *6*, e16591. [CrossRef]
25. Liew, M.F.; Siow, W.T.; Yau, Y.W.; See, K.C. Safe patient transport for COVID-19. *Crit. Care* **2020**, *24*, 1–13. [CrossRef]
26. Brown, A.S.; Hustey, F.M.; Reddy, A.J. Interhospital transport of patients with COVID-19: Cleveland Clinic approach. *Cleve Clin. J. Med.* **2020**. [CrossRef]
27. Macedo, M.C.; Pinheiro, I.M.; Carvalho, C.J.; Fraga, H.C.; Araujo, I.P.; Montes, S.S.; Araujo, O.A.; Alves, L.A.; Saba, H.; Araújo, M.L.; et al. Correlation between hospitalized patients' demographics, symptoms, comorbidities, and COVID-19 pandemic in Bahia, Brazil. *PLoS ONE* **2020**, *15*, e0243966. [CrossRef]

healthcare

MDPI

Review

Health, Economic and Social Development Challenges of the COVID-19 Pandemic: Strategies for Multiple and Interconnected Issues

Sigamani Panneer [1,*], Komali Kantamaneni [2,*], Udhayakumar Palaniswamy [1], Lekha Bhat [1], Robert Ramesh Babu Pushparaj [1], Kesavan Rajasekharan Nayar [3], Hilaria Soundari Manuel [4], F. X. Lovelina Little Flower [5] and Louis Rice [6]

1 Department of Social Work, School of Social Sciences and Humanities, Central University of Tamil Nadu, Thiruvarur 610005, Tamil Nadu, India; pudhayakumar@cutn.ac.in (U.P.); lekhabhatd@gmail.com (L.B.); robertrb19@students.cutn.ac.in (R.R.B.P.)
2 Faculty of Science and Technology, University of Central Lancashire, Preston PR1 2HE, UK
3 Global Institute of Public Health, Ananthapuri Hospitals and Research Institute, Thiruvananthapuram 695024, Kerala, India; krnayar@gmail.com
4 Centre for Applied Research, The Gandhigram Rural Institute, Deemed to be University, Gandhigram, Dindigul 624302, Tamil Nadu, India; m.hillariasoundari@ruraluniv.ac.in
5 Department of Social Work, Bharathiar University, Coimbatore 641046, Tamil Nadu, India; lovelina@buc.edu.in
6 Centre for Architecture and Built Environment Research, University of the West of England, Bristol BS16 1QY, UK; louis.rice@uwe.ac.uk
* Correspondence: sigamanip@cutn.ac.in (S.P.); kkantamaneni@uclan.ac.uk (K.K.)

Citation: Panneer, S.; Kantamaneni, K.; Palaniswamy, U.; Bhat, L.; Pushparaj, R.R.B.; Nayar, K.R.; Soundari Manuel, H.; Flower, F.X.L.L.; Rice, L. Health, Economic and Social Development Challenges of the COVID-19 Pandemic: Strategies for Multiple and Interconnected Issues. *Healthcare* **2022**, *10*, 770. https://doi.org/10.3390/healthcare10050770

Academic Editor: Krzysztof Goniewicz

Received: 24 March 2022
Accepted: 17 April 2022
Published: 21 April 2022

Abstract: The COVID-19-pandemic-related economic and social crises are leading to huge challenges for all spheres of human life across the globe. Various challenges highlighted by this pandemic include, but are not limited to, the need for global health cooperation and security, better crisis management, coordinated funding in public health emergencies, and access to measures related to prevention, treatment and control. This systematic review explores health, economic and social development issues in a COVID-19 pandemic context and aftermath. Accordingly, a methodology that focuses on identifying relevant literature with a focus on meta-analysis is used. A protocol with inclusion and exclusion criteria was developed, with articles from 15 December 2019 to 15 March 2022 included in the study. This was followed by a review and data analysis. The research results reveal that non-pharmaceutical measures like social distancing, lockdown and quarantine have created long-term impacts on issues such as changes in production and consumption patterns, market crashes resulting in the closure of business operations, and the slowing down of the economy. COVID-19 has exposed huge health inequalities across most countries due to social stratification and unequal distribution of wealth and/or resources. People from lower socio-economic backgrounds lack access to essential healthcare services during this critical time for both COVID-19 and other non-COVID ailments. The review shows that there is minimal literature available with evidence and empirical backup; similarly, data/studies from all countries/regions are not available. We propose that there is a need to conduct empirical research employing a trans-disciplinary approach to develop the most effective and efficient strategies to combat the pandemic and its aftermath. There is a need to explore the social and ecological determinants of this contagious infection and develop strategies for the prevention and control of COVID-19 or similar infections in future.

Keywords: COVID-19; global economy; healthcare; social development; low- and middle-income countries; transdisciplinary research

1. Introduction

This paper explores the challenges of the COVID-19 pandemic and the significance of non-pharmaceutical measures for global health and socio-economic development. The

COVID-19 pandemic introduced economic and social crises that are posing huge challenges across the globe. The most serious challenges related to the COVID-19 pandemic and post-COVID future are related to the employment and incomes of millions of people, social security, income support schemes, the burden on women, the plight of migrants and informal sector workers, mental health issues, and restrictions on economic activity, including halted production, with firms unable to sell their goods and services [1]. The pandemic has also sparked fear and anxiety due to economic shocks and recession [2]. In an attempt to "flatten the curve", various countries' governments have imposed international border shutdowns [3,4], internal travel constraints [5] and longer periods of quarantine [6,7]. Economists have predicted that the COVID-19 pandemic will slow down Gross Domestic Product (GDP) growth by one-half a percentage point for 2020, and this applies to all countries (from 2.9% to 2.4%) [8]. Social distancing, lockdown and quarantine have high economic and social costs associated with them because they introduce changes in production and consumption patterns, which caused financial markets to crash, resulting in the closure of business operations [9]. Furthermore, this pandemic also introduced the international community to various challenges relating to global health cooperation and security, crisis management (investment in emergency preparedness) and coordinated funding during public health emergencies. The global economy has been very badly affected, especially the agro-livestock industry, hitting their lowest growth rates across various countries [10]. A decrease in inputs availability and a decrease in agricultural production during the pandemic affected food security as well [11].

Globally 3.3 billion people, which constitutes 81% of the world's workforce, were affected by the lockdown. Of this lockdown-affected workforce, 61% were workers from the informal sector, and of this 90% were from low- and middle-income countries [12,13]. The nationwide lockdowns during the COVID-19 pandemic disunited and isolated much of the migrant populations. Due to the lack of job opportunities, millions of migrant workers were forced to return to their countries/counties/villages in a time when public transportation was closed or severely restricted. Migrants faced humanitarian and health security challenges and unusual logistical nightmares from the states where they migrated [14]. Furthermore, in many developing and underdeveloped countries, the available social security measures are weak, with a lack of access to health care and economic security [15]. As many state borders were closed, inter-country travel and trade were shut and more than 30 million people fell into poverty in the absence of active policies to protect or substitute income flows to vulnerable populations. These policies, decisions and actions severely impacted the health and wellbeing of a large section of the population [16]. With chronic low funding in rural healthcare and the economy, the pandemic has revealed the weaknesses of rural infrastructure in almost all countries [17].

2. Review Protocol

A systematic review has been selected for this study with exclusion and inclusion criteria applied to narrow down the literature search. A large number of academic literature and policy documents related to COVID-19 have been considered for this study. Google, Google Scholar, PubMed, Science Direct, Web of Science and Scopus were used to identify the relevant literature. Google has been used to search various policy reports and other associated documents that are not available in scientific search engines such as Science Direct, Web of Science and Scopus. This review attempted to find solutions to health, economic and social development challenges of the COVID-19 pandemic. The major objectives of the review were to understand the inter-linkages between health, economy and society, to assess the pandemic crisis, to explore health and development implications of COVID-19, to compile possible and easily workable strategies for solving problems of COVID-19, to understand the role of multi-stakeholders in time of crisis and to document innovative collaborative strategic directions to control the pandemic. Based on these objectives, the search was made to look through each database that contained the terms: COVID-19, health and development challenges, pandemics, multiple and interconnected issues, economic impact and strategies, prevention and recommendations. During the search, results from diverse sources identified some duplicate articles, especially those associated with COVID-19. Due to this, a unique combination of words was used to explore the relevant literature as follows:

COVID-19 and low- and middle-income countries
COVID-19 and developed countries
Stages of lockdown and health impacts
Lockdown and economic impact
COVID-19 and health impacts
COVID-19—disaster management
Post-pandemic context

Appropriate literature was identified from the diverse sources, based on data quality, focus area, rigourous methods, and removal of replicas; the subsequent works were scrutinised according to the exclusion and inclusion criteria listed in Table 1. This process was undertaken in different phases, with the date of publication, abstract and title considered for exclusion and inclusion. If the title and abstract did not fully reveal the scope of the study, the full article was examined to fully assess the entire information for that specific particular. Furthermore, some grey literature was considered for this study. Google and organization websites such as United Nations Development Programme (UNDP), World Health Organization (WHO), United Nations (UN), and United Nations Office for Outer Space Affairs (UNOOSA) were used to get the most up-to-date information. PICO was used as the strategy to undertake the systematic review.

Table 1. Criteria for the inclusion and exclusion.

Number	Inclusion	Exclusion
1	Literature published between December 2019 and March 2022	Literature published before December 2019. For the discussion and introduction and discussions, articles that were published before December 2019 were not considered
2	Literature available on COVID-19, developed and developing (low-and middle-income countries), COVID-19 and health impacts in post-pandemic context	Literature that are related but very complicated and some sensitive topics such as political decisions for the COVID-19 lockdown and vaccine development
3	Literature related to the search words	Literature that is not associated with the search words
4	Literature with novel results without any geographical remit	Literature that is highly technical in nature, and articles with incomplete, aggressive or biased results
5	Other disasters/pandemics related to the COVID-19 pandemic	Articles which were published in predatory journals and literature unrelated to the pandemics/disasters
6	Reports from various national and international organizations were also accessed apart from several non-academic sources (example: newspaper reports/online news sites). Only articles/reviews in the English language were included in the study.	The vast scope of COVID19 literature which did not give precise and accurate information related to the search words

Based on Google, Google Scholar, PubMed, Science Direct, Web of Science and Scopus, a total of 1825 relevant articles were identified. However, more than 600 (628) duplicates were identified and these were deleted. Moreover, literature that was not closely related to the search words led to the deletion of a further 426 articles. At this stage, 771 articles had been considered for assessment. After careful consideration of the titles and abstracts, a further 424 articles were removed. At this stage, 347 articles had been considered for the analysis. After reading these 347 papers, a further 202 articles were deleted, as they had either highly technical or overly sensitive issues. Finally, 145 papers were considered for the study. Of these 145 papers, Table 2 presents the top 10 papers, which are the most relevant and highly cited articles. Figure 1 provides information on the inclusion and exclusion criteria of the literature.

Table 2. Systematic analysis results—top 10 articles and their information.

No.	Title of the Article	Type of the Article	Article Description
1	"Social isolation in COVID-19: The impact of loneliness"	Review	Highlights the problem of loneliness due to social isolation due to COVID-19 and suggests ways to overcome loneliness
2	"Bouncing forward: a resilience approach to dealing with COVID-19 and future systemic shocks"	Review	Reviews the impact of COVID-19 on socio-economic development and suggests various policies, infrastructure, and systems to bounce back with a resilience approach. It addresses future similar issues with proactive strategies
3	"Challenges in ensuring global access to COVID-19 vaccines: production, affordability, allocation, and deployment"	Health Policy	Reveals the challenges involved in COVID-19 vaccines and suggests various policies to ensure global access to these vaccines
4	"The plight of essential workers during the COVID-19 pandemic"	Review	Identifies struggles of healthcare and essential workers situation during COVID-19
5	"Multivalue ethical framework for fair global allocation of a COVID-19 vaccine"	Ethical Framework	Analyzes the importance of global access to COVID-19 vaccines and presents an ethical framework to make sure it is globally accessible to everyone.
6	"The Great Lockdown in the Wake of COVID-19 and Its Implications: Lessons for Low and Middle-Income Countries"	Review	Reveals the impact created by the great lockdown imposed due to COVID-19 and presents lessons for low- and middle-income countries to fight against COVID-19
7	"COVID-19: Impact on the Indian economy"	Policy Document	Analyzes the impact of COVID-19 on the Indian economy and suggests various policies and recommendations for different sectors
8	"Guidelines for Responding to COVID-19 Pandemic: Best Practices, Impacts, and Future Research Directions"	Review	Based on the COVID-19 pandemic experience the study presents guidelines for the improvement of workforce-related issues, demand and supply chain, and insurance needs.
9	"Multistakeholder Participation in Disaster Management—The Case of the COVID-19 Pandemic"	Review	Presents the need, policies and strategies required to fight against the COVID-19 pandemic through multi-stakeholder participation
10	"The effect of control strategies to reduce social mixing on outcomes of the COVID-19 epidemic in Wuhan, China: a modelling study"	Review	Analyzes the effectiveness of the physical distance measures related to the COVID-19 pandemic

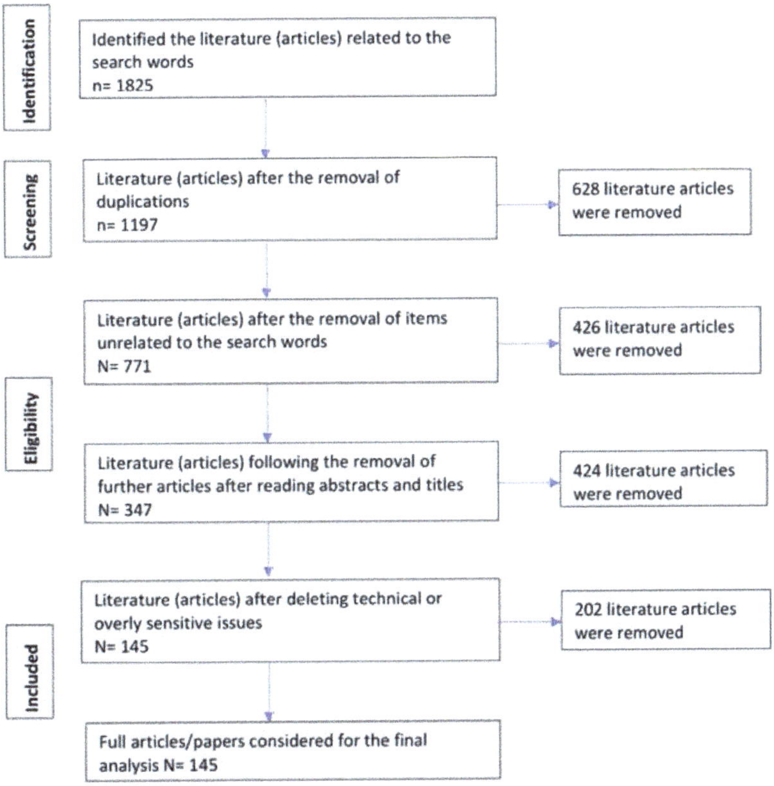

Figure 1. Systematic review—PRISMA model flow diagram (inclusion and exclusion criteria).

3. Review Results

3.1. Pandemics and Their Impact on Various Population Groups

Pandemics/disasters often leave a significant impact on human health and development. This includes, but is not limited to, loss of human lives, livelihood issues, and psycho-social problems. Pandemics can create long-term imbalances in societies and communities. The challenges confronted by the general public due to the pandemic have revealed inadequacies in the areas of managing health risks, injuries, diseases, disabilities, psychological problems and deaths [18]. The COVID-19 pandemic has affected all aspects of human life and the global economy [19]. The World Trade Organization (WTO) and Organization for Economic Cooperation and Development (OECD) marked the COVID-19 pandemic as the greatest peril to the world economy since the financial emergency of 2008–2009 [20]. Emerging issues related to jobs and income of millions of people, social safety net, future of income support schemes, the burden on women, and the plight of migrants and informal sector workers are some of the main challenges that the world is confronting [21]. Oxfam predicts that the economic crisis due to COVID-19 could push half a billion people into poverty [22]. Due to the lockdown, economic activities and livelihoods were affected in many ways, especially in the fields such as production and distribution, consumption, restriction on trade and business, large-scale uncertainties in the market, lack of access to the resources and sudden disappearance of the more informal sectors of employment/sector [23]. The global outbreak has resulted in developmental impacts on health, education, gender, economy, politics and the environment. The COVID-19 pandemic has exposed huge health inequalities across countries and within countries due to existing social stratification and resource sharing. People from lower socio-economic strata lack access to essential healthcare services during the pandemic time [24]. The economic decline during the pandemic has significantly affected people from the lower socio-economic stratum [23]. This pandemic has marked a significant impact on the lives of many vulnerable sections of society, including women and children. Across countries, the number of cases related to domestic violence has increased [25]. The pandemic has had an extensive impact on the education sector [26–28], and all educational institutions have been closed for several months, especially in countries where vaccination proceeded at a slower pace. The pandemic has forced a worldwide lockdown, with a huge number of citizens confined to their homes [29], often resulting in social isolation. Social isolation has led to chronic loneliness and boredom, which has affected mental health, human happiness and wellbeing [25].

The pandemic affected political systems across the globe, causing ideological differences, lack of need-based initiatives, geopolitical cooperation/dysfunctions, misinformation and misleading/false claims. The COVID-19 pandemic has affected religion in many ways, including cutting short pilgrimages and journeys related to religious practices and festivities [30]. People working in the informal sector, including migrant workers, are at a high risk of poverty as their income and livelihood options are limited [31,32]. Vulnerable populations have struggled to cope with the magnitude of problems and the incidence of suicide has increased due to loss of income, livelihood and other factors [33]. Challenges of immunization, nutrition, poverty, hunger, acute undernourishment, and health inequalities, especially amongst vulnerable groups, have posed severe health and economic challenges [31].

The pandemic's impact on social life, the economy and the financial sector has led millions of people to face an unprecedented situation related to poverty, wherein an average of 3.3 billion of the global workforce are at risk of losing their livelihoods [12,34]. Breadwinners working in the informal economy, particularly marginalized populations in low-income countries, which includes small-scale farmers and indigenous peoples, have been drastically affected [35]. According to a WHO survey, in May 2020, it was found that in 155 countries, the pandemic had severely curtailed people's ability to avail treatment services for Non-Communicable Diseases (NCDs). This situation is of significant concern because people living with non-communicable diseases tend to be at higher risk of severe COVID-19-related illness and death [36]. While the health systems of various countries are being challenged by the increasing demand for care of COVID-19 patients, it is imperative to maintain preventive and curative health care services, especially for the most vulnerable populations, such as children, women, older persons, people living with chronic conditions, minorities and people living with disabilities [37]. The pandemic has deepened pre-existing inequalities in social, political and economic systems, including access to health services and social protection. Women with care responsibilities, informal workers, low-income families and young people have been most adversely affected by the pandemic. There has also been a significant rise in domestic violence [38]. An increase in violence against women has resulted in a threat to public health and women's health across the globe. The health impacts of violence, particularly intimate partner or domestic violence, on women and children have significantly increased in various societies. Women who have been displaced, are refugees, and are living in conflict-affected areas are the most vulnerable [39]. Lack of education and economic insecurity has also increased the risk of gender-based violence. Without sufficient economic resources, women cannot escape from abusive partners and hence face a greater threat of sexual exploitation and trafficking [40]. Pandemic-induced poverty has also widened the gender poverty gap, pushing women into extreme poverty, as they earn less and hold less secure jobs than men [22,41]. The economic fallout for women has increased due to more unpaid care work, thereby compelling them to go back to traditional gender roles of more household and care workers [42].

Children are affected due to the pandemic and this is most visible in their health and education in various ways [43]. Children from marginalized sections have been the victims as inequalities in the teaching-learning system widened. Data show that 463 million children did not have access to the internet or digital devices for remote learning during the closure of schools [44]. Closures of schools have severely affected those children who rely on school-based nutrition programmes for their food and survival. Children suffering violence at home, refugee children, migrant children and children affected by conflict face appalling human rights violations and threats to their safety and well-being [45]. The additional stress and stigma that befall families struggling to cope have also impacted their children [45]. In the last two decades, there has been significant progress in the fight against child labour; however, the pandemic could significantly reverse this otherwise positive trend [46]. This reversal is because the crisis has enormously disrupted global education, and the lack of distance-learning solutions in many of the developing and underdeveloped countries has excluded children from online education for a very long duration. Furthermore, this trend has the potential to push millions of children into child labour [47]. Whilst the adverse socio-economic and financial impacts have fallen on the majority of households globally, there is significant inequality with some children impacted more severely, for example marginalized minority groups, disabled, street-connected and homeless populations, single or child-headed households, migrants, refugees, internally displaced persons, or people from conflict or disaster-affected areas, will be more vulnerable to child labour [48].

Beyond poverty and informality, the most explicit references to other vulnerable people and groups include older persons and people living with disabilities [49]. As the world struggles with an incomparable health crisis, older persons have become the topmost victims. The pandemic affected persons of all ages, yet older persons and those with underlying medical conditions tend to be at a higher risk of serious illness and death due to COVID-19 [50]. In the face of a life-threatening pandemic, especially during the first wave, many of the older persons faced challenges in accessing medical treatments and health care services for non-COVID ailments and chronic diseases. In developing countries, the prolonged lockdowns, weak health systems and healthcare facilities requiring out-of-pocket expenditure left millions of older people, especially those in the poorest groups, without access to basic health care, which ultimately increased their vulnerability to COVID-19 as well [51]. While older people often have been invisible in humanitarian action, the pandemic uncovered their exclusion. Older persons usually had to rely on multiple income sources, including paid work, savings, financial support from families and pensions. Additionally, for those older people living alone, isolation combined with other factors such as limited mobility creates greater risks [52]. Individuals living with disabilities represent 15% of the population [53], and their barriers related to accessing mobility, access to health services and appropriate communication have increased tremendously, which further increases their vulnerability [54]. The physical, social, economic and health impacts of COVID 19 on people with disabilities require empirical studies so that severity can be assessed and appropriate policies can be developed [55].

3.2. Governance Issues

The pandemic also put to test the efficiency and quality of governance and the political will of the leadership in each country. During a public health crisis, people naturally depend on their governments for security and support [56]. COVID-19 brought in a unique set of challenges to governments across the globe, such as a lack of post-crisis reconstruction and recovery, weak legal and institutional mechanisms, weak infrastructural facilities, including communication networks, a lack of systematic, periodic assessment and accounting of potential losses, and poorly managed financial, technical and human resources [57]. Spontaneous behavioural reactions such as generalized panic and rumours regarding the spread of COVID-19 were reported from across the countries and each country dealt with it using different levels of efficiency and effectiveness [58]. For example, in India, the most troubling aspect was the shortage of proper provision of safety nets (e.g., food safety) during the lockdown for the weakest and vulnerable sections of the population, which was tackled by providing free food grains and cash transfer support for three months [59]. The unprecedented pandemic situation has shown the inadequacies in the global governance structure [31]. Moreover, the spread of fake news and misinformation was a major unresolved challenge for many of the democratic governments [60].

3.3. *Strategies for Solving Multiple, Interconnected Problems of COVID-19*

The WHO report on global surveillance for human infection with novel coronavirus highlights the importance of research studies to understand the viral transmission from animals and animal handlers, which will serve as evidence to prevent outbreaks similar to COVID 19 in the future [61]. To effectively respond to a public health emergency, the health system of the country must engage and step up preparedness activities with active involvement and leadership of the health department/ministry. Public health systems play a crucial role in planning health responses to respond and recover from the threats and emergencies introduced by pandemics. In various countries, fragmentation of health services has led to limited timely interventions and responses to health crises, which shows the need to have a strong coordination mechanism in place [62]. Public health emergency preparedness requires planning and intervention activities to prevent the spread of the virus, protect against other diseases and environmental hazards, promote and encourage health-seeking behaviours, respond to the crisis, assist communities in recovery, ensure quality and accessibility of the essential health services. Highly active surveillance is needed in all countries using the WHO-recommended surveillance case definition [63]. Furthermore, epidemiologic and surveillance activities would enable the public health systems to choose the most efficient ways to control the pandemic [64]. Non-pharmaceutical interventions based on supported physical distancing have a strong potential to lower the epidemic peak [65]. Priority should be accorded to certain areas, including assessment of the global health landscape; to accepting and recognizing epidemiological, environmental and economic crisis; to ensuring health regulations, such as tobacco control; to upgrading healthcare service delivery systems; and to ensuring innovative infection control, global research collaboration, universal health coverage, and public health surveillance. To support contact tracing, governments must consider expanding the use of information technology and digital initiatives to find high-risk areas [66].

The role of effective public health surveillance is crucial both in the short term and long term because the disease may remain in isolated pockets and regions even if it ceases to be a pandemic anymore. Surveillance informs about reality on the ground and provides insights for policymakers, which is essential [67]. Exploring and using web-based open tools to modernize data reporting can help provide newer, faster insights about COVID-19 controls [68]. COVID-19 surveillance in low/middle-income countries for a longer period is a real challenge due to a lack of resources, expertise, skills, people's attitude to tackling these issues technology transfer, financial assistance and capacity-building support is to be ensured [69].

The disease load of the pandemic is inequitably distributed among vulnerable populations [70]. People living in low- and middle-income countries have reduced capacity for self-protection (due to poor housing, sanitation and living conditions) [71] a high risk of food insecurity [72], a widened gap in health care access [73], loss of livelihoods, and a decrease in dietary intake and health care consumption [74]. Public policy needs to reorient federal, state and local governments to handle health equity issues sensibly [75]. The relevance of integrating public health efforts with broader public policy and acknowledging the role of social determinants of health is important [76]. Developing universal schemes for food assurance, minimum incomes, reforming unemployment insurance, and investment in community development will help to address health-inequity-related issues in the post-pandemic era [77].

COVID-19 is unlikely to be controlled or eliminated until there is global coverage of the population with effective vaccination. Vaccine development itself is not adequate; its mass production, affordability, global availability and acceptability in local communities are also important [78]. Strategies are needed to ensure affordability by handling Intellectual Property Rights issues and increasing production [79]. Long-term massive investment in the vaccination is needed; however, if the regular health budget is diverted for this, it will lead to long-term adverse consequences for general health indicators and development [80]. Increasing government revenue and getting grants and aid from donors and international loan providers are important [81]. Uneven distribution of vaccination is always a major challenge [82]; hence, vaccines should be distributed in stages, giving priority to older persons, high-risk individuals and people with co-morbidities [83]. The distribution must adhere to the WHO framework for allocating COVID-19 vaccines internationally based on need [84]. Vaccine hesitancy is prevalent in low-income and high-income countries alike, with sceptics found in all socioeconomic, religious and ethnic groups [85]. Culturally tailored health communication measures [86], community engagement [87] and a robust pharmacovigilance system [88] are important strategies for addressing vaccine hesitancy.

3.4. Role of Multi-Stakeholders in Controlling the Pandemic and Promoting the Development

COVID-19 presents a set of significant challenges to health care providers worldwide [89]. Given the complexity of the problem and the requirement of inter-sectoral collaboration, formal multidisciplinary working groups are recommended to offer relevant, effective and pragmatic solutions [90]. The pandemic is a complex phenomenon, with multiple determinants and impacts across all spheres of life. The pandemic experience serves as evidence for the need to adopt a comprehensive trans-disciplinary approach, including several experts, not only from medical sciences but also from engineering, political science, economics, humanities, psycho-social and demographic disciplines [91], as well as media that raises public awareness about health promotion and prevention [92]. The care of patients with COVID-19 can be optimized by collaborating with various multi-stakeholders to meet the demands that are required to combat the deadly disease. Multiple stakeholder engagement is critical to address the public health crises resulting from the pandemic, including but not limited to: aid donors [93,94], international aid networks, legislative and regulatory arms of the state, logistics organizations, private health care sectors [95,96], direct suppliers, media, social media [97–99], local aid networks, private insurance companies [100], military and para-military forces [101], government and inter-government organizations. Inputs of experts from the field of management, economics, environmental health, disaster management and other specialized disciplines to be incorporated in policy formulation based on inter-sectoral collaboration, which in turn can create programs and policies that are more efficient and feasible [90]. The support of patients, healthcare professionals and the wider community in addition to the government is equally important to address this health crisis [60].

3.5. COVID-19 and Social Development

The innovative, collaborative and strategic directions proposed to control the pandemic by slowing down transmission and reducing mortality associated with the pandemic are presented in Table 3.

Table 3. Strategies for COVID-19 and beyond.

Strategies
Identify innovative and culturally acceptable measures to prevent similar public health crises which explores and accommodates strategies beyond conventional economic lockdowns [102,103]
Identify easily available, culturally adaptable local technology, which is easily accessible and affordable to everyone [104,105]
Ensure that the most vulnerable populations are consulted and included in planning and response [106,107]
Organise communities to ensure that essentials including alternative livelihood opportunities to cater to needs related to food, clean water, essential healthcare and other basic services [108–112]
Advocate and promote priority-based social welfare services and in a social policy environment that services adapt, remain open and pro-active in supporting communities and vulnerable populations particularly women, children, elderly and persons with special needs [113,114]

Table 3. *Cont.*

Strategies
Facilitate easily acceptable physical distancing with social solidarity advocating for the advancement and strengthening of social welfare services as an essential protection against the disaster [115]
Identify adaptable or easily doable strategies and remain open and adapt to the conditions based on available successful examples of best practices [116–118]
Respond to the pandemic situation with inputs from social and behavioural sciences to develop a vision beyond this crisis and translate fear, sorrow and loss into empowerment and social transformation [119]
Ensure realistic forecast, targets and goals for prevention [120,121] and control using integrated environmental and health management perspective
Promote and ensure community participation and empowerment [122,123]
Promote behavioural modification (build ownership) [124]
Work with public-private partnership modes in research, development and health care delivery [125,126]
Ensure social participation [127], long-term commitment and leadership [128–130]
Use and encourage e-reporting [131,132], community-controlled partnerships and intervention [133]
Develop capabilities at all levels for handling emergencies, pandemic prevention and management [134,135]
Ensure responsible and competent state leadership which includes a women's leadership component [136,137]
Promote greater participation and accountability of local communities and other stakeholders [138,139]
Strengthen inter-organizational coordination and local responsibility with centre's coordination [140–142]

4. Future Research: Moving beyond the Transdisciplinary Framework and Study Limitations

Trans-disciplinary health science research must be the prime approach to develop a universal response to COVID-19. Long-term research priorities must serve towards an evidence base for the public health system to plan or respond to future pandemics and to develop effective systems to reach out to the public [143]. The COVID-19 pandemic has been developed as a public health and developmental crisis for all countries, and this has revealed new challenges to the research community across the globe. Extensive research is needed to understand the COVID-19 crisis life cycle and its causes and consequences *(Recovery, Mitigation, Response and Preparation)*. Revisiting datasets, redefining relevant methodologies, facilitating access to online resources and exploring culturally relevant approaches is critical at this juncture. The search for relevant information sources and trying to compile proper data of active as well as closed COVID-19 cases is an important task for health researchers. Research studies are needed to explore the interconnection of climate change to the development of the virus and to understand the possible environmental factors that could influence virus diffusion [144]. Comprehensive scientific studies needed to be initiated to explore COVID-19's impact on human development, human happiness, the well-being of helping professionals, their families and others in the community. Synthesizing evidence more rapidly will help contribute towards provision of broad-ranging intervention guidelines and longer-term strategies for human happiness and well-being and social and economic recovery. Ensuring adequate quality research work, communicating thereof with multi-stakeholders and developing policy briefs for appropriate government action is a priority area. There is also a need to strengthen community-based crisis risk management, learn from the field with empirical evidence and replicate best practices. Transdisciplinary research is best suited to explore the new parameters that could be appropriate to explain COVID-19's initial diffusion and its development as a pandemic [144].

5. Recommendations

The widespread prevalence of the infection and high causalities has made pandemic policies a high priority. As a response to control the pandemic, the WHO has recommended countries to develop preparatory policies to fight against the pandemic as well as address pandemic-induced developmental problems [145]. Developing appropriate COVID-19 control policies is a huge public health concern for all countries, and this requires combined inter-sectoral collaboration and government agreements through various coalitions [90]. The policy response should be two-fold: address present critical health and livelihood issues and suggest an approach to deal with the long-term issues the pandemic has introduced. The public health sector must take the lead for the whole of society, with a welfare approach to minimize the negative impacts of COVID-19 and help people restore the balance in their lives and livelihoods. This includes responding with appropriate public health emergency actions, identifying economic impacts, identifying and dealing effectively with misinformation spread about the disease [146]. Governments need to focus on providing authoritative information via multiple sources to ensure accurate data and appropriate social behaviour. Increasing transparency, ensuring proper restrictions, designing suitable prioritization guidelines about how to allocate scarce resources and making use of effective technologies are important [146]. To recognize the potential of psychological burnout from long hours of work and potential demoralization from persistent stress among health care workers is also an area that needs the urgent attention of policy framers. Vaccine and therapeutic investment, as well as research and development on COVID-19 control/elimination, is another key area. Governments need to strike a balance between protecting health and respecting human rights [146]. Identifying a new set of priorities and reworking national spending priorities will help to utilise available resources most efficiently and facilitate the return of normality in people's lives. Governments should address the long-standing challenges of health and nutrition of low-income households, strengthen food supply chains and empower women in food chains [147]. In response to the COVID-19 crisis, the International Labour Organization (ILO) has structured the four-pillar policy framework based on international labour standards to tackle the socio-economic crisis, stimulate the economy and employment, protect workers in the workplace, and rely on social dialogue for solutions [148].

6. Conclusions

The world is facing unprecedented challenges due to COVID-19, and hence pragmatic and innovative approaches are needed for pandemic management. To contain the spread of the virus, public health surveillance needs to be strengthened, through research, capacity building and action. Inter-institutional collaborations can help in enhancing the quality of surveillance, preparedness and capacity building during public health emergencies. Working closely with inter-regional and national public health and emergency management plans will help to control virus transmission and other risk factors. Since the pandemic has profound and long-term economic and social impacts, an integrated model for sustainable development, the delivery of training courses, and strengthening institutional mechanisms are essential for sustainable recovery and restoring normality in people's lives. The complex problems of pandemic threats have to be handled proactively by formulating innovative strategies and protocols to respond to similar outbreaks in the future. Furthermore, it is necessary to implement practical, evidence-based public policy measures and innovative approaches to deal with pandemic management, including developing strong linkages between strategic partners, alternative resource mapping strategies, a robust institutional and legal framework, and promoting health equity across economies.

Author Contributions: Conceptualization, S.P.; methodology, S.P., K.K., R.R.B.P., L.B. and H.S.M.; validation, K.K., L.R. and H.S.M.; data analysis and data synthesis, S.P., R.R.B.P., L.B., H.S.M., F.X.L.L.F. and K.R.N.; writing—original draft preparation, S.P., U.P., L.B. and R.R.B.P.; writing—review and editing, K.R.N., R.R.B.P., L.B., H.S.M., F.X.L.L.F. and L.R.; visualization, S.P.; supervision, S.P., K.K. and U.P. All authors have read and agreed to the published version of the manuscript.

Funding: This research received no external funding.

Institutional Review Board Statement: Not applicable.

Informed Consent Statement: Not applicable.

Data Availability Statement: Not applicable.

Conflicts of Interest: The authors declare no conflict of interest.

References

1. Policy Response to COVID-19. Available online: https://www.imf.org/en/Topics/imf-and-covid19/Policy-Responses-to-COVID-19 (accessed on 1 January 2022).
2. Nicola, M.; Alsafi, Z.; Sohrabi, C.; Kerwan, A.; Al-Jabir, A.; Iosifidis, C.; Agha, M.; Agha, R. The socio-economic implications of the coronavirus pandemic (COVID-19): A review. *Int. J. Surg.* **2020**, *78*, 185–193. [CrossRef] [PubMed]
3. Wells, C.R.; Sah, P.; Moghadas, S.M.; Pandey, A.; Shoukat, A.; Wang, Y.; Wang, Z.; Meyers, L.A.; Singer, B.H.; Galvani, A.P. Impact of international travel and border control measures on the global spread of the novel 2019 coronavirus outbreak. *Proc. Natl. Acad. Sci. USA* **2020**, *117*, 7504–7509. [CrossRef] [PubMed]
4. Now, India Bans Entry of Indians from EU, Turkey and UK. *The Economic Times*. 18 March 2020. Available online: https://economictimes.indiatimes.com/news/politics-and-nation/government-prohibits-entry-of-passengers-from-eu-turkey-uk-from-march-18/articleshow/74657194.cms (accessed on 22 January 2021).
5. Kwok, K.; Lai, F.; Wei, V.; Tsoi, M.; Wong, S.; Tang, J. Comparing the impact of various interventions to control the spread of COVID-19 in twelve countries. *J. Hosp. Infect.* **2020**, *106*, 214. [CrossRef] [PubMed]
6. Jazeera, A. Travel Restrictions, Border Shutdowns by Country. Available online: https://www.aljazeera.com/news/2020/03/coronavirus-travel-restrictions-border-shutdowns-country-200318091505922.html (accessed on 25 December 2020).
7. Buck, T. Coronavirus Declared a Pandemic as Fears of Economic Crisis Mount. Available online: https://www.ft.com/content/d72f1e54-6396-11ea-b3f3-fe4680ea68b5 (accessed on 24 December 2020).
8. Gupta, M.; Abdelmaksoud, A.; Jafferany, M.; Lotti, T.; Sadoughifar, R.; Goldust, M. COVID-19 and economy. *Dermatol. Ther.* **2020**, *33*, e13329. [CrossRef] [PubMed]
9. Capurro, A.; Deagosto, G.; Ferro, F.; Ithurralde, S.; Oddone, G. Social and Economic Impact of COVID-19 and Policy Options in Uruguay. 2020. Available online: https://www.greengrowthknowledge.org/sites/default/files/downloads/resource/undp-rblac-CD19-PDS-Number10-EN-Uruguay.pdf (accessed on 15 October 2021).
10. Hashem, N.M.; Hassanein, E.M.; Hocquette, J.-F.; Gonzalez-Bulnes, A.; Ahmed, F.A.; Attia, Y.A.; Asiry, K.A. Agro-Livestock Farming System Sustainability during the COVID-19 Era: A Cross-Sectional Study on the Role of Information and Communication Technologies. *Sustainability* **2021**, *13*, 6521. Available online: https://www.mdpi.com/2071-1050/13/12/6521 (accessed on 11 February 2022).
11. Hashem, N.M.; González-Bulnes, A.; Rodriguez-Morales, A.J. Animal Welfare and Livestock Supply Chain Sustainability Under the COVID-19 Outbreak: An Overview. *Front. Vet. Sci.* **2020**, *7*, 582528. [CrossRef]
12. BBC. Coronavirus: Four out of Five People's Jobs Hit by Pandemic. *BBC NEWS*. 7 April 2020. Available online: https://www.bbc.com/news/business-52199888 (accessed on 15 October 2021).
13. Lancet, T. India under COVID-19 lockdown. *Lancet* **2020**, *395*, 1315. [CrossRef]
14. Puri, L. The Migrant Worker Crisis Needs a Multipronged Response. Available online: https://www.hindustantimes.com/analysis/the-migrant-worker-crisis-needs-a-multipronged-response/story-NRCjV7PFFnjJTqlOpi8bYJ.html (accessed on 23 December 2020).
15. Lancet, T. The plight of essential workers during the COVID-19 pandemic. *Lancet* **2020**, *395*, 1587. [CrossRef]
16. UNDP. COVID-19 and Human Development: Assessing the Crisis, Envisioning the Recovery 2020. Available online: http://hdr.undp.org/en/hdp-covid (accessed on 20 December 2020).
17. Iyengar, K.P.; Jain, V.K. COVID-19 and the plight of migrants in India. *Postgrad. Med. J.* **2021**, *97*, 471–472. [CrossRef]
18. Klemeš, J.J.; Van Fan, Y.; Tan, R.R.; Jiang, P. Minimising the present and future plastic waste, energy and environmental footprints related to COVID-19. *Renew. Sustain. Energy Rev.* **2020**, *127*, 109883. [CrossRef]
19. Chakraborty, I.; Maity, P. COVID-19 outbreak: Migration, effects on society, global environment and prevention. *Sci. Total Environ.* **2020**, *728*, 138882. [CrossRef] [PubMed]
20. UNDP The Social and Economic Impact of COVID-19 in Asia—Pacific Region. Available online: https://www.undp.org/publications/social-and-economic-impact-covid-19-asia-pacific-region (accessed on 13 January 2021).

21. Oxfam. Dignity not Destitution—An 'Economic Rescue Plan For All' to Tackle the Coronavirus Crisis and Rebuild a More Equal World 2020. Available online: https://www.oxfam.org/en/research/dignity-not-destitution (accessed on 8 December 2020).
22. Chakraborty, S. COVID-19 and Women Informal Sector Workers in India. *Econ. Political Wkly.* **2020**, *55*, 17–21. Available online: https://www.isstindia.org/pdf/1600241417_small_Com_ShineyChakraborty_29August2020_Pages_17-21.pdf (accessed on 16 December 2021).
23. Banerjee, D.; Rai, M. Social Isolation in COVID-19: The Impact of Loneliness. *Int. J. Soc. Psychiatry* **2020**, *66*, 525–527. [CrossRef]
24. Gopalan, H.S.; Misra, A. COVID-19 pandemic and challenges for socio-economic issues, healthcare and National Health Programs in India. *Diabetes Metab. Syndr. Clin. Res. Rev.* **2020**, *14*, 757–759. [CrossRef] [PubMed]
25. Crawford, J.; Butler-Henderson, K.; Rudolph, J.; Malkawi, B.; Glowatz, M.; Burton, R.; Magni, P.; Lam, S. COVID-19: 20 countries' higher education intra-period digital pedagogy responses. *J. Appl. Learn. Teach.* **2020**, *3*, 1–20.
26. Tamrat, W.; Teferra, D. COVID-19 poses a serious threat to higher education. *Univ. World News* **2020**, *9*. Available online: https://www.researchgate.net/profile/Wondwosen-Tamrat/publication/340663552_COVID-19_poses_a_serious_threat_to_higher_education/links/5e97e216299bf130799e4314/COVID-19-poses-a-serious-threat-to-higher-education.pdf (accessed on 19 November 2021).
27. Butler-Henderson, K.; Crawford, J.; Rudolph, J.; Lalani, K.; Sabu, K. COVID-19 in Higher Education Literature Database (CHELD V1): An open access systematic literature review database with coding rules. *J. Appl. Learn. Teach.* **2020**, *3*, 1–6.
28. Hellewell, J.; Abbott, S.; Gimma, A.; Bosse, N.I.; Jarvis, C.I.; Russell, T.W.; Munday, J.D.; Kucharski, A.J.; Edmunds, W.J.; Sun, F. Feasibility of controlling COVID-19 outbreaks by isolation of cases and contacts. *Lancet Glob. Health* **2020**, *8*, e488–e496. [CrossRef]
29. Burke, D. The Great Shutdown 2020: What Churches, Mosques and Temples Are Doing to Fight the Spread of Coronavirus? Available online: https://edition.cnn.com/2020/03/14/world/churches-mosques-temples-coronavirus-spread/index.html (accessed on 26 December 2020).
30. Challenges Confronting World Due to COVID-19 Put Forth Global Governance Inadequacies: Akbaruddin. Available online: https://economictimes.indiatimes.com/news/politics-and-nation/challenges-confronting-world-due-to-covid-19-put-forth-global-governance-inadequacies-akbaruddin/articleshow/75528828.cms (accessed on 12 December 2020).
31. Dodds, K.; Broto, V.C.; Detterbeck, K.; Jones, M.; Mamadouh, V.; Ramutsindela, M.; Varsanyi, M.; Wachsmuth, D.; Woon, C.Y. *The COVID-19 Pandemic: Territorial, Political and Governance Dimensions of the Crisis*; Taylor & Francis: Oxfordshire, UK, 2020. [CrossRef]
32. Panneer, S.; Kantamaneni, K.; Akkayasamy, V.S.; Susairaj, A.X.; Panda, P.K.; Acharya, S.S.; Rice, L.; Liyanage, C.; Pushparaj, R.R.B. The Great Lockdown in the Wake of COVID-19 and Its Implications: Lessons for Low and Middle-Income Countries. *Int. J. Environ. Res. Public Health* **2022**, *19*, 610. [CrossRef]
33. Bishop, J.; Roberts, A. *Challenges and Opportunities in the Post-COVID-19 World*; World Economic Forum: Geneva, Switzerland, 2020; Available online: https://www3.weforum.org/docs/WEF_Challenges_and_Opportunities_Post_COVID_19.pdf (accessed on 8 December 2021).
34. PS, A. Life of Wedding Photographers during COVID 19 Lockdown: A Study Conducted in Thiruvananthapuram District. 2021. Available online: http://digitallibrary.loyolacollegekerala.edu.in:8080/jspui/handle/123456789/2271 (accessed on 19 October 2021).
35. WHO, Impact of COVID-19 on People's Livelihoods, their Health and Our Food Systems. 2020. Available online: https://www.who.int/news/item/13-10-2020-impact-of-covid-19-on-people\T1\textquoterights-livelihoods-their-health-and-our-food-systems (accessed on 5 August 2021).
36. WHO. COVID-19 Significantly Impacts Health Services for Noncommunicable Diseases. 2020. Available online: https://www.who.int/news/item/01-06-2020-covid-19-significantly-impacts-health-services-for-noncommunicable-diseases (accessed on 23 March 2022).
37. WHO. Maintaining Essential Health Services: Operational Guidance for the COVID-19 Context: Interim Guidance, 1 June 2020; World Health Organization: 2020. Available online: https://www.who.int/emergencies/diseases/novel-coronavirus-2019/related-health-issues (accessed on 6 June 2021).
38. ILO. COVID-19: G7 Nations Need to Get Gender Equality Right for a Better Future for Women at Work. 2020. Available online: https://www.ilo.org/global/about-the-ilo/newsroom/news/WCMS_744753/lang--en/index.htm (accessed on 4 February 2022).
39. WHO. *COVID-19 and Violence against Women: What the Health Sector/System Can Do, 7 April 2020*; World Health Organization: Geneva, Switzerland, 2020. Available online: https://www.who.int/reproductivehealth/publications/emergencies/COVID-19-VAW-full-text.pdf (accessed on 16 April 2021).
40. UNWOMEN. COVID-19 and Its Economic Toll on Women: The Story behind the Numbers. Available online: https://www.unwomen.org/en/news/stories/2020/9/feature-covid-19-economic-impacts-on-women (accessed on 16 December 2020).
41. Shah, S.; Khurana, S. Gendered Impacts of the COVID-19 Pandemic on The Health And Financial Well-Being of Women: A Narrative Review With Recommendations. *Int. J.* **2021**, *1*, 831–867. Available online: https://ijpsl.in/wp-content/uploads/2021/09/Gendered-Impacts-of-the-COVID19-Pandemic-on-the-Health-and-Financial-Well-Being-of-Women_Sakshi-Shah-Shirley-Khurana.pdf (accessed on 12 January 2022).
42. UN. *WOMEN. Policy Brief: The Impact of COVID-19 on Women*; United Nations: New York, NY, USA, 2020. Available online: https://www.un.org/sexualviolenceinconflict/wp-content/uploads/2020/06/report/policy-brief-the-impact-of-covid-19-on-women/policy-brief-the-impact-of-covid-19-on-women-en-1.pdf (accessed on 15 October 2021).

43. UNICEF. *Addressing the Multiple Impacts of COVID-19 on Children Beyond Masks*; United Nations Children's Fund: New York, NY, USA, 9 November 2020. Available online: https://www.unicef-irc.org/article/2070-addressing-the-multiple-impacts-of-covid-19-on-children-beyond-masks.html (accessed on 17 November 2021).
44. UNICEF. COVID-19: At Least a Third of the world's Schoolchildren Unable to Access Remote Learning during School Closures, New UNICEF Report Says. 2020. Available online: https://www.unicef.org/indonesia/press-releases/covid-19-least-third-worlds-schoolchildren-unable-access-remote-learning-during (accessed on 18 November 2021).
45. UNICEF. Protecting the Most Vulnerable Children from the Impact of Coronavirus: An Agenda for Action. 3 April 2020. Available online: https://www.unicef.org/coronavirus/agenda-for-action#:~{}:text=Keep%20children%20healthy%20and%20well,way%20to%20fight%20the%20virus (accessed on 28 December 2021).
46. ILO. COVID-19: Protect Children from Child Labour, Now More than Ever! 2020. Available online: https://www.ilo.org/ipec/Campaignandadvocacy/wdacl/2020/lang--en/index.htm (accessed on 16 June 2021).
47. ILO. COVID-19 Impact on Child Labour and Forced Labour: The Response of the IPEC+Flagship Programme. 2020. Available online: https://www.ilo.org/wcmsp5/groups/public/@ed_norm/@ipec/documents/publication/wcms_745287.pdf (accessed on 21 April 2021).
48. UNICEF/ILO. COVID-19 and Child Labour: A Time of Crisis, a Time to Act. 2020. Available online: https://data.unicef.org/resources/covid-19-and-child-labour-a-time-of-crisis-a-time-to-act/ (accessed on 16 April 2021).
49. Paul Ladd, E.B. Protecting and Supporting Vulnerable Groups through the COVID-19 Crisis 2020. Available online: https://www.unrisd.org/80256B3C005BCCF9/(httpPublications)/0AC8BC84CFBB2D488025859F001EB3C3?OpenDocument (accessed on 7 July 2021).
50. Nations, U.; Ferre, J.; Rafeh, A.A. COVID-19 and Older Persons: A Defining Moment for an Informed, Inclusive and Targeted Response. United Nations, 2020. Available online: https://doi.org/10.18356/7eec92ae-en (accessed on 18 June 2021).
51. UNSDG. Secretary-General's Policy Brief: The Impact of COVID-19 on Older Persons 2020. Available online: https://unsdg.un.org/resources/policy-brief-impact-covid-19-older-persons (accessed on 7 June 2021).
52. UN-DESA. Older People's Livelihoods, Income Security and Access to Social Protection during COVID-19 and beyond. *March 2021*. Available online: https://www.un.org/development/desa/ageing/wp-content/uploads/sites/24/2021/02/Florian-Juergens_paper.pdf (accessed on 18 December 2021).
53. WHO. Disability and Health. Available online: https://www.who.int/news-room/fact-sheets/detail/disability-and-health (accessed on 16 June 2021).
54. Buchanan, J. Protect Rights of People with Disabilities During COVID-19. *Hum. Rights Watch N. Y.* **2020**. Available online: https://reliefweb.int/report/world/protect-rights-people-disabilities-during-covid-19-enarru (accessed on 12 January 2022).
55. Bezyak, J.L.; Sabella, S.; Hammel, J.; McDonald, K.; Jones, R.A.; Barton, D. Community participation and public transportation barriers experienced by people with disabilities. *Disabil. Rehabil.* **2020**, *42*, 3275–3283. [CrossRef]
56. Dev, S.M.; Sengupta, R. Covid-19: Impact on the Indian economy. *Indira Gandhi Inst. Dev. Res. Mumbai April* **2020**. Available online: http://www.igidr.ac.in/pdf/publication/WP-2020-013.pdf (accessed on 12 January 2022).
57. Rashid, S.F.; Theobald, S.; Ozano, K. Towards a socially just model: Balancing hunger and response to the COVID-19 pandemic in Bangladesh. *BMJ Glob. Health* **2020**, *5*, e002715. [CrossRef] [PubMed]
58. Naher, N.; Hoque, R.; Hassan, M.S.; Balabanova, D.; Adams, A.M.; Ahmed, S.M. The influence of corruption and governance in the delivery of frontline health care services in the public sector: A scoping review of current and future prospects in low and middle-income countries of south and south-east Asia. *BMC Public Health* **2020**, *20*, 880. [CrossRef]
59. Legido-Quigley, H.; Asgari, N.; Teo, Y.Y.; Leung, G.M.; Oshitani, H.; Fukuda, K.; Cook, A.R.; Hsu, L.Y.; Shibuya, K.; Heymann, D. Are high-performing health systems resilient against the COVID-19 epidemic? *Lancet* **2020**, *395*, 848–850. [CrossRef]
60. World Health Organization. *Global Surveillance for Human Infection with Novel Coronavirus (2019-nCoV): Interim Guidance, 31 January 2020*; World Health Organization: Geneva, Switzerland, 2020. Available online: https://apps.who.int/iris/handle/10665/330857 (accessed on 6 January 2022).
61. Armocida, B.; Formenti, B.; Ussai, S.; Palestra, F.; Missoni, E. The Italian health system and the COVID-19 challenge. *Lancet Public Health* **2020**, *5*, e253. [CrossRef]
62. World Health Organization. *COVID-19 Strategic Preparedness and Response Plan: Operational Planning Guideline: 1 February 2021 to 31 January 2022*; World Health Organization: Geneva, Switzerland, 2021. Available online: https://apps.who.int/iris/handle/10665/340073 (accessed on 12 February 2022).
63. Lipsitch, M.; Swerdlow, D.L.; Finelli, L. Defining the epidemiology of COVID-19—Studies Needed. *N. Engl. J. Med.* **2020**, *382*, 1194–1196. [CrossRef]
64. Prem, K.; Liu, Y.; Russell, T.W.; Kucharski, A.J.; Eggo, R.M.; Davies, N.; Flasche, S.; Clifford, S.; Pearson, C.A.; Munday, J.D. The effect of control strategies to reduce social mixing on outcomes of the COVID-19 epidemic in Wuhan, China: A modelling study. *Lancet Public Health* **2020**, *5*, e261–e270. [CrossRef]
65. Alqutob, R.; Al Nsour, M.; Tarawneh, M.R.; Ajlouni, M.; Khader, Y.; Aqel, I.; Kharabsheh, S.; Obeidat, N. COVID-19 crisis in Jordan: Response, scenarios, strategies, and recommendations. *JMIR Public Health Surveill.* **2020**, *6*, e19332. [CrossRef]
66. Razonable, R.R.; Pennington, K.M.; Meehan, A.M.; Wilson, J.W.; Froemming, A.T.; Bennett, C.E.; Marshall, A.L.; Virk, A.; Carmona, E.M. *A Collaborative Multidisciplinary Approach to the Management of Coronavirus Disease 2019 in the Hospital Setting*; Elsevier: Amsterdam, The Netherlands, 2020; pp. 1467–1481. [CrossRef]

67. Ng, Y.; Li, Z.; Chua, Y.X.; Chaw, W.L.; Zhao, Z.; Er, B.; Pung, R.; Chiew, C.J.; Lye, D.C.; Heng, D. Evaluation of the effectiveness of surveillance and containment measures for the first 100 patients with COVID-19 in Singapore—January 2–February 29, 2020. *Morb. Mortal. Wkly. Rep.* **2020**, *69*, 307. [CrossRef]
68. Peixoto, V.R.; Nunes, C.; Abrantes, A. Epidemic surveillance of COVID-19: Considering uncertainty and under-ascertainment. *Port. J. Public Health* **2020**, *38*, 23–29. [CrossRef]
69. Stockholm. Strategies for the Surveillance of COVID-19 2020. Available online: https://www.ecdc.europa.eu/sites/default/files/documents/COVID-19-surveillance-strategy-9-Apr-2020.pdf (accessed on 8 April 2021).
70. Van Dorn, A.; Cooney, R.E.; Sabin, M.L. COVID-19 exacerbating inequalities in the US. *Lancet* **2020**, *395*, 1243. [CrossRef]
71. Haque, M. Handwashing in averting infectious diseases: Relevance to COVID-19. *J. Popul. Ther. Clin. Pharmacol.* **2020**, *27*, e37–e52. [CrossRef] [PubMed]
72. Sharma, V.; Scott, J.; Kelly, J.; VanRooyen, M.J. Prioritizing vulnerable populations and women on the frontlines: COVID-19 in humanitarian contexts. *Int. J. Equity Health* **2020**, *19*, 66. [CrossRef] [PubMed]
73. Chen, T.; Wang, Y.; Hua, L. "Pairing assistance": The effective way to solve the breakdown of health services system caused by COVID-19 pandemic. *Int. J. Equity Health* **2020**, *19*, 68. [CrossRef]
74. Shadmi, E.; Chen, Y.; Dourado, I.; Faran-Perach, I.; Furler, J.; Hangoma, P.; Hanvoravongchai, P.; Obando, C.; Petrosyan, V.; Rao, K.D. Health equity and COVID-19: Global perspectives. *Int. J. Equity Health* **2020**, *19*, 104. [CrossRef]
75. Hooper, M.W.; Nápoles, A.M.; Pérez-Stable, E.J. COVID-19 and racial/ethnic disparities. *JAMA* **2020**, *323*, 2466–2467. [CrossRef]
76. Kim, J. Implications of the COVID-19 pandemic on health equity and healthy cities. *Korean J. Health Educ. Promot.* **2020**, *37*, 81–89. [CrossRef]
77. Berkowitz, S.A.; Cené, C.W.; Chatterjee, A. COVID-19 and health equity—Time to think big. *N. Engl. J. Med.* **2020**, *383*, e76. [CrossRef]
78. Wouters, O.J.; Shadlen, K.C.; Salcher-Konrad, M.; Pollard, A.J.; Larson, H.J.; Teerawattananon, Y.; Jit, M. Challenges in ensuring global access to COVID-19 vaccines: Production, affordability, allocation, and deployment. *Lancet* **2021**, *397*, 1023–1034. [CrossRef]
79. Findlay, S. Covid Vaccines Will Be Available for Private Purchase in India. Available online: https://www.ft.com/content/224b13fb-1d7d-4250-a6c6-1535b30496bc (accessed on 8 April 2021).
80. Duggan, J.; Morris, S.; Sandefur, J.; Yang, G.; Is the World Bank's COVID-19 crisis lending big enough, fast enough? New evidence on loan disbursements. *Cent. Glob. Dev. Work. Pap.* 2020, 554. Available online: https://mronline.org/wp-content/uploads/2021/04/world-banks-covid-crisis-lending-big-enough-fast-enough-new-evidence-loan-disbursements.pdf (accessed on 23 March 2022).
81. COVID 19: Debt Service Suspension Initiative. Available online: https://www.worldbank.org/en/news/factsheet/2020/05/11/debt-relief-and-covid-19-coronavirus (accessed on 12 January 2021).
82. World Health Organization. Report of the WHO Pandemic Influenza A (H1N1) Vaccine Deployment Initiative. 2012. Available online: https://apps.who.int/iris/bitstream/handle/10665/44795/9789241564427_eng.pdf (accessed on 15 March 2021).
83. WHO. Fair Allocation Mechanism for COVID-19 Vaccines through the COVAX Facility. Available online: https://www.who.int/publications/m/item/fair-allocation-mechanism-for-covid-19-vaccines-through-the-covax-facility (accessed on 16 April 2021).
84. Liu, Y.; Salwi, S.; Drolet, B.C. Multivalue ethical framework for fair global allocation of a COVID-19 vaccine. *J. Med. Ethics* **2020**, *46*, 499–501. [CrossRef]
85. Trogen, B.; Oshinsky, D.; Caplan, A. Adverse consequences of rushing a SARS-CoV-2 vaccine: Implications for public trust. *Jama* **2020**, *323*, 2460–2461. Available online: http://jamanetwork.com/article.aspx?doi=10.1001/jama.2020.8917 (accessed on 16 November 2021). [CrossRef] [PubMed]
86. Larson, H.J. *Stuck: How Vaccine Rumors Start-and Why They Don't Go Away*; Oxford University Press: Oxford, MS, USA, 2020; ISBN 9480190077259.
87. Chandler, R.E. Optimizing safety surveillance for COVID-19 vaccines. *Nat. Rev. Immunol.* **2020**, *20*, 451–452. [CrossRef] [PubMed]
88. Sam Halabi, J.D.; Andrew Heinrich, J.D.; Saad, B.; Omer, M.B. No-Fault Compensation for Vaccine Injury—The Other Side of Equitable Access to COVID-19 Vaccines. *N. Engl. J. Med.* **2020**, *383*, e125. Available online: https://www.nejm.org/doi/full/10.1056/NEJMp2030600 (accessed on 23 March 2022). [CrossRef] [PubMed]
89. Raoofi, A.; Takian, A.; Akbari Sari, A.; Olyaeemanesh, A.; Haghighi, H.; Aarabi, M. COVID-19 Pandemic and Comparative Health Policy Learning in Iran. *Arch Iran Med* **2020**, *23*, 220–234. Available online: http://www.aimjournal.ir/Article/aim-15740 (accessed on 15 May 2021). [CrossRef] [PubMed]
90. Bontempi, E. Commercial exchanges instead of air pollution as possible origin of COVID-19 initial diffusion phase in Italy: More efforts are necessary to address interdisciplinary research. *Environ. Res.* **2020**, *188*, 109775. [CrossRef]
91. Noshad, S.; Afarideh, M.; Heidari, B.; Mechanick, J.I.; Esteghamati, A. Diabetes Care in Iran: Where We Stand and Where We Are Headed. *Ann. Glob. Health* **2015**, *81*, 839–850. [CrossRef]
92. Holmes, E.A.; O'Connor, R.C.; Perry, V.H.; Tracey, I.; Wessely, S.; Arseneault, L.; Ballard, C.; Christensen, H.; Cohen Silver, R.; Everall, I.; et al. Multidisciplinary research priorities for the COVID-19 pandemic: A call for action for mental health science. *Lancet Psychiatry* **2020**, *7*, 547–560. [CrossRef]
93. Loayza, N. Aid Effectiveness during the COVID-19 Pandemic: This Time It Must Be Better. Available online: https://blogs.worldbank.org/developmenttalk/aid-effectiveness-during-covid-19-pandemic-time-it-must-be-better (accessed on 20 March 2021).

94. Kobayashi, Y.; Heinrich, T.; Bryant, K.A. Public support for development aid during the COVID-19 pandemic. *World Dev.* **2021**, *138*, 105248. [CrossRef]
95. Ihekweazu, C.; Agogo, E. Africa's response to COVID-19. *BMC Med.* **2020**, *18*, 151. [CrossRef]
96. Davalbhakta, S.; Sharma, S.; Gupta, S.; Agarwal, V.; Pandey, G.; Misra, D.P.; Naik, B.N.; Goel, A.; Gupta, L.; Agarwal, V. Private health sector in India-ready and willing, yet underutilized in the covid-19 pandemic: A cross-sectional study. *Front. Public Health* **2020**, *8*, 571419. [CrossRef]
97. Hussain, W. Role of social media in COVID-19 pandemic. *Int. J. Front. Sci.* **2020**, *4*, 59–60. [CrossRef]
98. Cuello-Garcia, C.; Pérez-Gaxiola, G.; van Amelsvoort, L. Social media can have an impact on how we manage and investigate the COVID-19 pandemic. *J. Clin. Epidemiol.* **2020**, *127*, 198. [CrossRef] [PubMed]
99. Latif, F.; Bashir, M.F.; Komal, B.; Tan, D. Role of electronic media in mitigating the psychological impacts of novel coronavirus (COVID-19). *Psychiatry Res.* **2020**, *289*, 113041. [CrossRef]
100. Roehr, B. The health of private insurance in the US during COVID-19. *bmj* **2020**, *370*, m2606. [CrossRef]
101. Sharma, K.; Pande, J. COVID-19: Critical Lessons for the Survival of Mankind from the Present and Future Pneumonic Viral Infections. *Ann. Natl. Acad. Med. Sci.* **2020**, *56*, 1–5. [CrossRef]
102. Kantamaneni, K.; Panneer, S.; Pushparaj, R.R.B.; Shekhar, S.; BHAT, L.; Rice, L. Multistakeholder Participation in Disaster Management. *Sch. Community Encycl.* **2021**. Available online: https://encyclopedia.pub/9117 (accessed on 22 November 2021).
103. Kapoor, H.; Ticku, A.; Tagat, A.; Karandikar, S. Innovation in isolation? COVID-19 lockdown stringency and culture-innovation relationships. *Front. Psychol.* **2021**, *12*, 83. [CrossRef]
104. WHO. Solidarity Call to Action: Making the Response to COVID-19 a Public Common Good. Available online: https://www.who.int/initiatives/covid-19-technology-access-pool/solidarity-call-to-action (accessed on 14 April 2022).
105. UN-UNCTAD. Technology and Innovation Report 2021—Catching Technological Waves Innovation with Equity 2021. Available online: https://unctad.org/system/files/official-document/tir2020_en.pdf (accessed on 16 June 2021).
106. UN. An UN Framework for the Immediate Socio-Economic Response to COVID-19 2020. p. 1–51. Available online: https://unsdg.un.org/sites/default/files/2020-04/UN-framework-for-the-immediate-socio-economic-response-to-COVID-19.pdf (accessed on 22 May 2021).
107. Nanda, L.Q.Y.A.S. In the Shadows of the COVID-19 Response: Informal Workers and the Rise of Gender-Based Violence. Available online: https://www.genderandcovid-19.org/editorial/in-the-shadows-of-the-covid-19-response-informal-workers-and-the-rise-of-gender-based-violence/ (accessed on 5 January 2022).
108. MHFW. Enabling Delivery of Essential Health Services during the COVID 19 Outbreak: Guidance Note 2020. Ministry of Health and Family Welfare New Delhi, India. 2020. Available online: https://www.mohfw.gov.in/pdf/EssentialservicesduringCOVID19updated0411201.pdf (accessed on 16 November 2021).
109. Food Security in a Pandemic. Available online: https://www.paho.org/disasters/dmdocuments/RespToolKit_14_Tool%2007_FoodSecurityinaPandemic.pdf (accessed on 17 August 2021).
110. Torero, M. *Without Food, There Can Be No Exit from the Pandemic*; Nature Publishing Group: New York, NY, USA, 2020. [CrossRef]
111. Lugo-Morin, D.R. Global Food Security in a Pandemic: The Case of the New Coronavirus (COVID-19). *World* **2020**, *1*, 171–190. [CrossRef]
112. Howard, G.; Bartram, J.; Brocklehurst, C.; Colford, J.M.; Costa, F.; Cunliffe, D.; Dreibelbis, R.; Eisenberg, J.N.S.; Evans, B.; Girones, R. COVID-19: Urgent actions, critical reflections and future relevance of 'WaSH': Lessons for the current and future pandemics. *J. Water Health* **2020**, *18*, 613–630. [CrossRef]
113. Vieira, C.M.; Franco, O.H.; Restrepo, C.G.; Abel, T. COVID-19: The forgotten priorities of the pandemic. *Maturitas* **2020**, *136*, 38–41. [CrossRef]
114. Moghanibashi-Mansourieh, A. Vulnerable Groups and COVID-19 Pandemic; How Appropriate Are Psychosocial Responses? In *Anxiety, Uncertainty, and Resilience During the Pandemic Period-Anthropological and Psychological Perspectives*; IntechOpen: London, UK, 2021. [CrossRef]
115. Panneer, S.; Kantamaneni, K.; Pushparaj, R.R.B.; Shekhar, S.; Bhat, L.; Rice, L. Multistakeholder Participation in Disaster Management—The Case of the COVID-19 Pandemic. *Healthcare* **2021**, *9*, 203. Available online: https://www.mdpi.com/2227-9032/9/2/203 (accessed on 7 July 2021). [CrossRef] [PubMed]
116. Peiris, D.; Sharma, M.; Praveen, D.; Bitton, A.; Bresick, G.; Coffman, M.; Dodd, R.; El-Jardali, F.; Fadlallah, R.; Flinkenflögel, M. Strengthening primary health care in the COVID-19 era: A review of best practices to inform health system responses in low-and middle-income countries. *WHO South East Asia J Public Health* **2021**, *10*, 6–25. [CrossRef]
117. Assaad, R.; El-adaway, I.H. Guidelines for Responding to COVID-19 Pandemic: Best Practices, Impacts, and Future Research Directions. *J. Manag. Eng.* **2021**, *37*, 06021001. [CrossRef]
118. Kuy, S.; Gupta, R.; Correa, R.; Tsai, R.; Vohra, S. Best practices for a COVID-19 preparedness plan for health systems. *NEJM Catal. Innov. Care Deliv.* **2020**, *1*.
119. Truell, R. As Social Workers Work through the COVID 19 Crisis We Work towards a Better World. Available online: https://www.ifsw.org/as-social-workers-work-through-the-covid-19-crisis-we-work-towards-a-better-world/ (accessed on 20 March 2022).
120. Perc, M.; Gorišek Miksić, N.; Slavinec, M.; Stožer, A. Forecasting covid-19. *Front. Phys.* **2020**, *8*, 127. [CrossRef]
121. Desai, A.N.; Kraemer, M.U.; Bhatia, S.; Cori, A.; Nouvellet, P.; Herringer, M.; Cohn, E.L.; Carrion, M.; Brownstein, J.S.; Madoff, L.C. Real-time epidemic forecasting: Challenges and opportunities. *Health Secur.* **2019**, *17*, 268–275. [CrossRef] [PubMed]

122. Gilmore, B.; Ndejjo, R.; Tchetchia, A.; De Claro, V.; Mago, E.; Lopes, C.; Bhattacharyya, S. Community engagement for COVID-19 prevention and control: A rapid evidence synthesis. *BMJ Glob. Health* **2020**, *5*, e003188. [CrossRef]
123. Al Siyabi, H.; Al Mukhaini, S.; Kanaan, M.; Al Hatmi, S.; Al Anqoudi, Z.; Al Kalbani, A.; Al Bahri, Z.; Wannous, C.; Al Awaidy, S.T. Community participation approaches for effective national covid-19 pandemic preparedness and response: An experience from Oman. *Front. Public Health* **2021**, *8*, 616763. [CrossRef]
124. Van Bavel, J.J.; Baicker, K.; Boggio, P.S.; Capraro, V.; Cichocka, A.; Cikara, M.; Crockett, M.J.; Crum, A.J.; Douglas, K.M.; Druckman, J.N. Using social and behavioural science to support COVID-19 pandemic response. *Nat. Hum. Behav.* **2020**, *4*, 460–471. [CrossRef]
125. Bolger, J.; Kelly, M.; Whelan, C.; Doyle, A.; Frizelle, H.; Boyd, W.; McEntee, G.; Conneely, J. Public-private partnership: Strategies for continuing urgent elective operative care during the COVID-19 pandemic. *J. Br. Surg.* **2020**, *107*, e320–e321. [CrossRef]
126. Ku, S.S.; Choe, Y.J. A public-private partnership model to build a triage system in response to a COVID-19 outbreak in Hanam City, South Korea. *Osong Public Health Res. Perspect.* **2020**, *11*, 339. [CrossRef] [PubMed]
127. Marston, C.; Renedo, A.; Miles, S. Community participation is crucial in a pandemic. *Lancet* **2020**, *395*, 1676–1678. [CrossRef]
128. LobdellKevin, W.; RoseGeoffrey, A. Improving health care leadership in the COVID-19 era. *NEJM Catal. Innov. Care Deliv.* **2020**.
129. Kaul, V.; Shah, V.H.; El-Serag, H. Leadership during crisis: Lessons and applications from the COVID-19 pandemic. *Gastroenterology* **2020**, *159*, 809. [CrossRef] [PubMed]
130. Wilson, S. Pandemic leadership: Lessons from New Zealand's approach to COVID-19. *Leadership* **2020**, *16*, 279–293. [CrossRef]
131. Garg, A. Preparedness of Hospitals Post COVID-19 Era. *Adv. Clin. Med. Res.* **2021**, *2*, 22–25. Available online: http://acmrjournal.com/index.php/acmr/article/view/17 (accessed on 3 January 2022).
132. Härmand, K. *Digitalisation before and after the Covid-19 Crisis*; ERA Forum; Springer: Berlin/Heidelberg, Germany, 2021; pp. 39–50.
133. Brewer, L.C.; Asiedu, G.B.; Jones, C.; Richard, M.; Erickson, J.; Weis, J.; Abbenyi, A.; Brockman, T.A.; Sia, I.G.; Wieland, M.L. Emergency preparedness and risk communication among African American churches: Leveraging a community-based participatory research partnership COVID-19 initiative. *Prev. Chronic Dis.* **2020**, *17*, E158. Available online: https://stacks.cdc.gov/view/cdc/100388 (accessed on 26 November 2021). [CrossRef]
134. Amengual, O.; Atsumi, T. COVID-19 pandemic in Japan. *Rheumatol. Int.* **2021**, *41*, 1–5. [CrossRef]
135. Tran, B.X.; Ha, G.H.; Nguyen, L.H.; Vu, G.T.; Hoang, M.T.; Le, H.T.; Latkin, C.A.; Ho, C.S.; Ho, R. Studies of novel coronavirus disease 19 (COVID-19) pandemic: A global analysis of literature. *Int. J. Environ. Res. Public Health* **2020**, *17*, 4095. [CrossRef]
136. Montiel, C.J.; Uyheng, J.; Dela Paz, E. The Language of Pandemic Leaderships: Mapping Political Rhetoric During the COVID-19 Outbreak. *Political Psychol.* **2021**, *42*, 747–766. [CrossRef]
137. Osland, J.S.; Mendenhall, M.E.; Reiche, B.S.; Szkudlarek, B.; Bolden, R.; Courtice, P.; Vaiman, V.; Vaiman, M.; Lyndgaard, D.; Nielsen, K.; et al. Perspectives on Global Leadership and the COVID-19 Crisis. In *Advances in Global Leadership*; Osland, J.S., Szkudlarek, B., Mendenhall, M.E., Reiche, B.S., Eds.; Emerald Publishing Limited: Bingley, UK, 2020; Volume 13, pp. 3–56. Available online: https://www.emerald.com/insight/content/doi/10.1108/S1535-120320200000013001/full/html (accessed on 17 August 2021).
138. Barnett, D.J.; Knieser, L.; Errett, N.A.; Rosenblum, A.J.; Seshamani, M.; Kirsch, T.D. Reexamining Health-Care Coalitions in Light of COVID-19. *Disaster Med. Public Health Prep.* **2020**, *4*, 1–5. [CrossRef] [PubMed]
139. Schaaf, M.; Boydell, V.; Van Belle, S.; Brinkerhoff, D.W.; George, A. Accountability for SRHR in the context of the COVID-19 pandemic. *Sex. Reprod. Health Matters* **2020**, *28*, 1779634. [CrossRef] [PubMed]
140. Belso-Martínez, J.A.; Mas-Tur, A.; Sánchez, M.; López-Sánchez, M.J. The COVID-19 response system and collective social service provision. Strategic network dimensions and proximity considerations. *Serv. Bus.* **2020**, *14*, 387–411. [CrossRef]
141. Liu, J.; Hao, J.; Shi, Z.; Bao, H.X. Building the COVID-19 Collaborative Emergency Network: A case study of COVID-19 outbreak in Hubei Province, China. *Nat. Hazards* **2020**, *104*, 2687–2717. [CrossRef]
142. Lu, Y.; Liu, T.; Wang, T. Dynamic Analysis of Emergency Inter-organizational Communication Network under Public Health Emergency: A case study of COVID-19 in Hubei Province of China. *Nat. Hazards* **2021**, *6*, 1–24. [CrossRef]
143. Bontempi, E.; Vergalli, S.; Squazzoni, F. Understanding COVID-19 diffusion requires an interdisciplinary, multi-dimensional approach. *Environ. Res.* **2020**, *188*, 109814. [CrossRef]
144. WHO. 2019 Novel Coronavirus (2019-nCoV): Strategic Preparedness and Response Plan 2020. Available online: https://www.who.int/docs/default-source/coronaviruse/srp-04022020.pdf (accessed on 12 December 2020).
145. Hynes, W.; Trump, B.; Love, P.; Linkov, I. Bouncing forward: A resilience approach to dealing with COVID-19 and future systemic shocks. *Environ. Syst. Decis.* **2020**, *40*, 174–184. [CrossRef]
146. How the Public Sector And Civil Society Can Respond to the Coronavirus Pandemic. Available online: https://www.hks.harvard.edu/faculty-research/policy-topics/health/how-public-sector-and-civil-society-can-respond-coronavirus (accessed on 26 January 2021).
147. Lele, U.; Bansal, S.; Meenakshi, J. Health and nutrition of India's labour force and COVID-19 challenges. *Econ. Political Wkly.* **2020**, *55*, 13. Available online: https://www.researchgate.net/profile/Uma-Lele-2/publication/341670761_Health_and_Nutrition_of_India\T1\textquoterights_Labour_Force_and_COVID-19_Challenges/links/5ece2cfb458515294514972d/Health-and-Nutrition-of-Indias-Labour-Force-and-COVID-19-Challenges.pdf (accessed on 12 November 2021).
148. ILO. A Policy Framework for Tackling the Economic and Social Impact of the COVID-19 Crisis. Available online: https://www.ilo.org/wcmsp5/groups/public/---dgreports/---dcomm/documents/briefingnote/wcms_745337.pdf (accessed on 8 January 2021).

International Journal of
Environmental Research and Public Health

MDPI

Article

The Associations between Evacuation Status and Lifestyle-Related Diseases in Fukushima after the Great East Japan Earthquake: The Fukushima Health Management Survey

Zhichao Sun [1,2], Hironori Imano [1,3], Eri Eguchi [4], Fumikazu Hayashi [4,5], Tetsuya Ohira [4,5], Renzhe Cui [6], Seiji Yasumura [5,7], Akira Sakai [5,8], Michio Shimabukuro [5,9], Hitoshi Ohto [5], Kenji Kamiya [5,10] and Hiroyasu Iso [1,11,*]

1 Public Health, Department of Social Medicine, Osaka University Graduate School of Medicine, Osaka 565-0871, Japan; szcsun@pbhel.med.osaka-u.ac.jp (Z.S.); imano@pbhel.med.osaka-u.ac.jp (H.I.)
2 Health Town Development Science Center, Yao City Health Center, Osaka 581-0006, Japan
3 Department of Public Health, Kindai University Faculty of Medicine, Osakasayama 589-8511, Japan
4 Department of Epidemiology, Fukushima Medical University School of Medicine, Fukushima 960-1295, Japan; e-eguchi@fmu.ac.jp (E.E.); fhayashi@fmu.ac.jp (F.H.); teoohira@fmu.ac.jp (T.O.)
5 Radiation Medical Science Center for the Fukushima Health Management Survey, Fukushima Medical University, Fukushima 960-1295, Japan; yasumura@fmu.ac.jp (S.Y.); sakira@fmu.ac.jp (A.S.); mshimabukuro-ur@umin.ac.jp (M.S.); hit-ohto@fmu.ac.jp (H.O.); kkamiya@hiroshima-u.ac.jp (K.K.)
6 Department of Internal Medicine, Okanami General Hospital, Iga 518-0842, Japan; cuirenzhe@hotmail.com
7 Department of Public Health, Fukushima Medical University School of Medicine, Fukushima 960-1295, Japan
8 Department of Radiation Life Sciences, Fukushima Medical University School of Medicine, Fukushima 960-1295, Japan
9 Department of Diabetes, Endocrinology and Metabolism, Fukushima Medical University School of Medicine, Fukushima 960-1295, Japan
10 Research Institute for Radiation Biology and Medicine, Hiroshima University, Hiroshima 734-8553, Japan
11 Institute for Global Health Policy Research, National Center for Global Health and Medicine, Tokyo 162-8655, Japan
* Correspondence: iso@pbhel.med.osaka-u.ac.jp; Tel.: +81-6-6879-3911

Citation: Sun, Z.; Imano, H.; Eguchi, E.; Hayashi, F.; Ohira, T.; Cui, R.; Yasumura, S.; Sakai, A.; Shimabukuro, M.; Ohto, H.; et al. The Associations between Evacuation Status and Lifestyle-Related Diseases in Fukushima after the Great East Japan Earthquake: The Fukushima Health Management Survey. *IJERPH* **2022**, *19*, 5661. https://doi.org/10.3390/ijerph19095661

Academic Editor: Krzysztof Goniewicz

Received: 28 March 2022
Accepted: 5 May 2022
Published: 6 May 2022

Abstract: Background: This study aimed to investigate the association between evacuation status and lifestyle-related disease risks among Fukushima residents following the Great East Japan earthquake. Methods: Fukushima health management survey respondents were classified into non-evacuees, returnees, evacuees in lifted areas, and evacuees in banned areas. During a seven-year follow-up, 22,234 men and 31,158 women were included. Those with a history of diabetes, hypertension, or dyslipidemia at baseline were excluded. The odds ratios of risk factors (ORs) and 95% confidence intervals (CIs) for diabetes, hypertension, and dyslipidemia were calculated using a logistic regression model. Spatial autocorrelation of the prevalence of these diseases in the Fukushima area in 2017, was calculated to detect the disease prevalence status. Results: The risks of diabetes, hypertension, and dyslipidemia were higher in evacuees in banned areas than in non-evacuees; the multivariable ORs were 1.32 (95% CI: 1.19–1.46), 1.15 (1.06–1.25), and 1.20 (1.11–1.30) for diabetes, hypertension, and dyslipidemia, respectively. Returnees and evacuees in lifted areas had no increased risk of diseases. The area analyzed had a non-uniform spatial distribution of diabetes, hypertension, and hyperlipidemia, with clusters around Fukushima and Koriyama. Conclusion: Our findings imply the need for continuous support for evacuees in banned areas.

Keywords: evacuation; Great East Japan earthquake; disaster; disease prevalence status; cardiovascular and metabolic diseases

1. Introduction

The Great East Japan earthquake occurred on 11 March 2011, causing a large tsunami [1] and a severe accident at the Fukushima Dai-ichi Nuclear Power Plant [2]. These serious disasters resulted in extensive damage to the coastal area adjacent to the east of Fukushima, infrastructure destruction, and potential ultra-low-dose level radioactive pollution. Thus, many residents needed to evacuate, as implemented by the national and Fukushima Prefecture governments [3].

Evacuation affects lifestyle and has been associated with increased alcohol consumption [4], high smoking prevalence [5], and impaired sleep quality [6]. Lifestyle changes, such as those mentioned above, have a strong effect on lifestyle-related diseases. Moreover, changes in the living environment and socio-economic factors [7,8] could affect the mental health of the evacuees. People who were forced to leave their homes were more likely to develop post-traumatic stress disorder [9,10], and approximately 4.7% of the residents in the Fukushima Prefecture lost or changed their job [11]. Previous studies have also shown that evacuees had higher risks of diabetes, heart disease, and sudden cardiac death [12,13] than non-evacuees.

To date, restrictions have been lifted in 67.8% of the previously restricted areas [14], and the national and prefectural governments have encouraged the evacuees to return to their homes. However, some people remained reluctant to return, although the areas were cleaned and declared safe [15]. Therefore, people who continued to evacuate have been forced to live in temporary houses and face new interpersonal relationships.

Evacuation status may impact lifestyle and cardiovascular risk factors, such as diabetes, hypertension, and dyslipidemia. In this study, we hypothesized that the evacuees forced to live outside their original houses in banned areas may have a higher risk of diabetes, hypertension, and dyslipidemia, and that returnees and evacuees in lifted areas do not have these increased risks. We used the database affiliated with the Fukushima health management survey to test this hypothesis.

2. Materials and Methods

2.1. Participants

We used the following three databases from the Fukushima health management survey (FHMS) in 2017 [16]: comprehensive health checks, mental health and lifestyle survey, and basic survey. Comprehensive health checks included two sets of respondents as follows: (1) people in the evacuation zone specified by the government and (2) people outside of the evacuation zone in the Fukushima Prefecture. The evacuation zone comprised Iitate Village (mura), Kawauchi Village, Katsurao Village, Hirono Town (machi), Naraha Town, Tomioka Town, Okuma Town, Futaba Town, Namie Town, Minamisoma City, and Tamura City. The mental health and lifestyle survey included these 13 areas.

Figure 1a presents a flow chart of the longitudinal analysis used in this study, with a follow-up for up to 7 years. Among the 89,571 participants of the comprehensive health check database, we excluded 27,334 who were aged <20 years and 12,321 who did not participate in the mental health and lifestyle survey. A total of 49,916 participants were included in the analysis. Subsequently, we excluded participants with a history of diabetes (n = 5224), hypertension (n = 21,754), or dyslipidemia (n = 25,522) at baseline. At follow-up, there were 11,693 participants with diabetes, 8234 with hypertension, and 7021 with dyslipidemia who never responded. Finally, we analyzed 32,999 participants with diabetes, 19,928 with hypertension, and 17,373 with hyperlipidemia.

For the spatial analysis, 53,094 individuals were included in the 2017 total comprehensive health check database. We excluded 4204 individuals aged <20 years. Finally, 48,890 individuals were included in the analysis (Figure 1b).

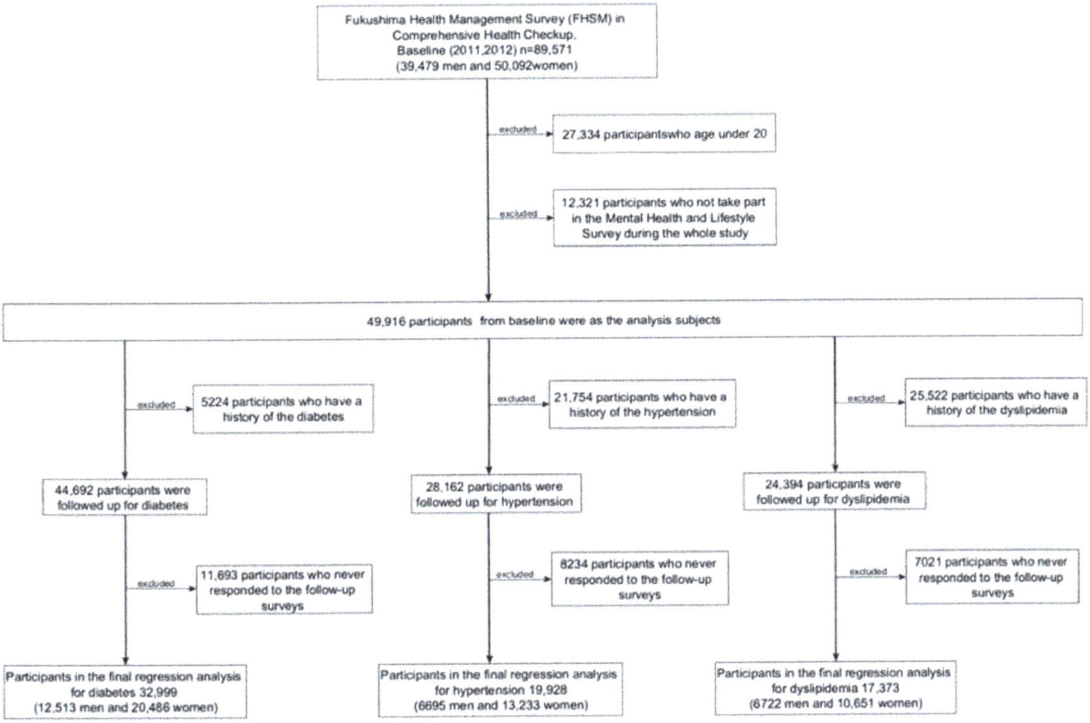

(a)

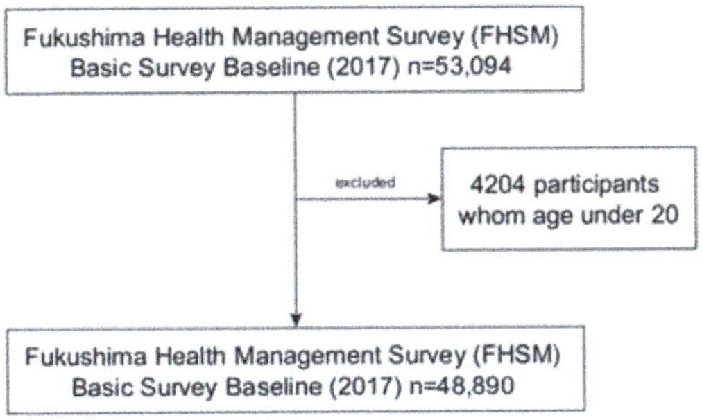

(b)

Figure 1. Flow diagram of the participant selection process: (**a**) longitudinal analysis; (**b**) spatial analysis.

2.2. Changes in Evacuation Status

Figure 2 shows the changes in the evacuation areas in the Fukushima Prefecture in 2017, based on the information provided by the national and local governments [14,17]. As of 2017, areas that still have restrictions were labeled as Area1 (red color); those that have lifted restrictions, Area 2 (orange color); those with a history of voluntary refuge [17], Area 3 (yellow color); and those outside of the Fukushima Prefecture, Area 4 (green color).

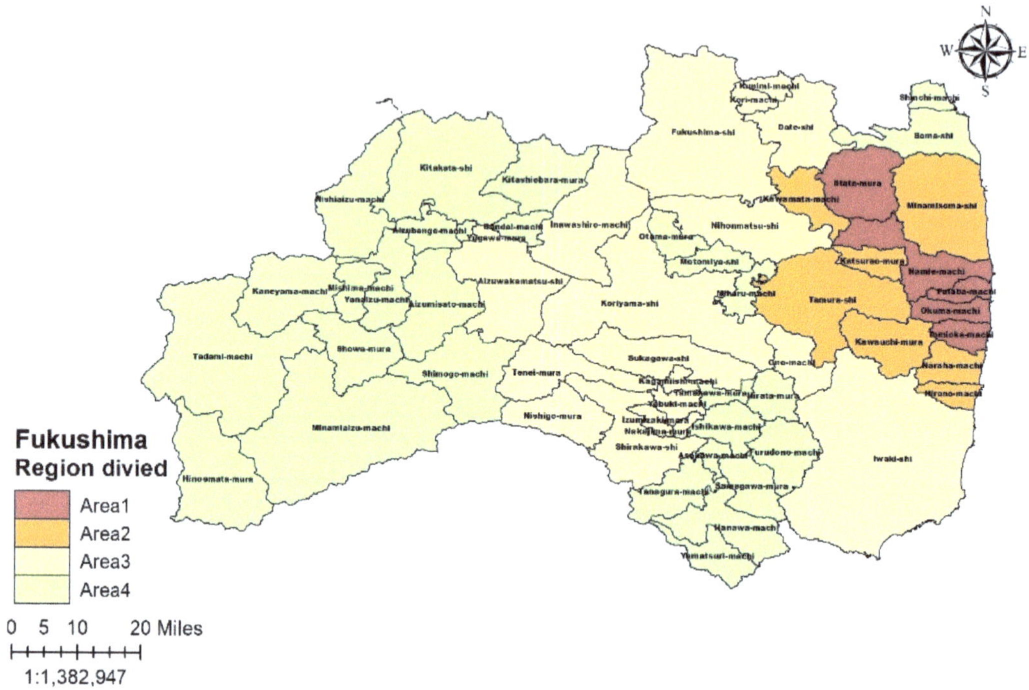

Figure 2. Group design based on the history of the Fukushima evacuation area and caution area. Area 1: still difficult to return at the time of the deadline; Area 2: where the evacuation alerts have been lifted at the time of the deadline; Area 3: near the evacuation area or with a history of voluntary evacuation; and Area 4: all other areas.

Evacuees were defined as follows: those who had lived in Area 2 or 3 before the earthquake and evacuated from lifted areas until 2017 were defined as evacuees from lifted areas, and those who lived in Area 1 before the earthquake were defined as evacuees from banned areas. Non-evacuees were defined as all individuals living in Areas 3 and 4 who never changed their residences. Returnees were defined as individuals who lived in Area 2 before the earthquake, evacuated to Area 3 or 4 after the earthquake, and returned to their homes in Area 2 before 2017.

2.3. Lifestyle Behaviors and Social Factors

Smoking and drinking behaviors, sleep, physical activity, job change, and education level were obtained from the mental health & lifestyle survey data. We assessed the smoking status of the participants using the question, "Do you smoke?" with the following options: "non-smoker", "ex-smoker", and "current smoker". Those who selected "current smoker" were considered as current smokers. Participants' alcohol intake was assessed using the question, "Do you consume alcohol?" with the following options: "non-drinker (less than once per month)", "ex-drinker", and "drinker (once or more per month)". Those who selected "drinker (once or more per month)" were considered as current drinkers. Sleep quality was evaluated using the question, "Are you satisfied with the length of sleep for the past month?" with the following options: "satisfied" and "not satisfied". Physical activity level was assessed using the question, "Do you exercise regularly?" with the following options: "≥daily", "2–4 times/week", "weekly", and "almost never". Those who selected "≥daily", "2–4 times/week", or "weekly" were considered to have a physical activity frequency of at least once a week. Education level was assessed by the question, "What is your last educational level?" with the following options: "elementary or junior high school", "high school", "vocational school or junior college", and "university or graduate school". Those who selected "university or graduate school" were considered to have received college or higher education. Change of job was assessed by the question, "Did you experience a change in work situation since the disaster?" with the following options: "yes" and "no". Psychological distress was evaluated using Kessler Psychological Distress (K6), and participants with a score of ≥13 were considered to have psychological distress.

Weight was measured in light indoor clothing without shoes, and height was recorded barefoot by well-trained staff. Weight and height measurements were obtained from comprehensive health check data. Body mass index (BMI) was calculated as weight (kg)/[height] (m)^2.

2.4. Onset of Diabetes, Hypertension, and Dyslipidemia

The onset of diabetes mellitus, hypertension, and dyslipidemia was acquired from the comprehensive health check data. Hypertension was defined as systolic blood pressure (SBP) ≥ 140 mmHg, diastolic blood pressure (DBP) ≥ 90 mmHg [18], and/or the use of antihypertensive medication. Diabetes was defined as a fasting plasma glucose (FPG) level ≥ 126 mg/dL (7.0 mmol/L), random blood glucose (RBG) level ≥ 200 (11.1 mmol/L), HbA1c ≥ 6.5% [19], and/or the use of insulin injection or hypoglycemic drugs. Dyslipidemia was defined as plasma triglyceride (TG) level ≥ 150 mg/dL (fasting time), high-density lipoprotein cholesterol (HDL-C) level ≤ 40 mg/dL, low-density lipoprotein cholesterol (LDL-C) level ≥ 140 mg/dL [20], and/or the use of lipid-lowering agents.

2.5. Addresses and Standardized Prevalence Ratios in the Fukushima Prefecture

We used the current postal code from the basic survey data for the spatial analysis to ensure reliability. Diabetes, hypertension, and hyperlipidemia were defined based on the comprehensive health check database of the whole prefecture. The standardized prevalence ratios (SPRs) for diabetes, hypertension, and dyslipidemia were used to avoid distortion due to inappropriate age adjustment. The SPRs for diabetes, hypertension, and hyperlipidemia in each municipality in the Fukushima Prefecture were calculated compared to the 1985 Japanese standard population model. Municipality SPRs were calculated by dividing the municipality observed cases by the municipality expected cases [21,22].

2.6. Statistical Analysis

First, we calculated the age-adjusted mean values and prevalence of risk factors using analysis of covariance. Multiple linear regression was performed to compare the returnees, evacuees in lifted areas, and evacuees in banned areas with the non-evacuees.

Using the logistic regression model, age- and multivariable-adjusted odds ratios (ORs) and 95% confidence intervals (CIs) for diabetes, hypertension, and hyperlipidemia among the returnees, evacuees in lifted areas, and evacuees in banned areas, compared with the non-evacuees were calculated. The adjustment variables included age (continuous), BMI (quintiles), cigarette smoking status (never-smoker, ex-smoker, current smoker), alcohol consumption (non-drinker, ex-drinker, current drinker), physical activity (≥once weekly or <once weekly), sleep satisfaction (satisfied or not satisfied), change of job (yes or no), and educational status (elementary or junior high school, high school, vocational school or junior college, university or graduate school). Statistical analyses were conducted using SAS version 9.4 (SAS Institute, Inc., Cary, NC, USA). Two-tailed p values < 0.05 were considered statistically significant.

The global Moran's index [23] was used to analyze regional spatial autocorrelation to identify geographic clustering. Hotspot analysis (Getis-Ord Gi*) [24] was used to determine the clusters. Hot spots represent a high-value spatial cluster of diabetes, hypertension, or dyslipidemia, whereas cold spots represent a low-value spatial cluster in the Fukushima Prefecture. Statistical significance was set at $p < 0.05$, and 90% CIs were dependent on the $z < -1.65$ or $z > +1.65$, whereas 95% CIs were dependent on the $z < -1.96$ or $z > +1.96$. All spatial analyses were conducted in ArcGis10.8.1 (Esri, Inc., Redlands, CA, USA).

3. Results

During a seven-year follow-up, 1822 participants had diabetes, 3609 had hypertension, and 4361 had dyslipidemia.

3.1. Characteristics of Participants at Baseline

Table 1 shows the age-adjusted mean values and characteristics at baseline according to the evacuation status. We found that 47.7% of the participants had been evacuated or were still evacuees. Compared with the non-evacuees, both evacuees in lifted areas and those in banned areas were younger and had a higher proportion of current smokers, current alcohol drinkers, dissatisfaction with sleep, change in their job, and university or graduate school education. Compared with the non-evacuees, the returnees were likely to have a lower average age and BMI and a higher proportion of dissatisfaction with sleep, change in their job, and university or graduate school education. Additionally, 11.6% of evacuees in banned areas had a K6 score of ≥13, which accounted for the highest proportion of individuals who had psychological distress.

Table 1. Characteristics of participants at baseline according to evacuation status (N = 49,916).

	Non-Evacuees (n = 26,115)	Returnees (n = 1573)	Evacuees in Lifted Areas (n = 5559)	Evacuees in Banned Areas (n = 16,669)
Age (years) Mean ± SD	57.4 ± 14.5	55.4 ± 14.1 ***	46.1 ± 16.5 ***	54.1 ± 15.2 ***
BMI (kg/m^2) Mean ± SD	23.8 ± 3.77	23.7 ± 3.52	23.2 ± 3.89 ***	23.9 ± 3.92 ***
Current alcohol drinker (%)	34.9	38.2 **	38.5 **	37.9 ***
Current smoker (%)	13.1	12.8	16.7 **	16.6 ***
Sleep, inadequate (%)	26.4	33.4 ***	33.2 ***	32.8 ***
Physical activity, ≥ once/week (%)	40.8	40.2	32.7 **	39.7 ***
Change of job, yes (%)	33.9	56.5 ***	48.7 ***	53.5 ***
Education attainment, i.e., university or graduate school (%)	4.8	6.7 ***	11.1 ***	7.1 ***
Psychological distress (K6 score of ≥13) (%)	6.7	10.9 ***	9.4 ***	11.6 ***

Difference from non-evacuees: ** $p < 0.01$; *** $p < 0.001$.

3.2. Associations between Evacuate Status and Diabetes, Hypertension, and Dyslipidemia

Table 2 presents the age- and multivariable-adjusted odds ratios (ORs) and 95% confidence intervals (95% CIs) for diabetes, hypertension, and dyslipidemia for the returnees, evacuees in lifted areas, and evacuees in the banned areas. The ORs for diabetes, hypertension, and dyslipidemia for evacuees in the banned areas were significantly higher than those for non-evacuees, and these associations remained statistically significant even after adjusting for confounders. The multivariable ORs (95% CIs) were 1.35 (1.22–1.51) for diabetes, 1.14 (1.05–1.24) for hypertension, and 1.22 (1.13–1.32) for dyslipidemia. The ORs for diabetes, hypertension, and dyslipidemia were higher in returnees than that in non-evacuees, albeit not statistically significantly. There was no statistically significant association between the evacuees in lifted areas and the non-evacuees. With additional adjustment for psychological distress, the results still showed the same associations. Multivariable ORs (95% CIs) were 1.35 (1.21–1.50) for diabetes, 1.14 (1.05–1.24) for hypertension, and 1.22 (1.13–1.32) for dyslipidemia.

Gender-specific analyses (Table 3) showed similar associations, except for hypertension in men. The multivariable ORs (95% CI) for diabetes, hypertension, dyslipidemia were 1.33 (1.15–1.55), 1.08 (0.95–1.23), and 1.31 (1.16–1.48) among male evacuees in banned area and 1.38 (1.19–1.61), 1.20 (1.08–1.35), and 1.21 (1.09–1.34) among female evacuees. Additional adjustment for psychological distress also showed the same associations. Multivariable ORs (95% CIs) for diabetes, hypertension, and dyslipidemia were 1.33 (1.15–1.54), 1.08 (0.94–1.23), and 1.31 (1.16–1.48), respectively, among male evacuees in banned areas and 1.38 (1.18–1.60), 1.20 (1.08–1.35), and 1.20 (1.09–1.33) among female evacuees in banned areas.

Table 2. Age-adjusted and multivariable odds ratios of diabetes, hypertension, and dyslipidemia according to evacuation status.

	Total			
	Non-Evacuees	Returnees	Evacuees in Lifted Areas	Evacuees in Banned Areas
No. at risk, *n*	16,784	1284	3207	11,724
Diabetes, *n*	875	63	118	766
Age-adjusted OR (95% CI)	Ref.	1.04 (0.80–1.35)	0.96 (0.79–1.17)	1.45 (1.30–1.59) ***
Multivariable OR (95% CI) §	Ref.	1.04 (0.79–1.35)	1.00 (0.82–1.22)	1.35 (1.22–1.51) ***
Multivariable OR (95% CI) §§	Ref.	1.03 (0.79–1.35)	0.99 (0.81–1.21)	1.35 (1.21–1.50) ***
No. at risk, *n*	9367	808	2417	7336
Hypertension, *n*	1828	146	267	1368
Age-adjusted OR (95% CI)	Ref.	1.07 (0.88–1.29)	0.84 (0.73–0.97) *	1.17 (1.08–1.27) ***
Multivariable OR (95% CI) §	Ref.	1.06 (0.87–1.29)	0.87 (0.75–1.00)	1.14 (1.05–1.24) **
Multivariable OR (95% CI) §§	Ref.	1.06 (0.87–1.29)	0.87 (0.75–1.00)	1.14 (1.05–1.24) **
No. at risk, *n*	8628	617	2031	6097
Dyslipidemia, *n*	2100	152	421	1688
Age-adjusted OR (95% CI)	Ref.	1.10 (0.91–1.33)	0.97 (0.86–1.10)	1.28 (1.18–1.38) ***
Multivariable OR (95% CI) §	Ref.	1.07 (0.88–1.30)	0.97 (0.86–1.10)	1.22 (1.13–1.32) ***
Multivariable OR (95% CI) §§	Ref.	1.07 (0.88–1.29)	0.97 (0.86–1.10)	1.22 (1.13–1.32) ***

CI, confidence interval; OR, odds ratio. * $p < 0.05$; ** $p < 0.01$;*** $p < 0.001$. § Adjust for age, body mass index, smoking status, alcohol consumption, sports time, sleep quality, education level, and change of job. §§ Adjusted further for psychological distress.

3.3. Spatial Distribution Characteristics

The global spatial autocorrelation showed that the prevalence of diabetes, hypertension, and hyperlipidemia was positively spatially autocorrelated in Fukushima (Supplementary Table S1). The global Moran's indexes for diabetes, hypertension, and dyslipidemia were 0.17, 0.16, and 0.34, respectively. The administrative region around the Fukushima and Koriyama cities were determined as clusters (Figure 3). However, Iwaki City is in the lower right corner of Fukushima Prefecture, so the spatial pattern may lack of significance.

Table 3. Gender-specific age-adjusted and multivariable odds ratios of diabetes, hypertension, and dyslipidemia according to evacuation status.

	Men				Women			
	Non-Evacuees	Returnees	Evacuees in Lifted Areas	Evacuees in Banned Areas	Non-Evacuees	Returnee	Evacuees in Lifted Areas	Evacuees in Banned Areas
No. at risk, *n*	6505	448	1062	4498	10,279	836	2145	7226
Diabetes, *n*	450	30	59	402	425	33	59	364
Age-adjusted OR (95% CI)	Ref.	1.06 (0.72–1.55)	1.01 (0.76–1.34)	1.46 (1.27–1.68) ***	Ref.	1.06 (0.74–1.52)	0.94 (0.71–1.24)	1.41 (1.22–1.63) ***
Multivariable OR (95% CI) §	Ref.	1.03 (0.70–1.52)	1.03 (0.77–1.37)	1.33 (1.15–1.55) ***	Ref.	1.06 (0.73–1.52)	0.97 (0.73–1.28)	1.38 (1.19–1.61) ***
Multivariable OR (95% CI) §§	Ref.	1.02 (0.69–1.51)	1.02 (0.77–1.37)	1.33 (1.15–1.54) ***	Ref.	1.05 (0.73–1.52)	0.96 (0.72–1.28)	1.38 (1.18–1.60) ***
No. at risk, *n*	3259	245	718	2473	6108	563	1699	4863
Hypertension, *n*	789	51	122	589	1039	95	145	779
Age-adjusted OR (95% CI)	Ref.	0.95 (0.69–1.33)	0.90 (0.72–1.12)	1.13 (0.99–1.28) *	Ref.	1.16 (0.91–1.47)	0.81 (0.67–0.99)	1.21 (1.08–1.34) **
Multivariable OR (95% CI) §	Ref.	0.92 (0.66–1.29)	0.93 (0.74–1.16)	1.08 (0.95–1.23)	Ref.	1.13 (0.89–1.45)	0.84 (0.69–1.02)	1.20 (1.08–1.35) **
Multivariable OR (95% CI) §§	Ref.	0.92 (0.66–1.28)	0.93 (0.74–1.16)	1.08 (0.94–1.23)	Ref.	1.13 (0.89–1.45)	0.84 (0.69–1.02)	1.20 (1.08–1.35) **
No. at risk, *n*	3612	225	627	2258	5016	392	1404	3839
Dyslipidemia, *n*	890	50	157	698	1210	102	264	990
Age-adjusted OR (95% CI)	Ref.	0.87 (0.63–1.20)	1.01 (0.83–1.23)	1.36 (1.21–1.53) ***	Ref.	1.28 (1.01–1.62)	0.97 (0.83–1.14)	1.24 (1.12–1.37) ***
Multivariable OR (95% CI) §	Ref.	0.85 (0.61–1.18)	1.01 (0.82–1.23)	1.31 (1.16–1.48) ***	Ref.	1.24 (0.98–1.58)	0.96 (0.82–1.13)	1.21 (1.09–1.34) ***
Multivariable OR (95% CI) §§	Ref.	0.85 (0.61–1.18)	1.01 (0.83–1.24)	1.31 (1.16–1.48) ***	Ref.	1.24 (0.97–1.57)	0.96 (0.82–1.23)	1.20 (1.09–1.33) ***

* $p < 0.05$; ** $p < 0.01$; *** $p < 0.001$. § Adjust for age, body mass index, smoking status, alcohol consumption, sports time, sleep quality, education level, and change of job. §§ Adjusted further for psychological distress.

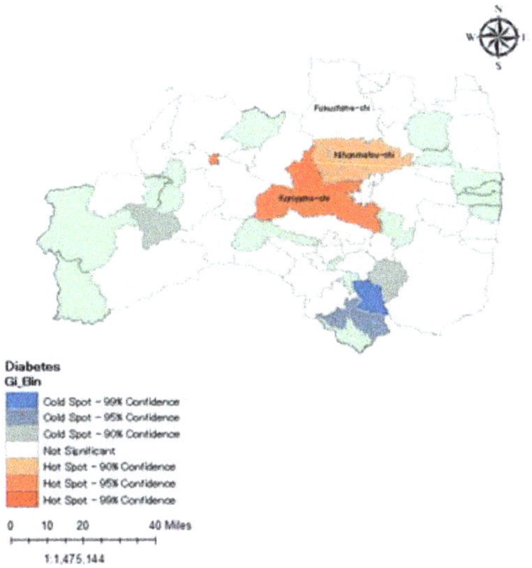

(a)

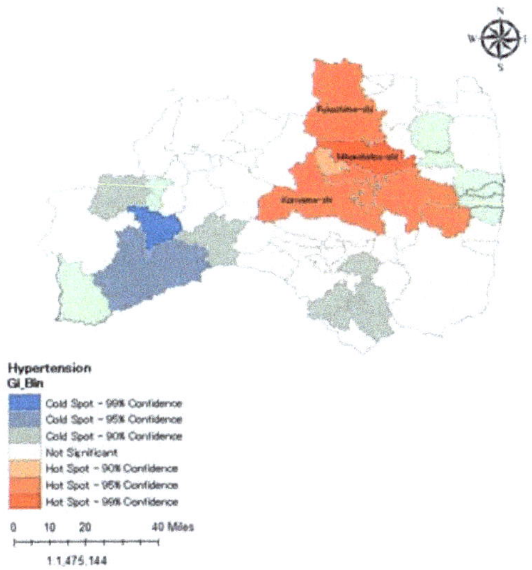

(b)

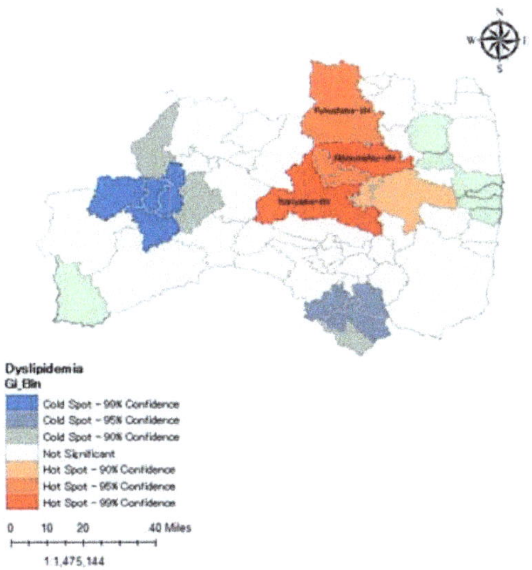

(c)

Figure 3. Hot spot analysis of spatial prevalence of lifestyle-related diseases among survey participants: (**a**) Spatial pattern of diabetes; (**b**) Spatial pattern of hypertension; (**c**) Spatial pattern of dyslipidemia.

4. Discussion

This study revealed that evacuees in banned areas had a higher risk of diabetes, hypertension, and dyslipidemia than non-evacuees, whereas returnees and evacuees in lifted areas did not have increased risks. These associations remained significant even after adjustment for selected lifestyles, education level, and change of job. Poor lifestyle factors including smoking, heavy alcohol consumption, physical inactivity, and inadequate sleep have been proven to enhance the incidence the lifestyle-related diseases [25,26]. Factors related to socioeconomic status such as low education level and change of job have also been confirmed as risk factors for the incidence of cardiovascular and metabolic diseases [7,27]. In addition, a high-high cluster of diabetes, hypertension, and dyslipidemia around the cities of Fukushima and Koriyama was noted. This study is the first to evaluate the risk of lifestyle-related diseases among returnees and evacuees in the lifted areas, and evacuees in the banned areas.

We attempted to explain why the evacuees in the banned areas had a higher risk of diabetes, hypertension, and hyperlipidemia than the other groups and the causes of spatial clustering in the discussion below.

First, in our study, the excess risks of diabetes, hypertension, and dyslipidemia among evacuees in banned areas were not altered after adjustment for psychological distress. However, this result in 2017 did not negate the possibility that that psychological distress confounded or mediated the excess risks probably because mental stress may temper over time [28].

Mental stress has been associated with an increased risks of diabetes [29], hypertension [30], and dyslipidemia [31,32]. Moreover, the incidence of diabetes increased [33,34] among evacuees immediately following the disaster. The hypothalamic–pituitary–adrenal axis [35,36] increases circulating cortisol levels, and under chronic stress conditions, the pituitary gland secretes vasopressin [35], which could affect glucose and lipid metabolism, leading to diabetes, hypertension, and dyslipidemia.

Second, diverse socio-economic factors may have influenced the incidence of lifestyle-related diseases. Evacuees in banned areas were closer to the center of the accident, were more vulnerable to the negative impact of the accident, and had no choice but to evacuate. Sugimoto et al. showed that long-term evacuation could lead to a poor perceived health status [35]. In addition, a recent report reported that evacuees in the banned area had less communication with others regarding their daily lives than those in the lifted areas [36]. These factors may have increased the risk of lifestyle-related disease onset.

Furthermore, the evacuees in the banned areas needed to leave their own houses and lose their material possessions and jobs, leading to a loss of purpose in life. Unemployment has been considered as a common factor that could increase the risk of delayed mental illness [37–39]. In addition, house damage, tsunami experience, nuclear power plant accident experience, and loss of family, realty, and close friends were associated with increased mental stress [40]. Moreover, we assumed that evacuees in the banned areas who were eager to return to their home but were unable to do so have a greater burden; thus, their risk of developing lifestyle-related diseases may be higher.

According to our findings, the prevalence clusters of hypertension, diabetes, and dyslipidemia were mainly located around the cities of Fukushima and Koriyama. Fukushima City is the provincial capital, whereas Koriyama City is one of the most populous commercial cities in the Fukushima province. Therefore, collective infrastructural resources are concentrated in Fukushima and Koriyama [41]. Additionally, after the disaster, these two cities, and the surrounding areas closest to the disaster site, quickly established emergency-relevant infrastructure and accepted many evacuees [42]. Therefore, this could partially explain why the spatial pattern of diabetes, hypertension, and dyslipidemia prevalence in the Fukushima and Koriyama cities were different from other cities.

Compared with other similar studies [13,43–45], this study has the following salient features. First, it analyzed a large population-based cohort, which not only included the residents in the affected areas of the Great East Japan earthquake, but also those throughout the entire Fukushima Prefecture. Second, over 70% of participants were followed-up for seven years from 2011–2017. Third, we adjusted for several potential confounders, including lifestyle and socioeconomic factors.

However, this study had some limitations. First, each participant may not have taken the comprehensive health checks and mental health and lifestyle surveys conducted annually. Therefore, we could not assess the impact of lifestyle changes on the incidence of diabetes, hypertension, and dyslipidemia. Second, we did not have data on the proportion of people who evacuated outside the Fukushima Prefecture and the prevalence of diseases in cities, towns, and villages in other prefectures around the Fukushima Prefecture. Third, regarding the spatial analysis, we only examined the prevalence of diabetes, hypertension, and dyslipidemia in 2017. Therefore, we could not examine the dynamic clustering process of each region. Lastly, the lifestyle parameters were based on a self-reported questionnaire and liable to misclassification.

Nevertheless, this is the first study to describe the prevalence and incidence of diabetes, hypertension, and dyslipidemia in the Fukushima area using both a cross-sectional design for the spatial dimension and a longitudinal design for the temporal dimension.

5. Conclusions

During a 7-year follow-up after the Great East Japan earthquake, evacuees in the banned areas had a higher incidence of diabetes, hypertension, and dyslipidemia than non-evacuees. Our findings imply the importance of continuous support for the prevention of lifestyle-related diseases for the evacuees in banned areas.

Supplementary Materials: The following supporting information can be downloaded at: https://www.mdpi.com/article/10.3390/ijerph19095661/s1, Table S1: Global Moran index of the spatial distribution of the prevalence of lifestyle-related diseases by administrative division among examinees.

Author Contributions: Z.S., R.C., H.I. (Hiroyasu Iso) and T.O. contributed to the study design; Z.S., E.E., F.H., T.O., S.Y., M.S., A.S., H.O. and K.K. were responsible for the data collection and overseeing the study procedures; The analysis was conducted by Z.S. and F.H.; The manuscript was written by Z.S.; H.I. (Hironori Imano), E.E., F.H., T.O., R.C., S.Y., A.S., M.S., H.O., K.K. and H.I. (Hiroyasu Iso) made significant contributions to the critically interpreted the results and provided intellectual content. All authors have read and agreed to the published version of the manuscript.

Funding: This survey was supported by the Japan National Health Fund for Children and Adults Affected by the Nuclear Incident; the Institute for Transdisciplinary Graduate Degree Programs of Osaka University, the Projects for Leading Graduate Schools on Interdisciplinary Program for Biomedical Science; the Network-type Joint Usage/Research Center for Radiation Disaster Medical Science, the Projects for Research on risk communication regarding radiation disasters; the Japan's Science and Technology Agency, Projects for Support for Pioneering Research Initiated by the Next Generation (grant number JPMJSP2138); and Research Project on Health Effects of Radiation organized by the Ministry of the Environment, Japan.

Institutional Review Board Statement: The study protocol was approved by the ethics committees of the Fukushima Medical University (IRB, approval number: 20018) and the Osaka University (IRB, approval number: 1319 and 2148). The target of this observational study was residents in the Fukushima Prefecture at the time of the disaster, and no intervention was implemented during the observation process. The study was conducted in accordance with the Declaration of Helsinki.

Informed Consent Statement: Informed consent was obtained from the community representatives to conduct an epidemiological study based on the guidelines of the Council for International Organizations of Medical Science.

Data Availability Statement: The datasets analyzed during the present study are not publicly available because the data from the Fukushima Health Management Survey belongs to the government of Fukushima Prefecture and can only be used within the organization.

Acknowledgments: We thank all the member who belongs to the Fukushima Health Management Survey for their support. The findings and conclusions of this article are solely the author's responsibility and do not represent the official views of the Fukushima Prefecture Government or the Japanese Government.

Conflicts of Interest: The authors declare no conflict of interest.

References

1. Fujiwara, T.; Kodaira, S.; No, T.; Kaiho, Y.; Takahashi, N.; Kaneda, Y. The 2011 Tohoku-Oki Earthquake: Displacement Reaching the Trench Axis. *Science* **2011**, *334*, 1240. [CrossRef] [PubMed]
2. Hirose, K. 2011 Fukushima Dai-ichi nuclear power plant accident: Summary of regional radioactive deposition monitoring results. *J. Environ. Radioact.* **2012**, *111*, 13–17. [CrossRef] [PubMed]
3. Ubaura, M. Changes in Land Use after the Great East Japan Earthquake and Related Issues of Urban Form. In *2011 Japan Earthquake and Tsunami: Reconstruction and Restoration: Insights and Assessment after 5 Years*; Springer: Berlin/Heidelberg, Germany, 2018; Volume 47, pp. 183–203. [CrossRef]
4. Ueda, Y.; Murakami, M.; Maeda, M.; Yabe, H.; Suzuki, Y.; Orui, M.; Yasumura, S.; Ohira, T.; Fukushima Hlth Management, S. Risk Factors for Problem Drinking among Evacuees in Fukushima following the Great East Japan Earthquake: The Fukushima Health Management Survey. *Tohoku J. Exp. Med.* **2019**, *248*, 239–252. [CrossRef] [PubMed]
5. Osaki, Y.; Maesato, H.; Minobe, R.; Kinjo, A.; Kuwabara, Y.; Imamoto, A.; Myoga, Y.; Matsushita, S.; Higuchi, S. Changes in smoking behavior among victims after the great East Japan earthquake and tsunami. *Environ. Health Prev. Med.* **2020**, *25*, 19. [CrossRef]
6. Zhang, W.; Ohira, T.; Maeda, M.; Nakano, H.; Iwasa, H.; Yasumura, S.; Ohtsuru, A.; Harigane, M.; Suzuki, Y.; Horikoshi, N.; et al. The association between self-reported sleep dissatisfaction after the Great East Japan Earthquake, and a deteriorated socioeconomic status in the evacuation area: The Fukushima Health Management Survey. *Sleep Med.* **2020**, *68*, 63–70. [CrossRef]
7. Zhang, W.; Ohira, T.; Yasumura, S.; Maeda, M.; Otsuru, A.; Harigane, M.; Horikoshi, N.; Suzuki, Y.; Yabe, H.; Nagai, M.; et al. Effects of socioeconomic factors on cardiovascular-related symptoms among residents in Fukushima after the Great East Japan Earthquake: A cross-sectional study using data from the Fukushima Health Management Survey. *BMJ Open* **2017**, *7*, e014077. [CrossRef]
8. Hagiwara, Y.; Yabe, Y.; Sugawara, Y.; Sato, M.; Watanabe, T.; Kanazawa, K.; Sonofuchi, K.; Koide, M.; Sekiguchi, T.; Tsuchiya, M.; et al. Influence of living environments and working status on low back pain for survivors of the Great East Japan Earthquake. *J. Orthop. Sci.* **2016**, *21*, 138–142. [CrossRef]
9. Li, X.Y.; Aida, J.; Hikichi, H.; Kondo, K.; Kawachi, I. Association of Postdisaster Depression and Posttraumatic Stress Disorder With Mortality Among Older Disaster Survivors of the 2011 Great East Japan Earthquake and Tsunami. *JAMA Netw. Open* **2019**, *2*, e1917550. [CrossRef]
10. Nagamine, M.; Giltay, E.J.; Shigemura, J.; van der Wee, N.J.; Yamamoto, T.; Takahashi, Y.; Saito, T.; Tanichi, M.; Koga, M.; Toda, H.; et al. Assessment of Factors Associated With Long-term Posttraumatic Stress Symptoms Among 56 388 First Responders After the 2011 Great East Japan Earthquake. *JAMA Netw. Open* **2020**, *3*, e2018339. [CrossRef]
11. Statistics Bureau. Labour Force Survey. 2011. Available online: https://www.stat.go.jp/data/roudou/rireki/gaiyou.html#ft_4hanki (accessed on 28 March 2022).
12. Takiguchi, M.; Ohira, T.; Nakano, H.; Yumiya, Y.; Yamaki, T.; Yoshihisa, A.; Nakazato, K.; Suzuki, H.; Ishikawa, T.; Yasumura, S.; et al. Trends in the Incidence of Sudden Deaths and Heart Diseases in Fukushima After the Great East Japan Earthquake. *Int. Heart J.* **2019**, *60*, 1253–1258. [CrossRef]
13. Satoh, H.; Ohira, T.; Nagai, M.; Hosoya, M.; Sakai, A.; Yasumura, S.; Ohtsuru, A.; Kawasaki, Y.; Suzuki, H.; Takahashi, A.; et al. Evacuation is a risk factor for diabetes development among evacuees of the Great East Japan earthquake: A 4-year follow-up of the Fukushima Health Management Survey. *Diabetes Metab.* **2019**, *45*, 312–315. [CrossRef] [PubMed]
14. Life Support Team for Nuclear Survivors. Situation in the Evacuation Zone. 2018. Available online: https://www.mext.go.jp/b_menu/shingi/chousa/kaihatu/016/shiryo/__icsFiles/afieldfile/2018/08/10/1408009_03_1.pdf (accessed on 28 March 2022).
15. Editorial Committee for the Paper on Decontamination Projects. Decontamination Projects for Radioactive Contamination Discharged by Tokyo Electric Power Company Fukushima Daiichi Nuclear Power Station Accident. 2018. Available online: http://josen.env.go.jp/en/policy_document/pdf/decontamination_report1807_01.pdf (accessed on 28 March 2022).
16. Yasumura, S.; Hosoya, M.; Yamashita, S.; Kamiya, K.; Abe, M.; Akashi, M.; Kodama, K.; Ozasa, K.; Fukushima Hlth Management Survey, G. Study Protocol for the Fukushima Health Management Survey. *J. Epidemiol.* **2012**, *22*, 375–383. [CrossRef] [PubMed]
17. Research Collaborators Conference. Voluntary Evacuation Related Data. 2011. Available online: https://www.mext.go.jp/b_menu/shingi/chousa/kaihatu/016/shiryo/__icsFiles/afieldfile/2011/11/25/1313502_3.pdf (accessed on 28 March 2022).
18. Unger, T.; Borghi, C.; Charchar, F.; Khan, N.A.; Poulter, N.R.; Prabhakaran, D.; Ramirez, A.; Schlaich, M.; Stergiou, G.S.; Tomaszewski, M.; et al. 2020 International Society of Hypertension global hypertension practice guidelines. *J. Hypertens.* **2020**, *38*, 982–1004. [CrossRef] [PubMed]
19. Araki, E.; Goto, A.; Kondo, T.; Noda, M.; Noto, H.; Origasa, H.; Osawa, H.; Taguchi, A.; Tanizawa, Y.; Tobe, K.; et al. Japanese Clinical Practice Guideline for Diabetes 2019. *J. Diabetes Investig.* **2020**, *11*, 1020–1076. [CrossRef] [PubMed]
20. Kinoshita, M.; Yokote, K.; Arai, H.; Iida, M.; Ishigaki, Y.; Ishibashi, S.; Umemoto, S.; Egusa, G.; Ohmura, H.; Okamura, T.; et al. Japan Atherosclerosis Society (JAS) Guidelines for Prevention of Atherosclerotic Cardiovascular Diseases 2017. *J. Atheroscler. Thromb.* **2018**, *25*, 846–984. [CrossRef] [PubMed]
21. Chan, C.K.; Feinstein, A.R.; Jekel, J.F.; Wells, C.K. The Value and Hazards of Standardization in Clinical Epidemiologic Research. *J. Clin. Epidemiol.* **1988**, *41*, 1125–1134. [CrossRef]
22. Tripepi, G.; Jager, K.J.; Dekker, F.W.; Zoccali, C. Stratification for Confounding—Part 2: Direct and Indirect Standardization. *Nephron Clin. Pract.* **2010**, *116*, C322–C325. [CrossRef]

23. Moran, P.A.P. Notes on Continuous Stochastic Phenomena. *Biometrika* **1950**, *37*, 17–23. [CrossRef]
24. Getis, A.; Ord, J.K. The Analysis of Spatial Association by Use of Distance Statistics. *Geogr. Anal.* **1992**, *24*, 189–206. [CrossRef]
25. Ketola, E.; Sipila, R.; Makela, M. Effectiveness of individual lifestyle interventions in reducing cardiovascular disease and risk factors. *Ann. Med.* **2000**, *32*, 239–251. [CrossRef]
26. Deng, X.R.; Wang, P.X.; Yuan, H.J. Epidemiology, risk factors across the spectrum of age-related metabolic diseases. *J. Trace Elem. Med. Biol.* **2020**, *61*, 126497. [CrossRef] [PubMed]
27. Nagai, M.; Ohira, T.; Zhang, W.; Nakano, H.; Maeda, M.; Yasumura, S.; Abe, M.; Fukushima Health Management Survey. Lifestyle-related factors that explain disaster-induced changes in socioeconomic status and poor subjective health: A cross-sectional study from the Fukushima health management survey. *BMC Public Health* **2017**, *17*, 340. [CrossRef] [PubMed]
28. Matsumoto, K.; Sakuma, A.; Ueda, I.; Nagao, A.; Takahashi, Y. Psychological trauma after the Great East Japan Earthquake. *Psychiatry Clin. Neurosci.* **2016**, *70*, 318–331. [CrossRef] [PubMed]
29. Hackett, R.A.; Steptoe, A. Type 2 diabetes mellitus and psychological stress—A modifiable risk factor. *Nat. Rev. Endocrinol.* **2017**, *13*, 547–560. [CrossRef] [PubMed]
30. Ushakov, A.V.; Ivanchenko, V.S.; Gagarina, A.A. Psychological Stress in Pathogenesis of Essential Hypertension. *Curr. Hypertens. Rev.* **2016**, *12*, 203–214. [CrossRef]
31. Devaki, M.; Nirupama, R.; Yajurvedi, H.N. Chronic stress-induced oxidative damage and hyperlipidemia are accompanied by atherosclerotic development in rats. *Stress Int. J. Biol. Stress* **2013**, *16*, 233–243. [CrossRef]
32. McCann, B.S.; Magee, M.S.; Broyles, F.C.; Vaughan, M.; Albers, J.J.; Knopp, R.H. Acute Psychological Stress and Epinephrine Infusion in Normolipidemic and Hyperlipidemic Men—Effects on Plasma-Lipid and Apoprotein Concentrations. *Psychosom. Med.* **1995**, *57*, 165–176. [CrossRef]
33. Satoh, H.; Ohira, T.; Hosoya, M.; Sakai, A.; Watanabe, T.; Ohtsuru, A.; Kawasaki, Y.; Suzuki, H.; Takahashi, A.; Kobashi, G.; et al. Evacuation after the Fukushima Daiichi Nuclear Power Plant Accident Is a Cause of Diabetes: Results from the Fukushima Health Management Survey. *J. Diabetes Res.* **2015**, *2015*, 627390. [CrossRef]
34. Satoh, H.; Ohira, T.; Nagai, M.; Hosoya, M.; Sakai, A.; Watanabe, T.; Ohtsuru, A.; Kawasaki, Y.; Suzuki, H.; Takahashi, A.; et al. Hypo-high-density Lipoprotein Cholesterolemia Caused by Evacuation after the Fukushima Daiichi Nuclear Power Plant Accident: Results from the Fukushima Health Management Survey. *Intern. Med.* **2016**, *55*, 1967–1976. [CrossRef]
35. Sugimoto, T.; Shinozaki, T.; Miyamoto, Y. Aftershocks associated with impaired health caused by the great East Japan disaster among youth across Japan: A national cross-sectional survey. *Interact. J. Med. Res.* **2013**, *2*, e31. [CrossRef]
36. Institute of Disaster Area Revitalization, Regrowth and Governance. National Survey on People Evacuated Due to the Nuclear Power Plant Accident. *Institute of Disaster Area Revitalization, Regrowth and Governance, Kwansei Gakuin University.* Available online: https://www.kwansei.ac.jp/fukkou/research/survey/detail/20210120.html (accessed on 28 March 2022).
37. Maehlisen, M.H.; Pasgaard, A.A.; Mortensen, R.N.; Vardinghus-Nielsen, H.; Torp-Pedersen, C.; Boggild, H. Perceived stress as a risk factor of unemployment: A register-based cohort study. *BMC Public Health* **2018**, *18*, 728. [CrossRef] [PubMed]
38. Morishima, R.; Ando, S.; Araki, T.; Usami, S.; Kanehara, A.; Tanaka, S.; Kasai, K. The course of chronic and delayed onset of mental illness and the risk for suicidal ideation after the Great East Japan Earthquake of 2011: A community-based longitudinal study. *Psychiatry Res.* **2019**, *273*, 171–177. [CrossRef] [PubMed]
39. Orpana, H.M.; Lemyre, L.; Gravel, R. Income and psychological distress: The role of the social environment. *Health Rep.* **2009**, *20*, 21–28. [PubMed]
40. Shiga, T.; Zhang, W.; Ohira, T.; Suzuki, Y.; Maeda, M.; Mashiko, H.; Yabe, H.; Iwasa, H.; Nakano, H.; Yasumura, S.; et al. Socioeconomic status, damage-related conditions, and PTSD following the Fukushima-daiichi nuclear power plant accident: The Fukushima Health Management Survey. *Fukushima J. Med. Sci.* **2021**, *67*, 71–82. [CrossRef] [PubMed]
41. Fukushima Prefectural Government. Overview of Fukushima Prefecture. 2021. Available online: https://www.pref.fukushima.lg.jp/sec/11045b/r3youran.html (accessed on 28 March 2022).
42. Disaster Countermeasures Office. Progress of Emergency Temporary Housing, Rented Housing, and Public Housing. 2022. Available online: https://www.pref.fukushima.lg.jp/site/portal/ps-nyuukyojoukyou.html (accessed on 28 March 2022).
43. Ohira, T.; Hosoya, M.; Yasumura, S.; Satoh, H.; Suzuki, H.; Sakai, A.; Ohtsuru, A.; Kawasaki, Y.; Takahashi, A.; Ozasa, K.; et al. Evacuation and Risk of Hypertension After the Great East Japan Earthquake The Fukushima Health Management Survey. *Hypertension* **2016**, *68*, 558–564. [CrossRef]
44. Shiba, K.; Hikichi, H.; Aida, J.; Kondo, K.; Kawachi, I. Long-Term Associations Between Disaster Experiences and Cardiometabolic Risk: A Natural Experiment From the 2011 Great East Japan Earthquake and Tsunami. *Am. J. Epidemiol.* **2019**, *188*, 1109–1119. [CrossRef] [PubMed]
45. Takahashi, S.; Yonekura, Y.; Tanno, K.; Shimoda, H.; Sakata, K.; Ogawa, A.; Kobayashi, S.; Kawachi, I. Increased incidence of metabolic syndrome among older survivors relocated to temporary housing after the 2011 Great East Japan earthquake & tsunami. *Metab. Open* **2020**, *7*, 100042. [CrossRef]

healthcare

Article

Unmanned Aerial Vehicle in the Logistics of Pandemic Vaccination: An Exact Analytical Approach for Any Number of Vaccination Centres

Adnan Benayad [1,2,*], Olaf Malasse [3], Hicham Belhadaoui [1,2] and Noureddine Benayad [4]

1 Laboratory of Computer Networks, Telecommunications and Multimedia, ESTC, Hassan II University, B.P. 8012 Oasis, Casablanca 20000, Morocco
2 National School of Electricity and Mechanics, Hassan II University, B.P. 8118 Oasis, Casablanca 20000, Morocco
3 Laboratoire LCFC, National School of Arts and Crafts, ParisTech, 57070 Metz, France
4 Laboratory of PHEMaC, Faculty of Sciences-Ain Chock, Hassan II University, B.P. 5366 Maarif, Casablanca 20000, Morocco
* Correspondence: adnanbenayad12@gmail.com; Tel.: +212-628-632-944

Abstract: While the development and manufacture of pandemic vaccines is a daunting task, the greatest challenge lies in how to deliver these vaccines to billions of people around the world. This requires an efficient strategy of deliveries, at constrained costs and deadlines. This paper proposes an exact analytical approach and operational strategy to the logistics of any pandemic vaccination efforts, applicable both to sparsely populated areas or deficient infrastructure, and to very dense urban fabrics where mobility is highly constrained. Our strategy consists in dividing the territory concerned into zones and districts in a concentric way. We opt for the use of unmanned aerial vehicles to free ourselves from land constraints. This involves serving, from a logistics centre (central depot), any number n of vaccination centres, while optimizing costs and deadlines. We have determined all equivalent and optimal flight path plans for a fixed and optimal number of drones, which depend on domain D(d); d being the demand of vaccination centers. The analysis of the results led us to define what we will call the "degeneracy of domain D". All our results are expressed as a function of the parameter n.

Keywords: pandemic vaccination; exact analytical approach; unmanned aerial vehicle (UAV); drone delivery; route planning problem; optimal flight path; equivalent graphs; degeneracy

Citation: Benayad, A.; Malasse, O.; Belhadaoui, H.; Benayad, N. Unmanned Aerial Vehicle in the Logistics of Pandemic Vaccination: An Exact Analytical Approach for Any Number of Vaccination Centres. *Healthcare* **2022**, *10*, 2102. https://doi.org/10.3390/healthcare10102102

Academic Editors: Amir Khorram-Manesh and Krzysztof Goniewicz

Received: 11 August 2022
Accepted: 11 October 2022
Published: 20 October 2022

1. Introduction

Until recently, Unmanned Aerial Vehicles (UAVs) or drones have primarily been used in the military. Recently, they are becoming more present in many civilian sectors. This will open new possibilities for further research and development of UAVs. They are considered as one of the technological innovations which may trigger a revolutionary reshaping of transportation industry, since they have the potential to significantly reduce the cost and time required to deliver packages. By performing these tasks autonomously, drones may be faster than traditional delivery vehicles such as trucks since they are not limited by established infrastructure such as roads, and generally face less complex obstacle avoidance scenarios which complies with current trends in the transport industry [1].

It is noteworthy that a lot of pilot projects have been launched to exploit the potentials of drones in logistics applications. Examples of large organisations experimenting with drones are Google, DHL, and Amazon Indeed, in 2013, Amazon announced Prime Air [2,3], a service that utilizes multirotor drones to deliver packages from Amazon to customers. German logistics company Deutsche Post DHL also started its Parcelcopter project in 2013; the Parcelcopter has transported medicine to the island of Juist in the North Sea [4]. Google revealed Project Wing in 2014 to produce drones that can deliver larger items than Prime

Air and Parcelcopter [5]. A startup called Matternet has partnered with Swiss Post to test a lightweight package delivery quadcopter [6]. Next to large-scaled projects of multi-national firms, also smaller-scaled projects of drone delivery systems have been successfully put into practice [7].

Non-military UAVs come in various shapes and sizes and typically contain a main airframe, navigation system and propulsion systems [8]. In medicine we use two primary types (i) fixed-wing aircraft and (ii) helicopter-like drones with single or multiple rotors.

For logistical applications, the speed, payload capacity and radius of operation are the most important technical parameters. They vary greatly among different drone models. Primarily models with payload capacity up to 5 kg are used [9,10]. However, also heavy-load UAVs are available with a payload capacity of up to 40 kg [11]. Drones, such as those produced by Zipline (Half Moon Bay, CA, USA), can fly at a speed of up to 128 km/h (80 mph) and have a range of 160 km (99 miles) round trip [12].

Developments in numerous technologies have enabled the above organizations to improve drone deliveries. Carbon fibre manufacturing costs have decreased significantly over the last years [13,14], enabling the development of strong, lightweight airframes. Lithium polymer batteries, known by their relatively high energy density [15] have improved the flight times of the drones compared to alternative technologies such as nickel-cadmium and nickel-metal hydride. UAVs typically use GPS to determine their location, and they are also able to take advantage of DGPS and localization techniques [16,17] to improve accuracy. Obstacles can be avoided through many techniques such as LIDAR and image processing [18,19]. Architectures and protocols have been developed that enable drones to form ad-hoc networks and to wirelessly communicate with other entities [20,21].

Other technological issues to be considered in logistical UAV applications are the launching and landing concept in addition to the autonomous control capability. Meanwhile, most commercial UAV models also provide fully automatic launching stations [22]. For B2C concepts, however, the UAV must be able to land on 'rough' ground. Further, some detachment technology like ropes (Flirty, Google) or parachutes (Zipline) could be available. In a B2C application scenario, it is reasonable to assume that UAVs must wait hovering until all prerequisites for detaching the cargo are fulfilled (e.g., waiting for the customer's approval or a clear detachment area).

Drones' systems have also been reported in other practical applications in emergency and disaster management situations where the crucial feature is the drone's ability to travel directly between several points of interest [23] over hazardous terrain during a crisis. These include intelligence, surveillance and reconnaissance (ISR) missions to visit a n set of locations [24]; and in emergency aid in order to reduce the worker's exposure to danger and also for emergency response in the event of forest fires, oil spills, and earthquakes [25]. UAVs equipped with cameras allow for viewing disaster scenes promptly, collecting critical data including aerial photograph, air quality or radiation levels. They can deploy wireless sensors to provide immediate updates on the event to the teams on the ground. On the other hand, in the healthcare sector, especially in developing countries [26], UAVs have already been used in different aspects, including transfer of blood product. They can also be used to transport diagnostic samples and various medical purposes [8,27]. Finally, we note that such drones are also used in agriculture (monitoring crop production), construction (surveying land), industry (warehouse management), public safety (law enforcement and traffic surveillance), and environmental conservation efforts (deforestation monitoring),

In a world where logistics has become a vital function, as we were able to verify during the COVID-19 health crisis, but where the margins of the various players in the supply chain are increasingly tight and prices constantly drawn down, the drone is a solution to consider and seriously study for all those who want to increase their operational efficiency and stand out for their quality of service.

The purpose of the paper is to offer an exact analytical approach and operational strategy to the logistics of any pandemic vaccination effort. Our study gives an answer to the following question: How to use drones in order to deliver pandemic vaccines to large areas (densely populated city or sparsely populated rural region) whatever the number of the population living there. Indeed, this paper primarily studies the route planning problem of the UAVs during distribution. The application scenario is the vaccines delivery from the distribution centre to the vaccination centres, and to determine all equivalent and optimum flight path plans for drones that need to serve multiple positions for any number of vaccination centres.

The structure of this paper is as follows. Section 2 provides a review on the relevant literature. In Section 3, we formally introduce the strategy, hypotheses and used notations. Section 4 describes the drone routing problem for fixed numbers of vaccination centres. In Section 5, we provide a generalization of the drone routing problem, i.e., for any number of vaccination centres. This problem leads us to define what can be called "the degree of degeneracy" of the vaccination centres demand. Section 6 concludes the paper.

2. Literature Review: Use of Drones in Healthcare

Research on employing drones in delivery operations has gained a lot of attention in recent years. There is an exploding body of literature on potential application scenarios concerning this subject. An extensive overview about civil applications of UAVs can be found in reference [28].

Drones have been used in several sectors of healthcare. Preliminary reports have indicated the feasibility of drone related transfer of biological samples (for instance, blood product) during short flights at room temperatures or colder with no significant influence on the accuracy of routine chemistry, haematology and coagulation analyses [29,30]. In this sector, we must notice that Rwanda was the first country to successfully use drones into health services at the national level. A drone delivery programme also known as 'Uber for blood' was launched in 2016. It uses battery-powered fixed-wing drones designed and built by Zipline capable of flying up to 150 km in a round trip and carrying up to 1.5 kg of blood. We note here that Rwandan patients have never received blood quickly and so efficiently: Indeed, blood delivery times have plummeted from approximately 4 h to only 15–45 min in remote areas. More than 18,000 life-saving delivery flights containing blood products were carried out in August 2019 [31].

In 2016, UNICEF and the Government of Malawi initiated an important programme in order to explore whether sample transportation by UAV is a cost-effective intervention to reduce time-to-result for human immunodeficiency virus testing in infants [32]. Drone have been also used in another sector of healthcare. In Papua New Guinea, where the prevalence of tuberculosis is one of the highest in the world (nearly 6/1000 population/year), drones were used to transport sputum samples of individuals with suspected tuberculosis from dispersed health centres to Kerema General Hospital, which circumvented the need to use road transport that was hampered during the rainy months [33].

On the hand, in 2017, Switzerland paved the way for the transport of specimens by drone in Europe by authorizing flights of autonomous drones for healthcare services over cities at any time. Swiss Post and Matternet have developed a medical transport network using quadcopter drones (20-km range, average speed 36 km/h, 2-kg maximum payload), with more than 3000 successful flights in Lugano, Bern and Zurich in April 2019 [27,34].

A drone programme has also been successfully implemented in Tanzania, a country with one of the highest maternal mortality rates in the world (556 deaths/100 000 deliveries). The drones were much faster than ground transportation, delivering on-demand blood, vaccines, and antiretroviral and malaria drugs via biodegradable parachutes to more than 1000 health facilities [35].

In April 2019, Gavi, the Vaccine Alliance, announced the launch of the largest drone healthcare project. Delivery of blood, medicines and vaccines is now available for 2000 health facilities serving 12 million people across Ghana. Distribution centres can deliver up to 600 on-demand drone transports per day with potential for further expansion to up to 2000 flights/day [36].

The economic and operational value concerning vaccine deliveries was recently assessed using a computational model [7]. Compared with traditional land transport, drone delivery increased vaccine availability and decreased costs ($0.05 to $0.21 per dose administered), proving that drones are cost-effective and useful in a variety of circumstances and settings if used frequently enough to overcome the system installation and maintenance costs [37]. We note that drone delivery has been successfully piloted in Vanuatu (a Pacific archipelago) where most villages are not easily reachable and often have no electricity to store vaccines, leaving nearly 20% of Vanuatu's 35,000 children under 5 years not fully vaccinated [37].

The World Health Organization has designated COVID-19 as a pandemic. Currently, over 140 million cases of COVID-19 have been confirmed worldwide, including more than 3,000,000 deaths. There is a dire need for therapeutics and vaccines to fight such pandemic. Distributing an effective vaccine to billions of people around the world is likely the greatest logistical challenge since the Second World War. First, to satisfy the high-demands during the COVID-19, some models have been developed [38] in order to increase the production of vaccines. On the other hand, they should be transported, from the manufacturing sites to distributors. These latter must deliver the vaccines to vaccination centres, which have to be adequately and uniformly distributed in urban and rural areas. This is not an easy task, especially if we know that maintaining the cold chain will be a crucial issue for such vaccines, which poses a significant problem in many parts of the world. Low temperatures must be maintained whether vaccines are being delivered to densely populated cities or sparsely populated rural areas. We must note that the pandemic vaccines have to be stored within appropriate and efficient conditions. This is the health guidelines state that even small deviations can render a vaccine ineffective. According to a 2019 report by the International Air Transport Association (IATA), approximately 25% of vaccines shipped are at risk due to poor temperature management in transportation vehicles. The report estimates that the associated damage costs the healthcare industry more than $34 billion annually. For the people and economies that depend on the prevention of COVID-19, inefficient cold chain management will be particularly costly. Thus, healthcare distributors and providers must operate in a specialized, temperature-controlled supply chain. It is worthy to note that in the context of the COVID-19 pandemic that Zipline is deploying its ingenious logistics. Faced with problems relatively identical to those of Rwanda, the Ghanaian government has also chosen to call on the Californian start-up for the delivery, initially of tests, then now of Covid vaccines. About 2.5 million doses are expected to be delivered in Ghana using these drones [31]. Not only does this make Ghana the first country in the world to deploy drones nationwide for the delivery of COVID-19 vaccines, but it is also a mammoth effort to ensure equitable access and enable Ghana to use fully its healthcare infrastructure to deliver vaccines," Zipline CEO Keller Rinaudo said in a statement.

3. Strategy, Hypotheses and Notations

3.1. Strategy

In this paper, we are interested in the use of drones in logistics of any pandemic vaccination. The strategy we adopt to vaccinate the population of a given territorial area (urban or rural) is clearly shown in Figure 1. Indeed,

(i) We divide the territorial area into M zones constituting M concentric circular bands with the same width.
(ii) Each band is divided into n isometric districts where the centre of each one of them is chosen as the vaccination center Thus, the set of vaccination centres in a given zone, are located on the vertices of a regular n-polygon.
(iii) Each vaccination centre deals with the vaccination of people living in its own district.
(iv) All vaccination centres belonging to the same zone (circular band, see Figure 1), are served independently from the others.

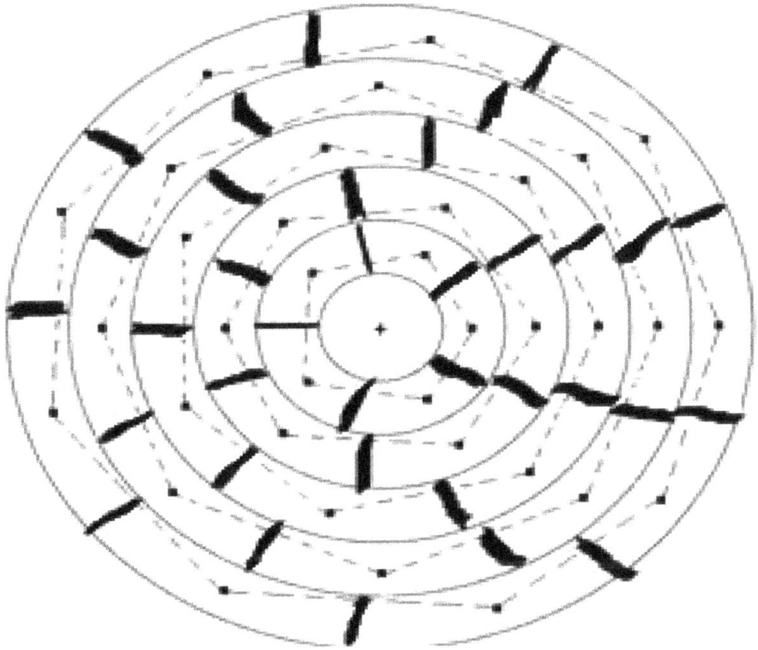

Figure 1. Localization of all vaccination centres belonging to the concerned territorial area.

3.2. Hypotheses

In order to perform such vaccination operation using drones, we have to study the route planning problem of the UAVs distribution. To this end, we consider the following assumptions:

1- The drones' platform, namely the starting and finishing points of the drones, is located on the centre of the considered territorial area which coincides with the common circumcenter of the circumcircles of regular polygons locating all the vaccination centres.
2- The drone is a single model. So, the load capacity is the same and fixed.
3- The drone batteries are fully charged before leaving the platform. The charge is enough to satisfy the maximum centres, according to the drone load capacity.
4- The vaccination centres make the same demands.
5- The vaccines are stored within appropriate and efficient conditions during the transportation.
6- Each trip is composed of segments (edges and radius of the n-polygon) interconnecting the locations, measured by the Euclidean distance between them. They are crossed at constant speed by the drone which is independent of its load capacity.
7- Each vaccination centre must be served only by one drone.
8- For a given range of vaccination centres demands, only optimum numbers of drones are used to cover the entire demands.
9- For a given range of vaccination centres demands, there is at least one drone that satisfies a maximum number of centres.

3.3. Notation

We define the different sets needed for modelling the problem in addition to the parameters and variables.

M	Number of zones (circular bands) covering the entire territorial area concerned by vaccination.
n	number of vaccination centres belonging to the same zone.
d	Quantity of vaccines demanded by vaccination centre.
C	Load capacity of the drone
N	optimum number of drones used for the logistic distribution.
$(k_1, k_2, \ldots, k_N)/k_1 \geq k_2 \geq, \ldots, \geq k_N$, with $\sum_{i=1}^{N} k_i = n$, where k_i is the number of vaccinations centres visited by the *i*th drone.	
$k_1(d)$	denotes the maximum number of vaccination centres that one drone can serve, according to the domain D of d.
G = {n, N, $(k_1, k_2, \ldots, k_N)$}	Graph defining the set of paths followed by the N drones in order to deliver vaccines to the n vaccinations centres belonging the same zone. For instance, the path described by the *i*th drone is formed by the set of locations or vertices to be visited and the set of directed links connecting them.
2 r	The radius of the first zone. It represents also the width of circular bands.

4. Drone Routing Problem for Fixed Number of Vaccination Centres

4.1. Optimum Number of Drones and Vaccination Centre Demands

Before giving our general formulation of logistics distribution for any number n of vaccination centres and valid for any zone, we give in this section, a detailed presentation of the model in the case of small, fixed values of n = 5,6,7,8, and 9.

First, we represent the correlation between the optimum number of drones necessary to use for logistics distribution and the needs of the vaccination centres. The cases n = 7,8, and 9 are presented in Table 1. The other cases corresponding to n = 5 and 6, are presented in Appendix A.

Table 1. Domains of d, corresponding graphs and lengths *L* (*n*, *N*) of the paths travelled by the set of optimum number of drones necessary for the logistics distribution, when zone contains n = 7, 8, and 9 vaccination centres, respectively.

n = 7				
d/C	$k_1(d)$	N	Graphs	$L(n, N)$
$\frac{d}{C} \leq \frac{1}{7}$	7	1	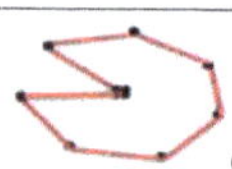 G = {n = 7, N = 1, (7)}	50.446 r
$\frac{1}{7} < \frac{d}{C} \leq \frac{1}{6}$	6	2	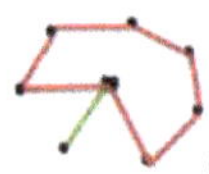 G = {n = 7, N = 2, (6, 1)}	58.371 r
$\frac{1}{6} < \frac{d}{C} \leq \frac{1}{5}$	5	2	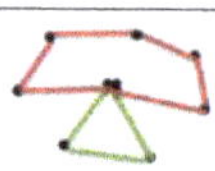 G = {n = 7, N = 2, (5, 2)}	

Table 1. *Cont.*

d/C	$k_1(d)$	N	Graphs	$L(n,N)$
$\frac{1}{5} < \frac{d}{C} \leq \frac{1}{4}$	4	2	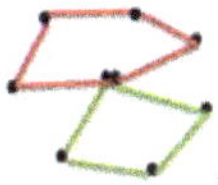 G = {n = 7, N = 2, (4, 3)}	
$\frac{1}{4} < \frac{d}{C} \leq \frac{1}{3}$	3	3	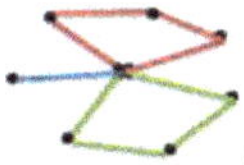 G = {n = 7, N = 3, (3, 2, 2)} 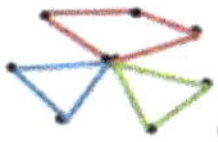 G = {n = 7, N = 3, (3, 3, 1)}	66.297 r
$\frac{1}{3} < \frac{d}{C} \leq \frac{1}{2}$	2	4	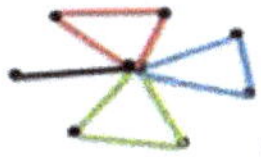 G = {n = 7, N = 4, (2, 2, 2, 1)}	74.223 r
$\frac{1}{2} < \frac{d}{C} \leq 1$	1	7	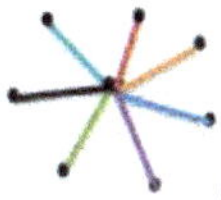 G = {n = 7, N = 7, (1, 1, 1, 1, 1, 1, 1)}	98 r
		n = 8		
d/C	$k_1(d)$	N	Graphs	$L(n,N)$
$\frac{d}{C} \leq \frac{1}{8}$	8	1	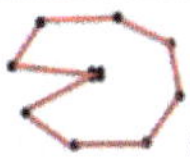 G = {n = 8, N = 1, (8)}	66.218 r
$\frac{1}{8} < \frac{d}{C} \leq \frac{1}{7}$	7	2	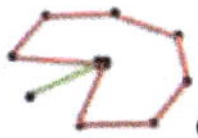 G = {n = 8, N = 2, (7, 1)}	77.329 r
$\frac{1}{7} < \frac{d}{C} \leq \frac{1}{6}$	6	2	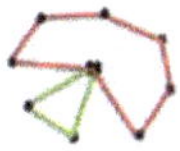	
$\frac{1}{6} < \frac{d}{C} \leq \frac{1}{5}$	5	2	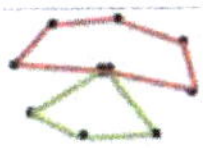	
$\frac{1}{5} < \frac{d}{C} \leq \frac{1}{4}$	4	2	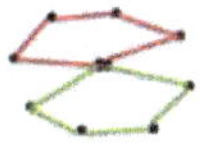	
$\frac{1}{4} < \frac{d}{C} \leq \frac{1}{3}$	3	3	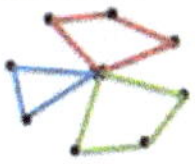	88.441 r
$\frac{1}{3} < \frac{d}{C} \leq \frac{1}{2}$	2	4	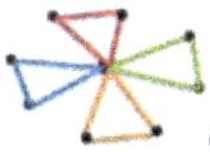 G = {n = 8, N = 4, (2, 2, 2, 2)}	99.553 r
$\frac{1}{2} < \frac{d}{C} \leq 1$	1	8	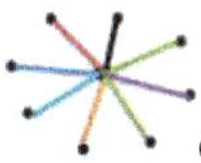 G = {n = 8, N = 8, (1, 1, 1, 1, 1, 1, 1, 1)}	144 r
		n = 9		
d/C	$k_1(d)$	N	Graphs	$L(n,N)$
$\frac{d}{C} \leq \frac{1}{9}$	9	1	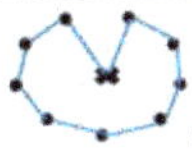 G = {n = 9, N = 1, (9)}	82.195 r

Table 1. *Cont.*

$\frac{1}{9} < \frac{d}{C} \leq \frac{1}{8}$	8	2	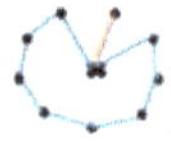 G = {n = 9, N = 2, (8, 1)}	96.6711 r
$\frac{1}{8} < \frac{d}{C} \leq \frac{1}{7}$	7	2	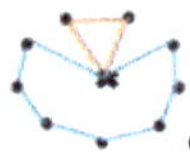 G = {n = 9, N = 2, (7, 2)}	
$\frac{1}{7} < \frac{d}{C} \leq \frac{1}{6}$	6	2	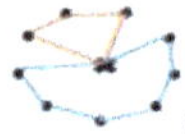 G = {n = 9, N = 2, (6, 3)}	
$\frac{1}{6} < \frac{d}{C} \leq \frac{1}{5}$	5	2	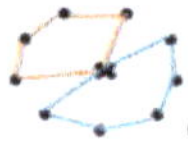 G = {n = 9, N = 2, (5, 4)}	
$\frac{1}{5} < \frac{d}{C} \leq \frac{1}{4}$	4	3	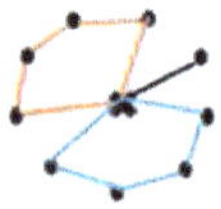 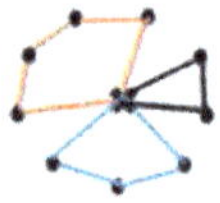 G = {n = 9, N = 3, (4, 4, 1)} G = {n = 9, N = 3, (4, 3, 2)}	111.146 r
$\frac{1}{4} < \frac{d}{C} \leq \frac{1}{3}$	3	3	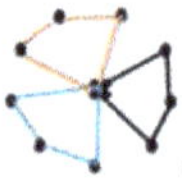 G = {n = 9, N = 3, (3, 3, 3)}	
$\frac{1}{3} < \frac{d}{C} \leq \frac{1}{2}$	2	5	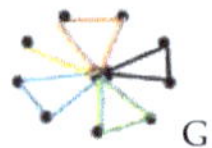 G = {n = 9, N = 5, (2, 2, 2, 2, 1)}	140.097 r
$\frac{1}{2} < \frac{d}{C} \leq 1$	1	9	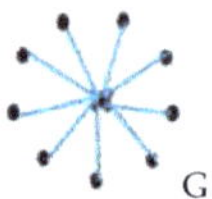 G = {n = 9, N = 9, (1, 1, 1, 1, 1, 1, 1, 1, 1)}	198 r

In the first column, we have considered all possible ratios d/C between the demand d of each vaccination centre and the load capacity C of the drone. In the second column, we indicate the maximum number $k_1(d)$ of vaccination centres that one drone can serve. In the third column, we note optimum number N of drone we should use for each logistics distribution, according to the various ranges of vaccination centres demands. In the fourth column, we represent the exact graphs calculated in the frame of our approach.

In all Tables, we represent the length *L* (*n*, *N*) of the paths travelled by the set of the optimal number of drones necessary for logistics distribution. Its general expression for any n and N is given by the following relation:

$$L(\mathrm{n}, \mathrm{N}) = (\mathrm{n} - \mathrm{N})a_n + 2\mathrm{N}r_n \tag{1}$$

where a_n is the distance between two nearest vaccination centres belonging to the same n-polygon (zone) and r_n is its circumradius. They are given by:

$$a_n = 2(2\mathrm{n} - 7)sin\left(\frac{\pi}{\mathrm{n}}\right)r$$

$$r_n = (2\mathrm{n} - 7)r$$

It is important to notice that this length is constant for any fixed N and therefore it does not depend on the corresponding intervals, although these latter correspond to various graphs.

In order to give an elegant formulation of the results demonstrated in the above Tables, we represent in Figure 2, the variation of optimum number N of drones as function of vaccination centre demands. This is done for different number n of centres. As is observed in these figures, this variation can be described by a function which can be called "ceiling function with unequal steps".

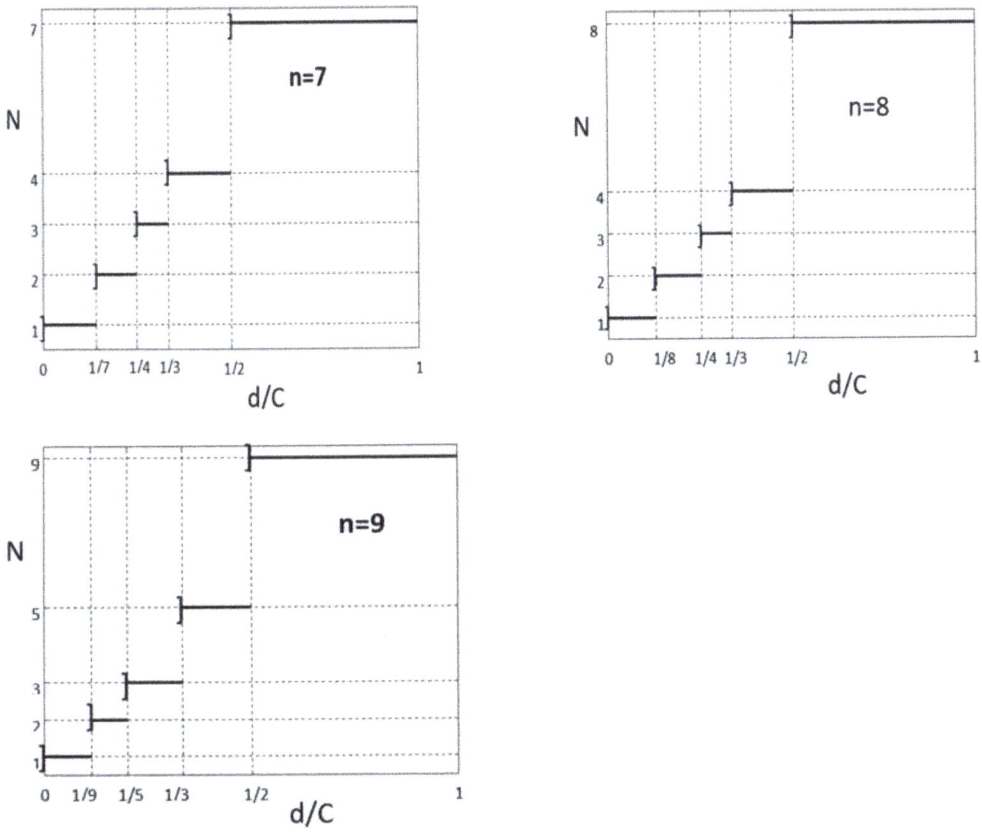

Figure 2. The variation of optimum number N of drones as function of vaccination centre demands, for n = 7, 8, and 9.

The other cases corresponding to n = 5 and 6 are presented in Appendix A.

4.2. Degeneracy of the Domains of Vaccination Centres Demands

In the rest of our investigation, we are interested in the study of the domains (intervals) of d/C where the set of vaccination centre demands, belonging to the same zone, are served by a fixed optimum number N of drones.

It is worthy to notice an interesting behaviour related to the topology of the graphs. It concerns the existence of multiple graphs for a defined range of vaccination centre demands satisfying a well-defined maximum number of centres. For instance, this is observed in the case N = 3 for n = 7 and 9 when d/C belongs to ranges $\left[\frac{1}{4}, \frac{1}{3}\right]$ and $\left[\frac{1}{5}, \frac{1}{4}\right]$, respectively. The corresponding variety of graphs can be called "equivalent graphs" in the sense that they have the same length of paths taken by the N drones but different topologies. Therefore, they use the same energy consumption during logistics distribution. This behaviour can be called the degeneracy of the corresponding domain. In the present paper, we focus our study to two cases, namely: (i) N = 2 and (ii) N = 3.

In Figures 3 and 4, we draw for various zones which contain respectively different centres (n = 12, 13, and 15), the set of possible graphs corresponding to the various domains D of d/C.

(i) For N = 2, we obtain

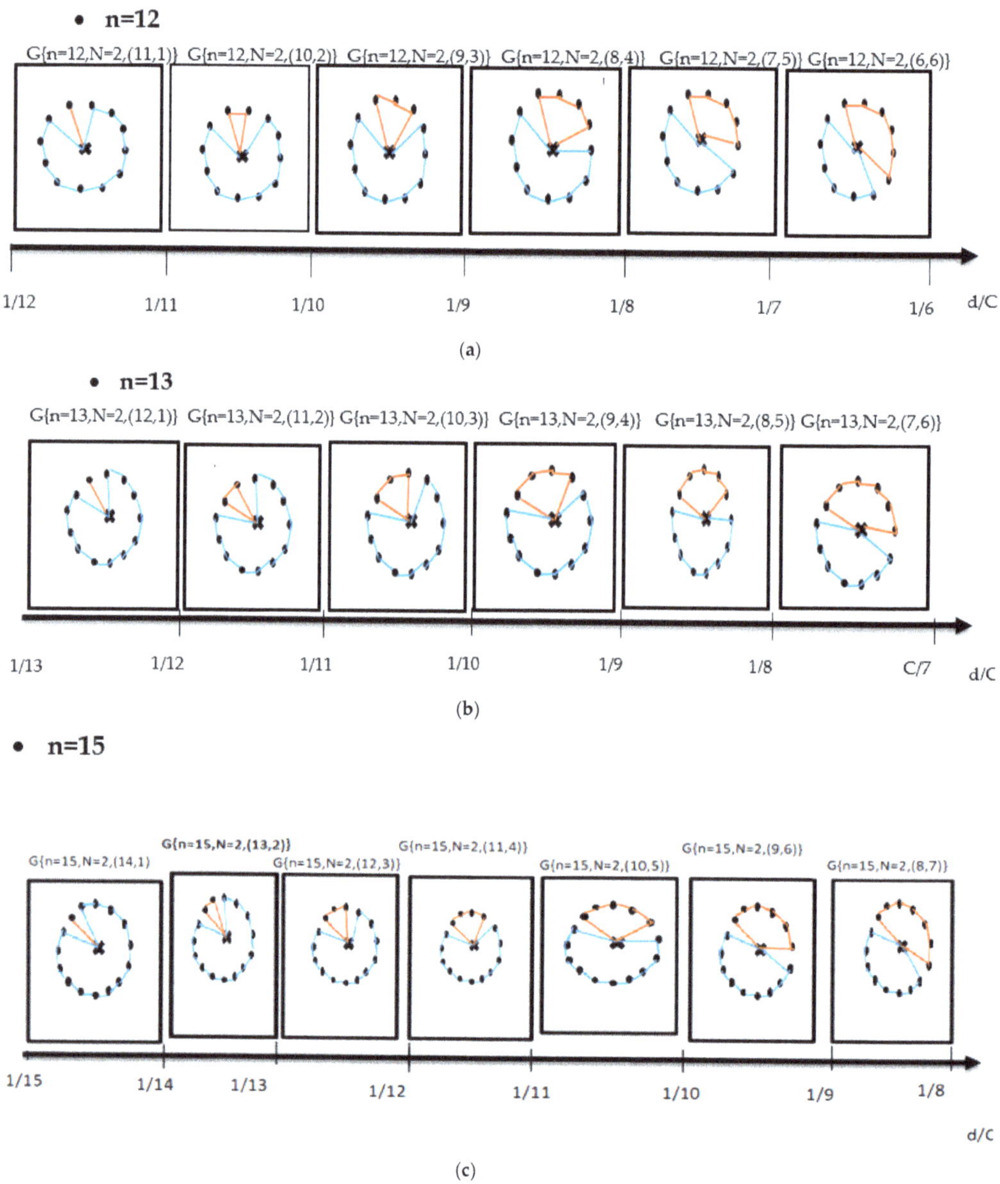

Figure 3. Set of possible graphs corresponding to the various domains of d/C for N = 2, (**a**) n = 12, (**b**) n = 13, and (**c**) n = 15.

As is observed from Figure 3, we note that, in every range of d/c, there is one and only one graph. We note that all graphs corresponding to N = 2 have different topologies which depend on the maximum number of vaccination centres that can be satisfied by one drone.

(ii) For N = 3, we obtain

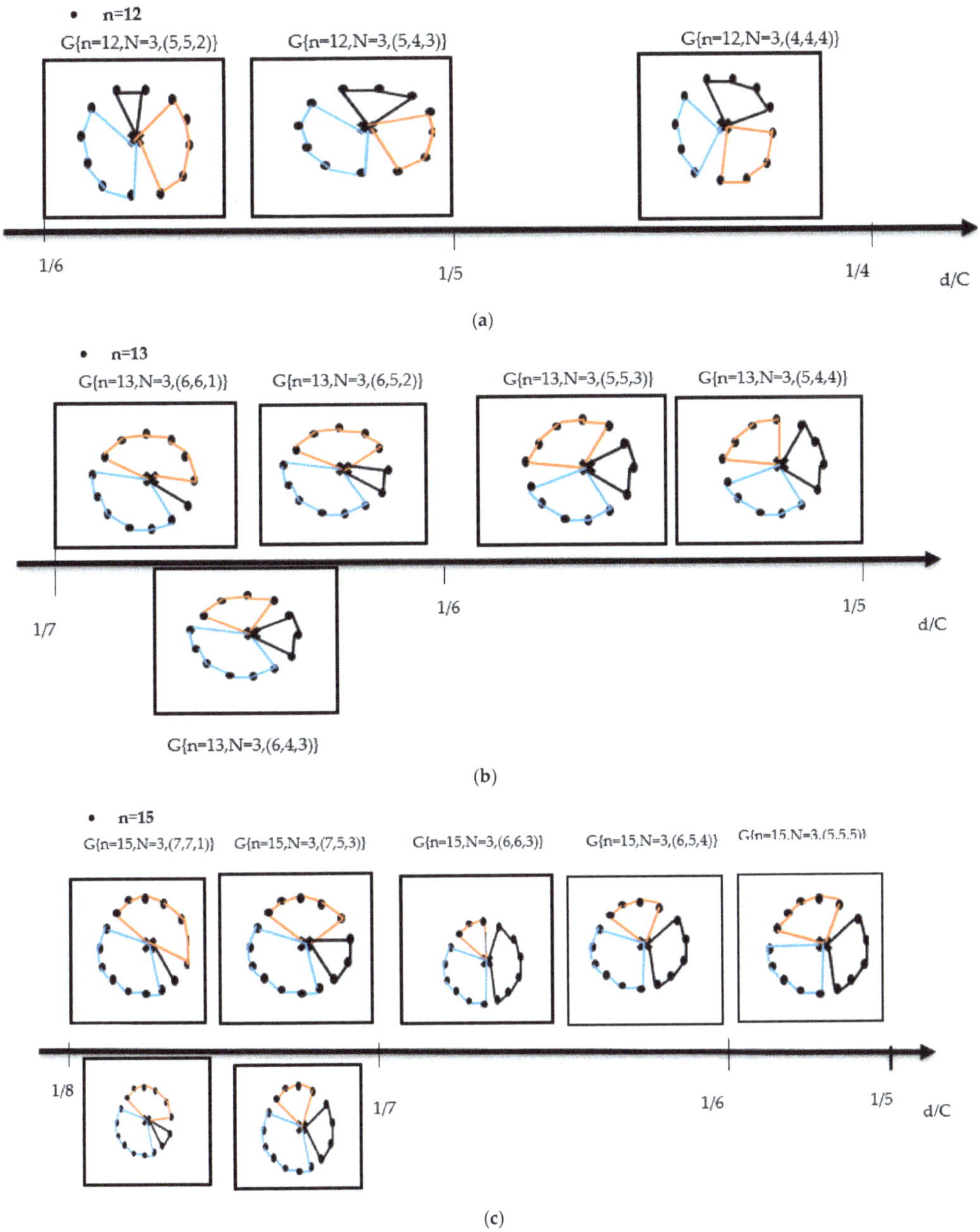

Figure 4. Set of possible graphs corresponding to the various domains of d/C for N = 3, (**a**) n = 12, (**b**) n = 13, and (**c**) n = 15.

In Figure 4, we represent all possible graphs for N = 3, according to each domain of vaccination centre demands. We note the existence of multitude graphs in well-defined domains of d/C. For instance, in the case (n = 15, N = 3), when d/C belongs to $\frac{1}{8} < \frac{d}{C} \leq \frac{1}{7}$, we have 4 equivalent graphs which they have the same global length and therefore the same "global" cost and the same delivery time.

In order to give a precise description to the above interesting behaviour, we suggest a new nomenclature describing this variety of equivalent graphs. To this end, we introduce the following definition: We define the degeneracy of a domain $D(\alpha < \frac{d}{C} \leq \beta)$ by the number of equivalent graphs existing in the specified range $(\alpha < \frac{d}{C} \leq \beta)$. In addition to the degeneracies expressed in Figure 4, we have calculated the degeneracy of domains corresponding to N = 3 for zones containing large numbers of vaccination centres (n = 18, 21, 24, and 27). Below, we give their degrees and corresponding graphs.

Deg(n = 18, N = 3, D($\frac{1}{9} < \frac{d}{C} \leq \frac{1}{8}$)) = 4,	G{n = 18, N = 3, (8, 8, 2)}, G{n = 18, N = 3, (8, 7, 3)},
	G{n = 18, N = 3, (8, 6, 4)},G{n = 18, N = 3, (8, 5, 5)}.
Deg(n = 18, N = 3, D($\frac{1}{8} < \frac{d}{C} \leq \frac{1}{7}$)) = 2,	G{n = 18, N = 3, (7, 7, 4)}, G{n = 18, N = 3, (7, 6, 5)}.
Deg(n = 18, N = 3, D($\frac{1}{7} < \frac{d}{C} \leq \frac{1}{6}$)) = 1,	G{n = 18, N = 3, (6, 6, 6)}.
Deg(n = 21, N = 3, D($\frac{1}{11} < \frac{d}{C} \leq \frac{1}{10}$)) = 5,	G{n = 21, N = 3, (10, 10, 1)}, G{n = 21, N = 3, (10, 9, 2)},
	G{n = 21, N = 3, (10, 8, 3)}, G{n = 21, N = 3, (10, 7, 4)},
	G{n = 21, N = 3, (10, 6, 5)}.
Deg(n = 21, N = 3, D($\frac{1}{10} < \frac{d}{C} \leq \frac{1}{9}$)) = 4,	G{n = 21, N = 3, (9, 9, 3)}, G{n = 21, N = 3, (9, 8, 4)},
	G{n = 21, N = 3, (9, 7, 5)}, G{n = 21, N = 3, (9, 6, 6)}
Deg(n = 21, N = 3, D($\frac{1}{9} < \frac{d}{C} \leq \frac{1}{8}$)) = 2,	G{n = 21, N = 3, (8, 8, 5)}, G{n = 21, N = 3, (8, 7, 6)}.
Deg(n = 21, N = 3, D($\frac{1}{8} < \frac{d}{C} \leq \frac{1}{7}$)) = 1,	G{n = 21, N = 3, (7, 7, 7)}.
Deg(n =24, N = 3, D($\frac{1}{12} < \frac{d}{C} \leq \frac{1}{11}$)) = 5,	G{n = 24, N = 3, (11, 11, 2)}, G{n = 24, N = 3, (11, 10, 3)},
	G{n = 24, N = 3, (11, 9, 4)}, G{n = 24, N = 3, (11, 8, 5)},
	G{n = 24, N = 3, (11, 7, 6)}.
Deg(n = 24, N = 3, D($\frac{1}{11} < \frac{d}{C} \leq \frac{1}{10}$)) = 4,	G{n = 24, N = 3, (10, 10, 4)}, G{n = 24, N = 3, (10, 9, 5)},
	G{n = 24, N = 3, (10, 8, 6)}, G{n = 24, N = 3, (10, 7, 7)}
Deg(n = 24, N = 3, D($\frac{1}{10} < \frac{d}{C} \leq \frac{1}{9}$)) = 2,	G{n = 24, N = 3, (9, 9, 6)}, G{n = 24, N = 3, (9, 8, 7)}.
Deg(n = 24, N = 3, D($\frac{1}{9} < \frac{d}{C} \leq \frac{1}{8}$)) = 1,	G{n = 24, N = 3, (8, 8, 8)}.
Deg(n =27, N = 3, D($\frac{1}{14} < \frac{d}{C} \leq \frac{1}{13}$)) = 7,	G{n = 27, N = 3, (13, 13, 1)}, G{n = 27, N = 3, (13, 12, 2)},
	G{n = 27, N = 3, (13, 11, 3)},G{n = 27, N = 3, (13, 10, 4)},
	G{n = 27, N = 3, (13, 9, 5)}, G{n = 27, N = 3, (13, 8, 6)},
	G{n = 27, N = 3, (13, 7, 7)}.
Deg(n=27, N = 3, D($\frac{1}{13} < \frac{d}{C} \leq \frac{1}{12}$)) = 5,	G{n = 27, N = 3, (12, 12, 3)}, G{n = 27, N = 3, (12, 11, 4)},
	G{n = 27, N = 3, (12, 10, 5)}, G{n = 27, N = 3, (12, 9, 6)},
	G{n = 27, N = 3, (12, 8, 7)}.
Deg(n= 27, N = 3, D($\frac{1}{12} < \frac{d}{C} \leq \frac{1}{11}$)) = 4,	G{n = 27, N = 3, (11, 11, 5)}, G{n = 27, N = 3, (11, 10, 6)},
	G{n = 27, N = 3, (11, 9, 7)}, G{n = 27, N = 3, (11, 8, 8)}.
Deg(n = 27, N = 3, D($\frac{1}{11} < \frac{d}{C} \leq \frac{1}{10}$)) = 2,	G{n = 2, N = 3, (10, 10, 7)}, G{n = 27, N = 3, (10, 9, 8)}.
Deg(n = 27, N = 3, D($\frac{1}{10} < \frac{d}{C} \leq \frac{1}{9}$)) = 1,	G{n = 27, N = 3, (9, 9, 9)}.

5. Drone Routing Problem for Any Number of Vaccination Centres

In this section, we reformulate our model for any number ($n \in \mathbb{N}$) of vaccination centres. The optimum number of drones that can be used to perform the distribution is N = 2 and 3.

Consider a zone and let n be the number of vaccination centres located on the sites (vertices) of the regular n-polygon inscribed in that zone. The drone's platform is situated on the centre of the circumcircle of the polygon.

5.1. General Expressions of Demand Domains and Their Corresponding Graphs

First, let us find for any fixed n, the set of domains D $(\alpha < \frac{d}{C} \leq \beta)$ defined in the previous section. The domains concerned by our generalization are those where the vaccination centres are served by an optimal number of drones equal to 3 (N = 3). To this end, it should be noted that these domains depend on the parity of n.

(a) For odd numbers $n \geq 3$

The possible domains and corresponding graphs are given by:

Domains: D	Equivalent graphs
$D_0(\frac{1}{\frac{n+1}{2}} < \frac{d}{C} \le \frac{1}{\frac{n-1}{2}})$ $k_1(d) = \frac{n-1}{2}$	G{n, N = 3, $(\frac{n-1}{2}, \frac{n-1}{2}, 1)$} G{n, N = 3, $(\frac{n-1}{2}, \frac{n-3}{2}, 2)$} I, with m = $\{\begin{smallmatrix} \frac{n}{4} - \frac{3}{4}, & n \in \{3+4k/k \in IN\} \\ \frac{n}{4} - \frac{5}{4}, & n \in \{5+4k/k \in IN\} \end{smallmatrix}$ G{n, N = 3, $(\frac{n-1}{2}, \frac{n-1}{2} - m, 1+m)$}
$D_1(\frac{1}{\frac{n-1}{2}} < \frac{d}{C} \le \frac{1}{\frac{n-3}{2}})$ $k_1(d) = \frac{n-3}{2}$	G{n, N = 3, $(\frac{n-3}{2}, \frac{n-3}{2}, 3)$} G{n, N = 3, $(\frac{n-3}{2}, \frac{n-5}{2}, 4)$} I, with m = $\{\begin{smallmatrix} \frac{n}{4} - \frac{9}{4}, & n \in \{9+4k\ /k \in IN\} \\ \frac{n}{4} - \frac{11}{4}, & n \in \{11+4k\ /k \in IN\} \end{smallmatrix}$ G{n, N = 3, $(\frac{n-3}{2}, \frac{n-3}{2} - m, 3+m)$}
$D_2(\frac{1}{\frac{n-3}{2}} < \frac{d}{C} \le \frac{1}{\frac{n-5}{2}})$ $k_1(d) = \frac{n-5}{2}$	G{n, N = 3, $(\frac{n-5}{2}, \frac{n-5}{2}, 5)$} G{n, N = 3, $(\frac{n-5}{2}, \frac{n-7}{2}, 6)$} I, with m = $\{\begin{smallmatrix} \frac{n}{4} - \frac{15}{4}, & n \in \{15+4k\ /k \in IN\} \\ \frac{n}{4} - \frac{17}{4}, & n \in \{17+4k\ /k \in IN\} \end{smallmatrix}$ G{n, N =3, $(\frac{n-5}{2}, \frac{n-5}{2} - m, 5+m)$}
$D_3(\frac{1}{\frac{n-5}{2}} < \frac{d}{C} \le \frac{1}{\frac{n-7}{2}})$ $k_1(d) = \frac{n-7}{2}$	G{n, N = 3, $(\frac{n-7}{2}, \frac{n-7}{2}, 7)$} G{n, N = 3, $(\frac{n-7}{2}, \frac{n-9}{2}, 8)$} I, with m = $\{\begin{smallmatrix} \frac{n}{4} - \frac{21}{4}, & n \in \{21+4k\ /k \in IN\} \\ \frac{n}{4} - \frac{23}{4}, & n \in \{23+4k\ /k \in IN\} \end{smallmatrix}$ G{n, N = 3, $(\frac{n-7}{2}, \frac{n-7}{2} - m, 7+m)$}
$D_p(\frac{1}{\frac{n-1}{2}-p+1} < \frac{d}{C} \le \frac{1}{\frac{n-1}{2}-p})$ $k_1(d) = \frac{n-1}{2} - p$	G{n, N = 3, $(\frac{n-1}{2} - p, \frac{n-1}{2} - p, 2p+1)$} G{n, N = 3, $(\frac{n-1}{2} - p, \frac{n-3}{2} - p - 1, 2p+2)$} I, with m = $\{\begin{smallmatrix} \frac{n}{4} - \frac{3(2p+1)}{4}, & n \in \{3+6p+4k\ /k \in IN\} \\ \frac{n}{4} - \frac{3(2p+1)}{4} - \frac{1}{2}, & n \in \{5+6p+4k\ /k \in IN\} \end{smallmatrix}$ G{n, N = 3, $(\frac{n-1}{2} - p, \frac{n-1}{2} - p - m, 2p+1+m)$}

where p is the smallest integer value satisfying the following inequality:

$$3\left(\frac{n-1}{2} - p - 1\right) < \text{n}.$$

It follows that p is given by:

$$p = floor\left(\frac{n-9}{6}\right) + 1 \quad (2)$$

which can be expressed by the following expression:

$$p = \begin{cases} \frac{n-9}{6} - \frac{1}{\pi} arccot\left[cot\left(\frac{n-9}{6}\pi\right)\right] + 1, & \text{n} \ne 12k + 15/k \in IN \\ \frac{n-9}{6} + 1, & n = 12k + 15/k \in IN \end{cases}$$

(b) For even numbers n $\geq$ 6

We note that for n = 2 or 4, there is no domains and equivalent graphs corresponding to N = 3. For even numbers n $\geq$ 6, the possible domains $\overline{D}$ and corresponding graphs are given by:

Domains: $\overline{D}$	Equivalent graphs
$\overline{D}_1(\frac{1}{\frac{n}{2}} < \frac{d}{C} \le \frac{1}{\frac{n}{2}-1})$ $k_1(d) = \frac{n}{2} - 1$	G{n, N = 3, $(\frac{n}{2}-1, \frac{n}{2}-1, 2)$} G{n, N = 3, $(\frac{n}{2}-1, \frac{n}{2}-2, 3)$} I, with m = $\{\begin{matrix} \frac{n}{4}-\frac{3}{2}, n \in \{6+4k\ /k \in IN\} \\ \frac{n}{4}-2, n \in \{8+4k\ /k \in IN\} \end{matrix}$ G{n, N = 3, $(\frac{n}{2}-1, \frac{n}{2}-1-m, 2+m)$}
$\overline{D}_2(\frac{1}{\frac{n}{2}-1} < \frac{d}{C} \le \frac{1}{\frac{n}{2}-2})$ $k_1(d) = \frac{n}{2} - 2$	G{n, N = 3, $(\frac{n}{2}-2, \frac{n}{2}-2, 4)$} G{n, N = 3, $(\frac{n}{2}-2, \frac{n}{2}-3, 5)$} I, with m = $\{\begin{matrix} \frac{n}{4}-3, n \in \{12+4k\ /k \in IN\} \\ \frac{n}{4}-\frac{7}{2}, n \in \{14+4k\ /k \in IN\} \end{matrix}$ G{n, N = 3, $(\frac{n}{2}-2, \frac{n}{2}-2-m, 4+m)$}
$\overline{D}_3(\frac{1}{\frac{n}{2}-2} < \frac{d}{C} \le \frac{1}{\frac{n}{2}-3})$ $k_1(d) = \frac{n}{2} - 3$	G{n, N = 3, $(\frac{n}{2}-3, \frac{n}{2}-3, 6)$} G{n, N = 3, $(\frac{n}{2}-3, \frac{n}{2}-4, 7)$} I, with m = $\{\begin{matrix} \frac{n}{4}-\frac{9}{2}, n \in \{18+4k\ /k \in IN\} \\ \frac{n}{4}-5, n \in \{20+4k\ /k \in IN\} \end{matrix}$ G{n, N = 3, $(\frac{n}{2}-3, \frac{n}{2}-3-m, 6+m)$}
$\overline{D}_q(\frac{1}{\frac{n}{2}-q+1} < \frac{d}{C} \le \frac{1}{\frac{n}{2}-q})$ $k_1(d) = \frac{n}{2} - q$	G{n, N = 3, $(\frac{n}{2}-q, \frac{n}{2}-q, 2q)$} G{n, N = 3, $(\frac{n}{2}-q, \frac{n}{2}-q-1, 2q+1)$} I, with m = $\{\begin{matrix} \frac{n}{4}-\frac{3q}{2}, n \in \{6q+4k\ /k \in IN\} \\ \frac{n}{4}-\frac{(3q+1)}{2}, n \in \{6q+2+4k\ /k \in IN\} \end{matrix}$ G{n, N = 3, $(\frac{n}{2}-q, \frac{n}{2}-q-m, 2q+m)$}

where q is the smallest integer value satisfying the following inequality:

$$3\left(\frac{n}{2} - q - 1\right) < n$$

It follows that q is given by:

$$q = floor\left(\frac{n}{6}\right) \tag{3}$$

which can be written in the following expression:

$$q = \begin{Bmatrix} \frac{n}{6} - \frac{1}{\pi}arccot\left[cot\left(\frac{n\pi}{6}\right)\right], & n \neq 12k + 6/k \in IN \\ \frac{n}{6}, & n = 12k + 6/k \in IN \end{Bmatrix}$$

We note that for any odd (or even) n, each domain D_i ($\overline{D}_i$) corresponds to certain number of equivalent graphs. This later represents the degeneracy of the domain D_i ($\overline{D}_i$).

5.2. General Expressions of the Domain Degeneracy

The detailed analysis of the domains and their corresponding graphs presented in Section 5.1: (a) and (b) of this section, allow us to establish general expressions of their degeneracy for both odd and even numbers n of vaccination centres. We have indicated that the defined degeneracy deg(n, N, D_ℓ (or $\overline{D}_i$)) depends on four sets covering all possible integer values. Thus,

(i) For $n \in \{3 + 4k/\ k \in IN\}$

$$\deg(\mathrm{n},\ \mathrm{N} = 3,\ \mathrm{D}_\ell) = \begin{Bmatrix} \frac{n}{4} - \frac{3}{4}(2\ell + 1) + 1, & if\ \ell\ is\ even \\ \frac{n}{4} - \frac{3}{4}(2\ell + 1) + \frac{1}{2}, & if\ \ell\ is\ odd \end{Bmatrix} \tag{4}$$

D_ℓ denotes the domain: $\frac{1}{\frac{n+1}{2}-\ell} < \frac{d}{C} \le \frac{1}{\frac{n-1}{2}-\ell}$ where

$$\ell \in \left\{0, 1,\ 2,\ 3, \ldots, floor\left(\frac{n-9}{6}\right) + 1\right\} \tag{5}$$

(ii) For $n \in \{5 + 4k/\ k \in IN\}$

$$\deg(\mathrm{n},\ \mathrm{N} = 3,\ \mathrm{D}_\ell) = \begin{Bmatrix} \frac{n}{4} - \frac{3}{4}(2\ell + 1) + 1, & if\ \ell\ is\ odd \\ \frac{n}{4} - \frac{3}{4}(2\ell + 1) + \frac{1}{2}, & if\ \ell\ is\ even \end{Bmatrix} \tag{6}$$

D_ℓ denotes the domain: $\frac{1}{\frac{n+1}{2}-\ell} < \frac{d}{C} \leq \frac{1}{\frac{n-1}{2}-\ell}$ where $\ell \in \{0, 1, 2, 3, \ldots, floor(\frac{n-9}{6}) + 1\}$.

In Appendix B, we represent the variation of domain degeneracy as a function of vaccination centre demands «site needs» for selected odd values of n. Furthermore, we plot in Figure 5, a generalization making possible to find the variation of such degeneracy for any odd number of vaccination centres.

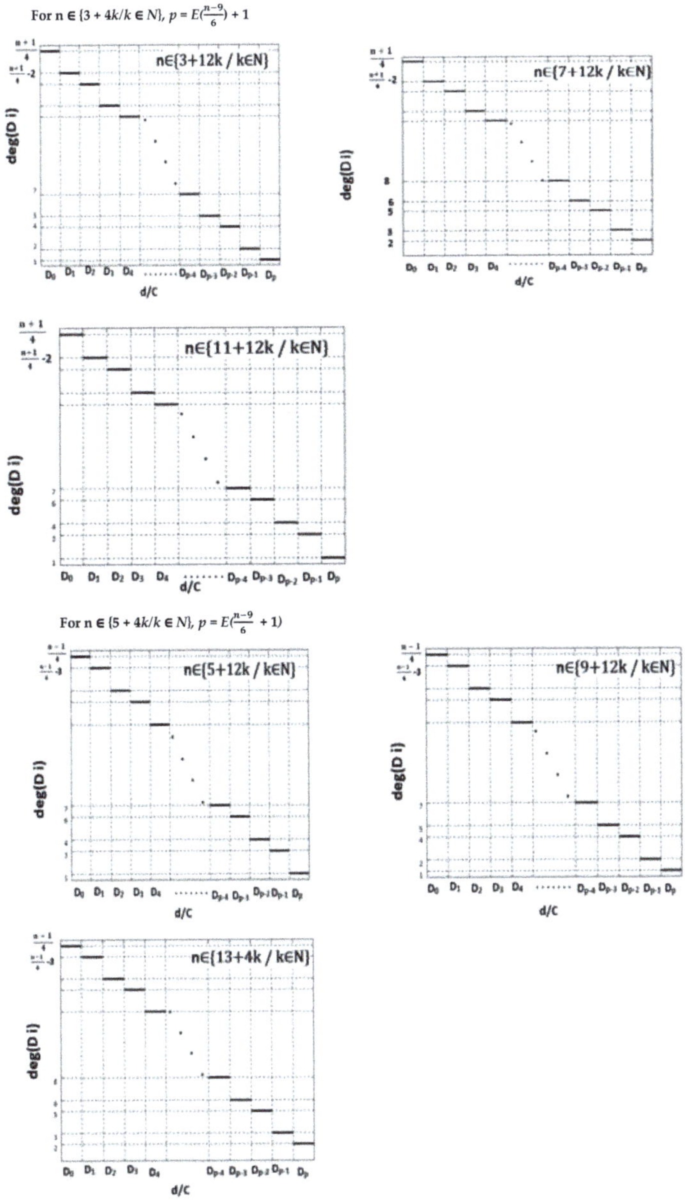

Figure 5. A generalization making possible to find the variation of domain degeneracy for any odd number of vaccination centres.

(i) For n $\in \{6 + 4k/\ k \in IN\}$

$$\deg(\mathrm{n}, \mathrm{N} = 3,\ \overline{D}_\ell) = \left\{ \begin{array}{l} \frac{n}{4} - \frac{3\ell}{2} + 1,\ if\ \ell\ is\ odd \\ \frac{n}{4} - \frac{(3\ell+1)}{2} + 1,\ if\ \ell\ is\ even \end{array} \right\} \quad (7)$$

$\overline{D}_\ell$ denotes the domain: $\frac{1}{\frac{n}{2}-\ell+1} < \frac{d}{C} \le \frac{1}{\frac{n}{2}-\ell}$ where

$$\ell \in \left\{1,\ 2,\ 3, \ldots, floor\left(\frac{n}{6}\right)\right\} \quad (8)$$

(ii) For n $\in \{8 + 4k/\ k \in IN\}$

$$\deg(\mathrm{n}, \mathrm{N} = 3,\ \overline{D}_\ell) = \left\{ \begin{array}{l} \frac{n}{4} - \frac{3\ell}{2} + 1,\ if\ \ell\ is\ even \\ \frac{n}{4} - \frac{(3\ell+1)}{2} + 1,\ if\ \ell\ is\ odd \end{array} \right\} \quad (9)$$

$\overline{D}_\ell$ denotes the domain: $\frac{1}{\frac{n}{2}-\ell+1} < \frac{d}{C} \le \frac{1}{\frac{n}{2}-\ell}$ where $\ell \in \left\{1,\ 2,\ 3, \ldots, floor\left(\frac{n}{6}\right)\right\}$.

In Appendix C, we represent the variation of domain degeneracy as a function of the vaccination centres demands for selected even values of n. Furthermore, we plot in Figure 6, a generalization making possible to find the variation of such degeneracy for any even number of vaccination centres.

For n ∈ {6 + 4k/k ∈ N}, $q = E(\frac{n}{6})$

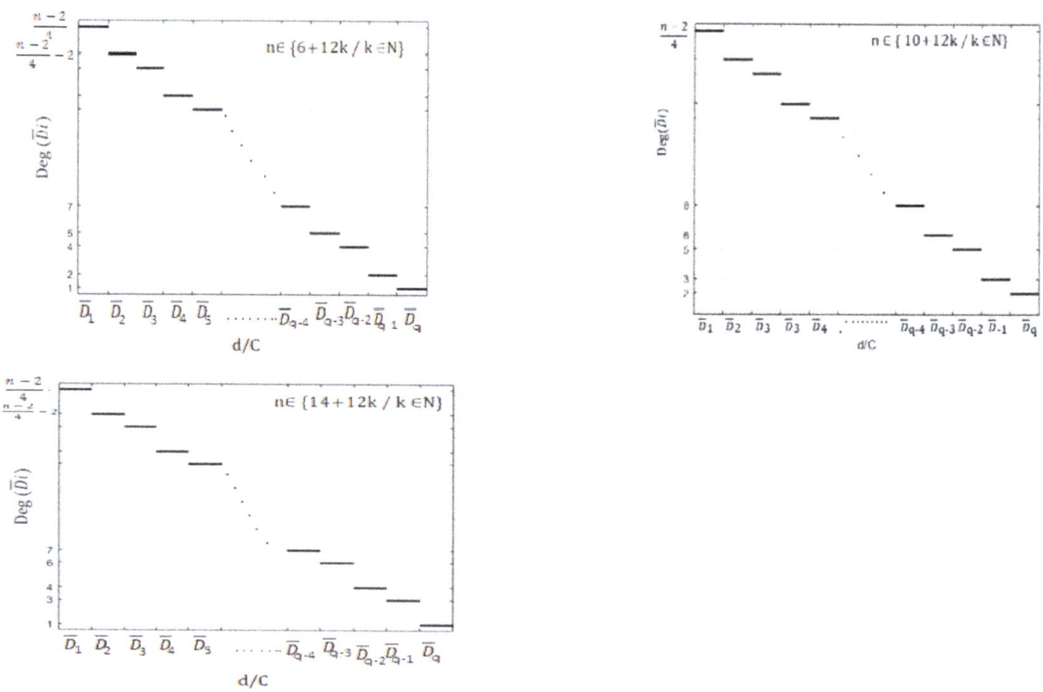

Figure 6. *Cont.*

For n ∈ {8 + 4*k*/*k* ∈ *N*}, *P* = *E*($\frac{n}{6}$)

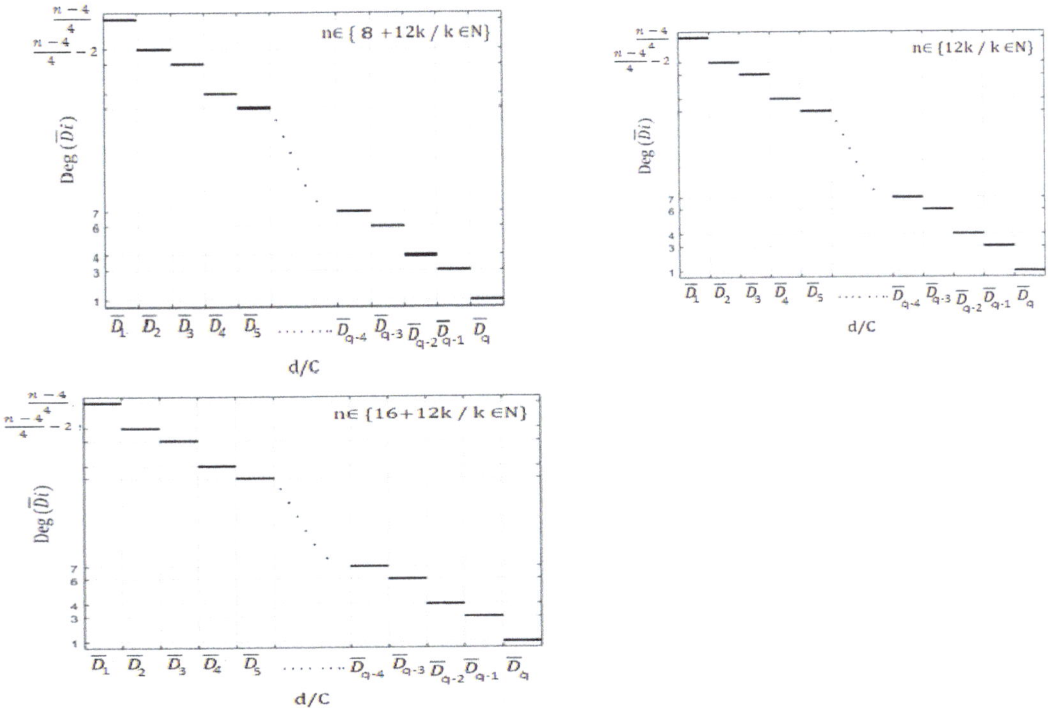

Figure 6. A generalization making possible to find the variation of domain degeneracy for any even number of vaccination centres.

As is observed in Appendices B and C and in Figures 5 and 6, these variations are represented by what we can call "descending ceiling functions".

In Figure 8, we reported the variation of the degrees of degeneracy deg(D_0) and deg($\overline{D}_1$). They correspond to the most degenerate domains for odd and even numbers of vaccination centres.

On the other hand, in Figure 7, we plot the variation of the degrees of degeneracy deg(D_p) and deg($\overline{D}_q$) corresponding to the least degenerate domains for odd n and even n, respectively. They can be expressed by the following functions:

$$\deg(D_p) = 1 \text{or} \deg(\overline{D}_q) = 1, \text{ if n} \in \{3k/k \in IN^*\} \cup \{5 + 3k/k \in IN\},$$

$$\deg(D_p) = 2 \text{or} \deg(\overline{D}_q) = 2, \text{ if n } \in \{7 + 3k/k \in IN\},$$

where $p = floor\left(\frac{n-9}{6}\right) + 1$, and $q = floor\left(\frac{n}{6}\right)$.

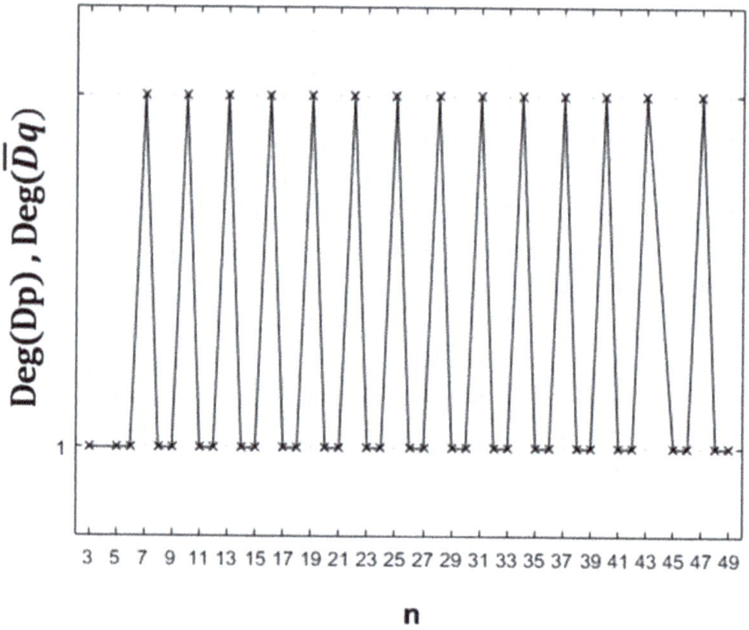

Figure 7. Variation of the degrees of degeneracy deg(D_p) and deg($\overline{D}_q$) corresponding to the least degenerate domains.

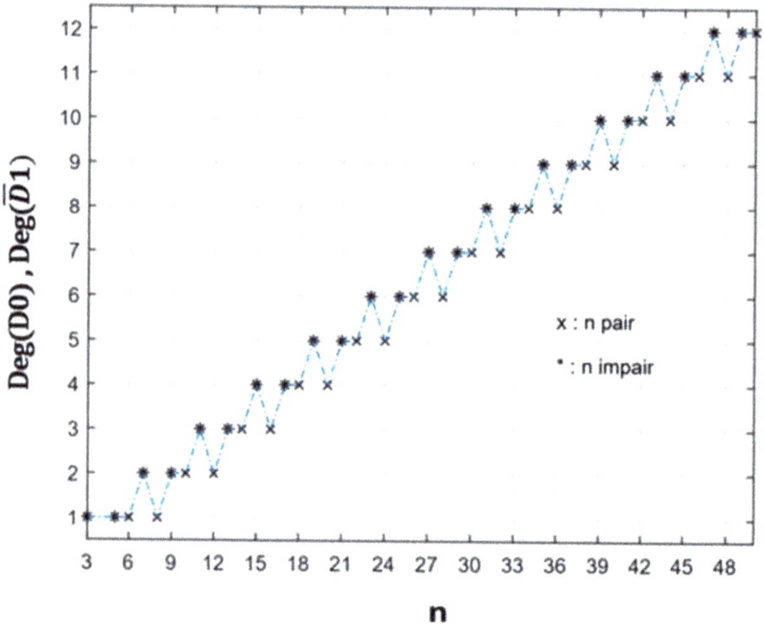

Figure 8. Variation of degree of degeneracy deg(D_0) and deg($\overline{D}_1$) with n.

5.3. General Expressions of the Number of Graphs (Different Paths) Using an Optimum Number N of Drones for Logistics Distribution

Let us first note that for the trivially case, namely $\frac{d}{C} \leq \frac{1}{n}$, delivery can be realized only by one drone. In this case, it is obvious that the drone has only one path to follow to accomplish the task, and therefore there exist only one graph which can be noted G{n, N = 1,(n)}, according to the adopted notation.

(a) General expressions of the number of graphs (paths) when the optimal number of drones is 2 (N = 2)

In the case N = 2 as optimum number of drones satisfying the maximum vaccination centres according to their demands, the corresponding domains and graphs are defined by the following intervals:

(i) For odd n

Domain	Corresponding graph
$D_1(\frac{1}{n} < \frac{d}{C} \leq \frac{1}{n-1})$	G{n, N = 2, (n − 1,1)}
$D_2(\frac{1}{n-1} < \frac{d}{C} \leq \frac{1}{n-2})$	G{n, N = 2, (n − 2,2)}
$D_3(\frac{1}{n-2} < \frac{d}{C} \leq \frac{1}{n-3})$	G{n, N = 2, (n − 3,3)}
$D_{\frac{n-1}{2}}(\frac{1}{\frac{n+3}{2}} < \frac{d}{C} \leq \frac{1}{\frac{n+1}{2}})$	G{n, N = 2, $(\frac{n+1}{2}, \frac{n-1}{2})$}

(ii) For even n

Domain	Corresponding graph
$\overline{D}_1(\frac{1}{n} < \frac{d}{C} \leq \frac{1}{n-1})$	G{n, N = 2, (n − 1,1)}
$\overline{D}_2(\frac{1}{n-1} < \frac{d}{C} \leq \frac{1}{n-2})$	G{n, N = 2, (n − 2,2)}
$\overline{D}_3(\frac{1}{n-2} < \frac{d}{C} \leq \frac{1}{n-3})$	G{n, N = 2, (n − 3,3)}
$\overline{D}_{\frac{n}{2}}(\frac{1}{\frac{n}{2}+1)} < \frac{d}{C} \leq \frac{1}{\frac{n}{2}})$	G{n, N = 2, $(\frac{n}{2}, \frac{n}{2})$}

For $N = 2$, each domain D_i or $\overline{D}_i$ corresponds to one and only one graph. This means that the domains are not degenerated for any number n of vaccination centres and for any demands using necessary two drones. We have to note that, in this case and for a given zone with n centres, all graphs constructed for any domain have the same length $L(\text{n}, \text{N} = 2)$. This later is given by:

$$L(\text{n}, \text{N} = 2) = (2\text{n} - 7)\left[4 + 2(\text{n} - 2)\sin\left(\frac{\pi}{\text{n}}\right)\right]r. \tag{10}$$

Therefore, it does not depend on the topology of the graph and the vaccination centre demands when this later belongs to the ranges:

(i) $\left[\frac{C}{n}, \frac{C}{\frac{n+1}{2}}\right]$ for odd n

(ii) $\left[\frac{C}{n}, \frac{C}{\frac{n}{2}}\right]$ for even n.

From the above ranges, we deduce that the total number *NG* (*n, N* = 2) of graphs, which correspond to N = 2 and for any number n of vaccination centres belonging to the same zone, is given by:

$$NG(\text{n}, \text{ N} = 2) = \frac{n-1}{2}, \text{for odd n} \tag{11a}$$

$$NG(\text{n}, \text{ N} = 2) = \frac{n}{2}, \text{for even n} \tag{11b}$$

which is represented in Figure 9.

(b) General expressions of the number of graphs (paths) when the optimal number of drones is 3 (N = 3)

Let us first note that when we have to use three UAVs to deliver vaccines to vaccination centres belonging to same zone, all graphs constructed for any domain D_i or $\overline{D}_i$ have the same length which is given by:

$$L(\text{n}, \text{N} = 3) = (2\text{n} - 7)\left[6 + 2(\text{n} - 3)\sin\left(\frac{\pi}{\text{n}}\right)\right]r. \tag{11c}$$

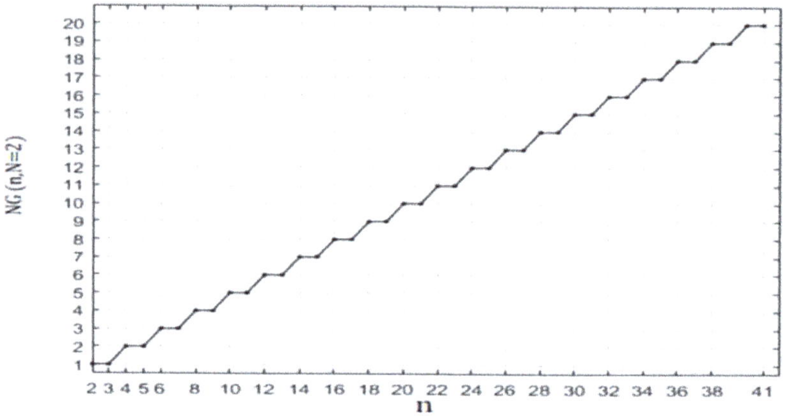

Figure 9. Dependence of the number of graphs *NG* (n, N = 2) as a function of n.

Thus, it does not depend on the structure of the graph. As demonstrated in Section 4.1, in order to satisfy the vaccination centres with N = 3 as optimum number of drones and according to our assumptions, the centre demands d have to belong to the following ranges:

(i) $\left[\frac{C}{\frac{n+1}{2}}, \frac{C}{\frac{n-1}{2}-p}\right]$, for odd n$\geq$ 3, with $p = floor\left(\frac{n-9}{6}\right)$+1

(ii) $\left[\frac{C}{\frac{n}{2}}, \frac{C}{\frac{n}{2}-q}\right]$, for even n$\geq$ 6, with $q = floor\left(\frac{n}{6}\right)$.

So, the total number *NG* (n, N = 3) of graphs corresponding to N = 3 depends on the parity of the number n of vaccination centres. Thus,

- For odd n

$$NG(\text{n},\ \text{N}=3) = \sum_{\ell=0}^{p} \deg(\text{n},\ \text{N}=3,\ D_\ell)$$

Using expressions Equations (4)–(6), we have demonstrated that *NG*(n, N = *3)* also depends on the parity of *p*. Its expression is given by:

- $\left\{\begin{matrix} \text{n} \in \{2k+1/\ k \in IN\} \\ floor\left(\frac{n-9}{6}\right)+1,\ \text{odd} \end{matrix}\right\}$,

$$NG(\text{n},\ \text{N}=3) = \frac{1}{4}\left[floor\left(\frac{n-9}{6}\right)+2\right]\left[n-3floor\left(\frac{n-9}{6}\right)-3\right]. \quad (12)$$

- $\left\{\begin{matrix} n \in \{3+4k/\ k \in IN\} \\ floor\left(\frac{n-9}{6}\right)+1,\ \text{even} \end{matrix}\right\}$,

$$NG(\text{n},\ \text{N}=3) = \left[floor\left(\frac{n-9}{6}\right)+2\right]\left[\frac{n}{4}+1\right]-\frac{1}{4}\left[floor\left(\frac{n-9}{6}\right)+1\right]\left[3floor\left(\frac{n-9}{6}\right)+10\right]-\frac{3}{4}. \quad (13)$$

- $\left\{\begin{matrix} \text{n} \in \{5+4k/\ k \in IN\} \\ floor\left(\frac{n-9}{6}\right)+1,\ \text{even} \end{matrix}\right\}$,

$$NG(\text{n},\ \text{N}=3) = \frac{1}{4}\left[floor\left(\frac{n-9}{6}\right)+2\right]\left[n-3floor\left(\frac{n-9}{6}\right)-3\right]-\frac{1}{4}. \quad (14)$$

In Figure 10, we represent the evolution of the number of graphs *NG*(n, N = 3) in zones containing odd numbers of vaccination centres.

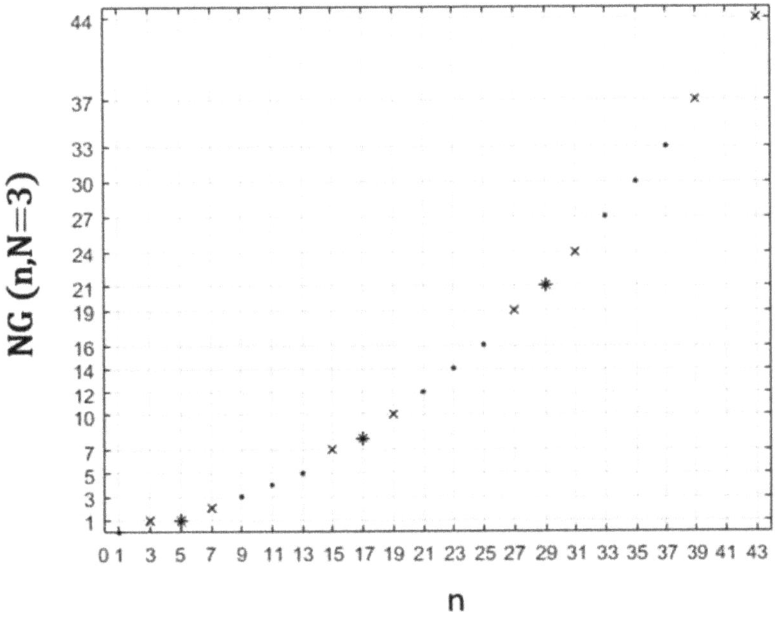

Figure 10. Dependence of the number of graphs NG(n, N = 3) as a function of odd n. •: (n $\in \{2k+1/\ k \in IN\}$, odd p); x: (n $\in \{3+4k/\ k \in IN\}$, even p); *: (n$\in$ $\{5+4k/k \in IN\}$, even p).

- For even n

$$NG(\mathrm{n},\ \mathrm{N}=3) = \sum_{\ell=1}^{q} \deg(\mathrm{n},\ \mathrm{N}=3,\ \overline{D}_\ell)$$

Using Equations (7)–(9), we have demonstrated that NG(n, N = 3) also depends on the parity of q. Its expression is given by:

(iii) $\left\{ \begin{array}{c} \mathrm{n} \in \{2k/\ k \in IN\} \\ floor\left(\frac{n}{6}\right) \text{ even} \end{array} \right\}$,

$$NG(\mathrm{n},\ \mathrm{N}=3) = \frac{n}{4}\left[floor\left(\frac{n}{6}\right)\right] - \frac{1}{4}floor\left(\frac{n}{6}\right)\left[3floor\left(\frac{n}{6}\right)+4\right] + floor\left(\frac{n}{6}\right) \quad (15)$$

(iv) $\left\{ \begin{array}{c} \mathrm{n} \in \{6+4k/\ k \in IN\} \\ floor\left(\frac{n}{6}\right), \text{ odd} \end{array} \right\}$,

$$NG(\mathrm{n},\ \mathrm{N}=3) = \frac{n}{4}\left[floor\left(\frac{n}{6}\right)\right] - \frac{1}{4}\left[floor\left(\frac{n}{6}\right)-1\right]\left[3floor\left(\frac{n}{6}\right)+1\right] - \frac{1}{2}floor\left(\frac{n}{6}\right) \quad (16)$$

(v) $\left\{ \begin{array}{c} \mathrm{n} \in \{8+4k/\ k \in IN\} \\ floor\left(\frac{n}{6}\right), \text{ odd} \end{array} \right\}$,

$$NG(\mathrm{n},\ \mathrm{N}=3) = \frac{n}{4}\left[floor\left(\frac{n}{6}\right)\right] - \frac{1}{4}\left[3floor\left(\frac{n}{6}\right)+1\right]\left[floor\left(\frac{n}{6}\right)+1\right] + floor\left(\frac{n}{6}\right) \quad (17)$$

In Figure 11, we plot the variation of the number of graphs NG(n, N = 3) in zones containing even numbers of vaccination centres.

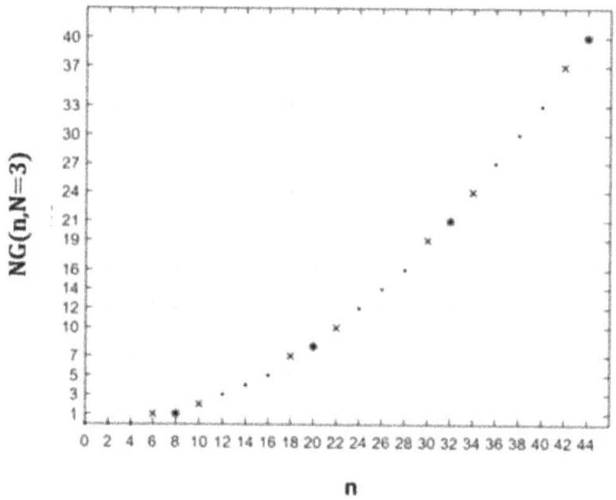

Figure 11. Dependence of the number of graphs NG(n, N = 3) as a function of even n. •: (n ∈ $\{2k/\ k \in IN\}$, even q); x: (n ∈ $\{6+4k/\ k \in IN\}$, odd q); *: (n ∈ $\{8+4k/k \in IN\}$, odd q).

6. Conclusions

Over the last years, the use of drones is leading to new working models in a variety of logistic scenarios. This happens in both developed and developing countries. Currently, fascinating pilot and implementation projects, especially in Africa and Asia, reveal their true potential. By some predictions, the commercial drone market will triple by 2023.In healthcare section, the potential for drone use is vast, and hopefully drones are able to fill some niches where our performance needs improvement. Drones may significantly increase access to healthcare for individuals and large populations, particularly those who do not benefit from appropriate care due to remoteness and lack of infrastructure or funds. In this paper, we have proposed an exact analytical approach and operational strategy to the logistics of any pandemic vaccination effort. Using Unmanned Aerials vehicles (drones), our approach developed a procedure which can be used to deliver pandemic vaccines to densely populated cities or sparsely populate rural areas, whatever the number of population living there. Our strategy consists of dividing the concerned territorial area into zones in the form of circular bands. Each zone is divided into several isometric districts where each of them contains a vaccination centre. We have been interested in the route planning problem of the drones during the distribution. This latter concern the vaccines delivery from central depot to any number of vaccination centres. In the case of fixed and optimal number of the used drones, we have determined all equivalent and optimal flight path plans (graphs). This depends on the domain D of vaccination centre demand d. The existence of equivalent graphs, corresponding to a well-known domain d, incites us to define what we called "degeneracy of the domain Dd". The equivalent graphs (paths) have de same length, the same global cost and the same delivery time. It is worthy to note that, the existence of such degeneracy gives us the possibility to choose the most appropriate paths according to the emergency states of the vaccination centres. Then, using the notion, of degeneracy of the domain D for all domains, we have calculated the total number of graphs (paths) corresponding to the fixed and optimal number of the used drones. In our present investigation all relations has been expressed for any number of vaccination centres.

Author Contributions: Conceptualization, A.B, O.M., H.B. and N.B.; methodology, A.B., H.B. and N.B; investigation, A.B and H.B.; writing—original draft preparation, and co-wrote the manuscript, A.B., H.B. and N.B.; revised the manuscript and approved the final version, A.B, O.M., H.B. and N.B.; writing—review and editing, A.B. and N.B. All authors have read and agreed to the published version of the manuscript.

Funding: This research received no external funding.

Institutional Review Board Statement: Not applicable.

Informed Consent Statement: Not applicable.

Data Availability Statement: Not applicable.

Conflicts of Interest: The authors declare no conflict of interest.

Appendix A

Table A1. Domains of d, corresponding graphs and lengths L (n, N) of the paths travelled by the set of optimum number of drones necessary for the logistics distribution, when zone contains n = 5, and 6 vaccination centres, respectively.

		n = 5		
d/C	$k_1(d)$	N	Graphs	$L(n,N)$
$\frac{d}{C} \le \frac{1}{5}$	5	1	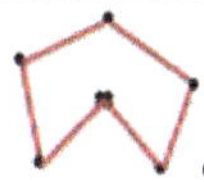 G = {n = 5, N = 1, (5)}	20.106 r
$\frac{1}{5} < \frac{d}{C} \le \frac{1}{4}$	4	2	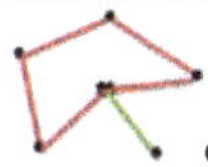 G = {n = 5, N = 2, (4, 1)}	22.580 r
$\frac{1}{4} < \frac{d}{C} \le \frac{1}{3}$	3	2	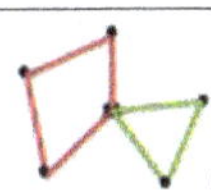 G = {n = 5, N = 2, (3, 2)}	
$\frac{1}{3} < \frac{d}{C} \le \frac{1}{2}$	2	3	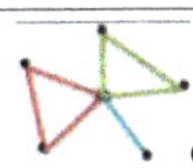 G={n = 5, N = 3, (2, 2, 1)}	25.053 r
$\frac{1}{2} < \frac{d}{C} \le 1$	1	5	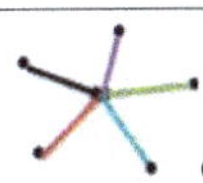 G = {n = 5, N = 5, (1, 1, 1, 1, 1)}	30 r
		n = 6		
d/C	$k_1(d)$	N	Graphs	$L(n,N)$
$\frac{d}{C} \le \frac{1}{6}$	6	1	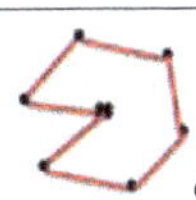 G = {n = 6, N = 1,(6)}	35 r
$\frac{1}{6} < \frac{d}{C} \le \frac{1}{5}$	5	2	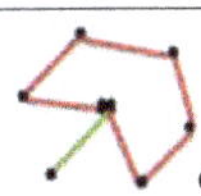 G = {n = 6,N = 2, (5, 1)}	40 r
$\frac{1}{5} < \frac{d}{C} \le \frac{1}{4}$	4	2	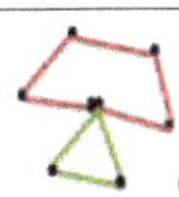 G = {n = 6, N = 2, (4, 2)}	
$\frac{1}{4} < \frac{d}{C} \le \frac{1}{3}$	3	2	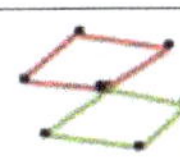 G = {n = 6, N = 2, (3, 3)}	
$\frac{1}{3} < \frac{d}{C} \le \frac{1}{2}$	2	3	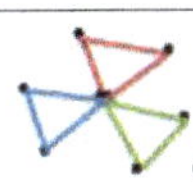 G = {n = 6, N = 3, (2, 2, 2)}	45 r
$\frac{1}{2} < \frac{d}{C} \le 1$	1	6	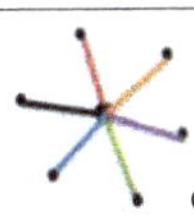 G = {n = 6, N = 6, (1, 1, 1, 1, 1, 1)}	60 r

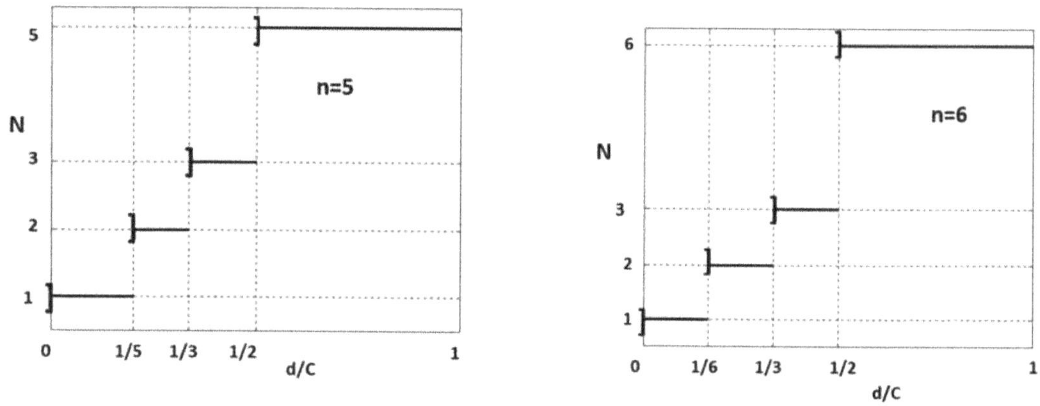

Figure A1. The variation of optimum number N of drones as function of vaccination centre demands, for n = 5, and 6.

Appendix B

$$n \in \{3 + 4k/k \in N\},\ p = E(\frac{n-9}{6}) + 1$$

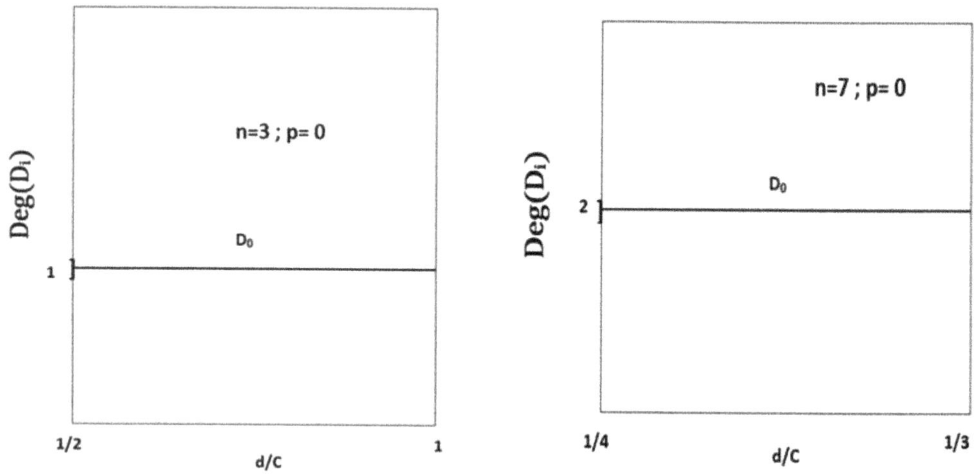

Figure A2. *Cont.*

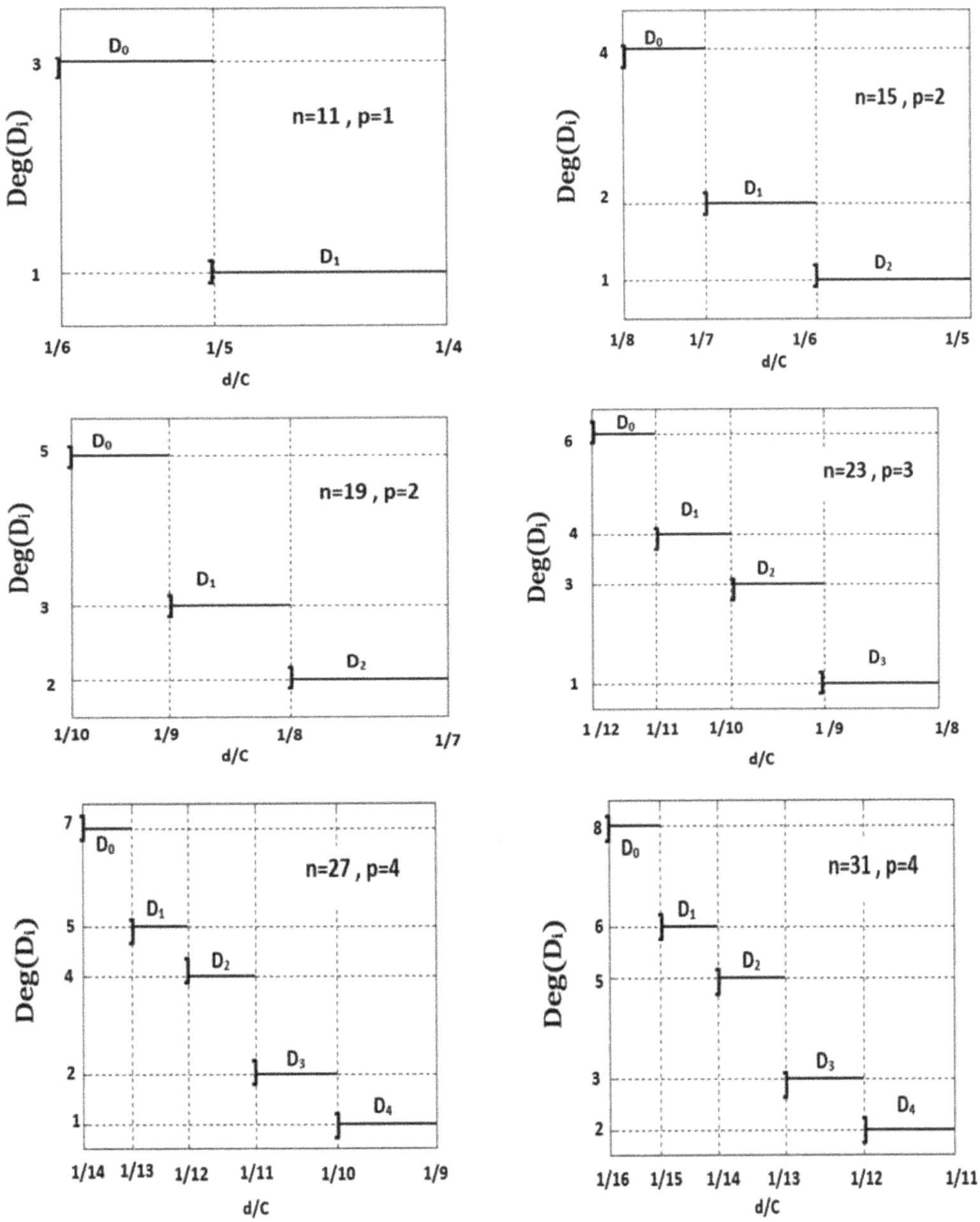

Figure A2. *Cont.*

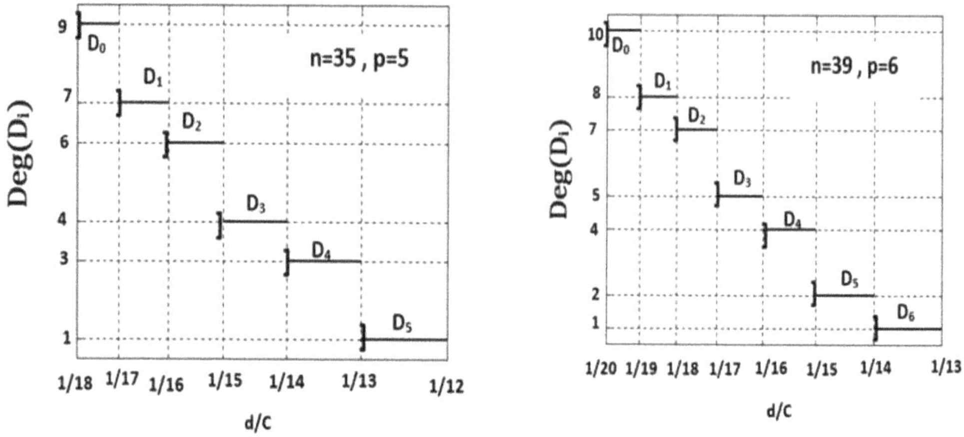

n ∈ {5 + 4k/k ∈ N}, $p = E(\frac{n-9}{6}) + 1$

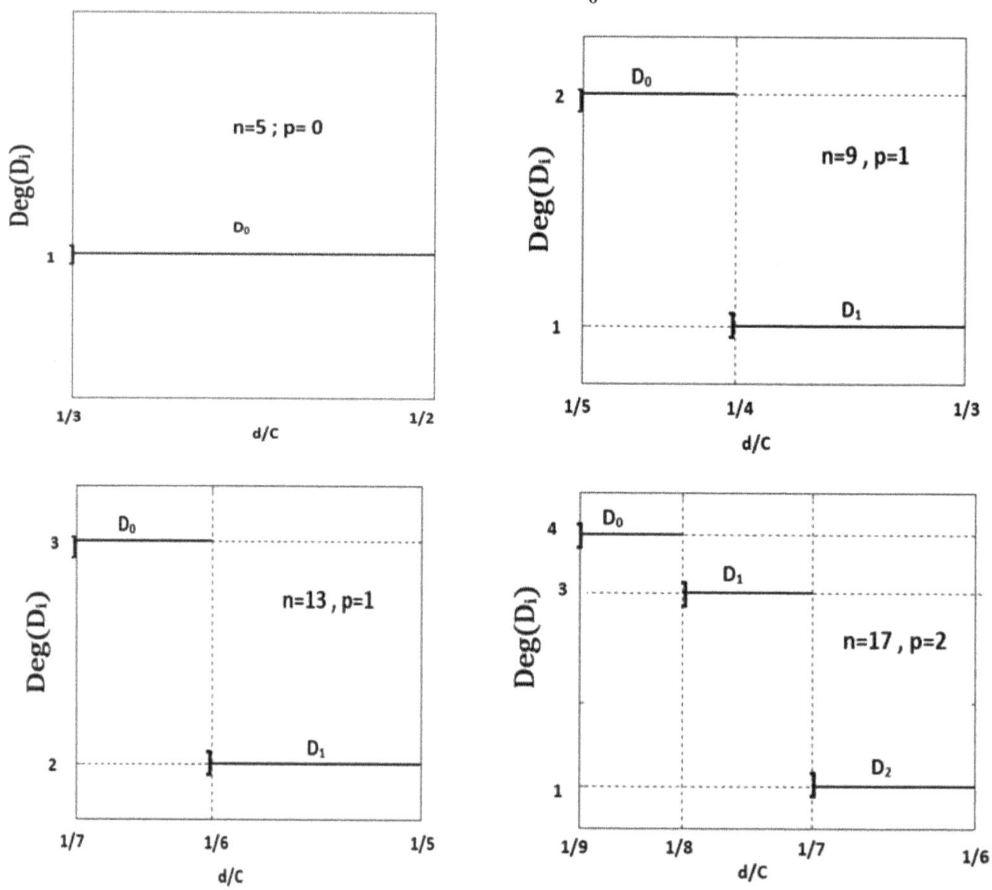

Figure A2. *Cont.*

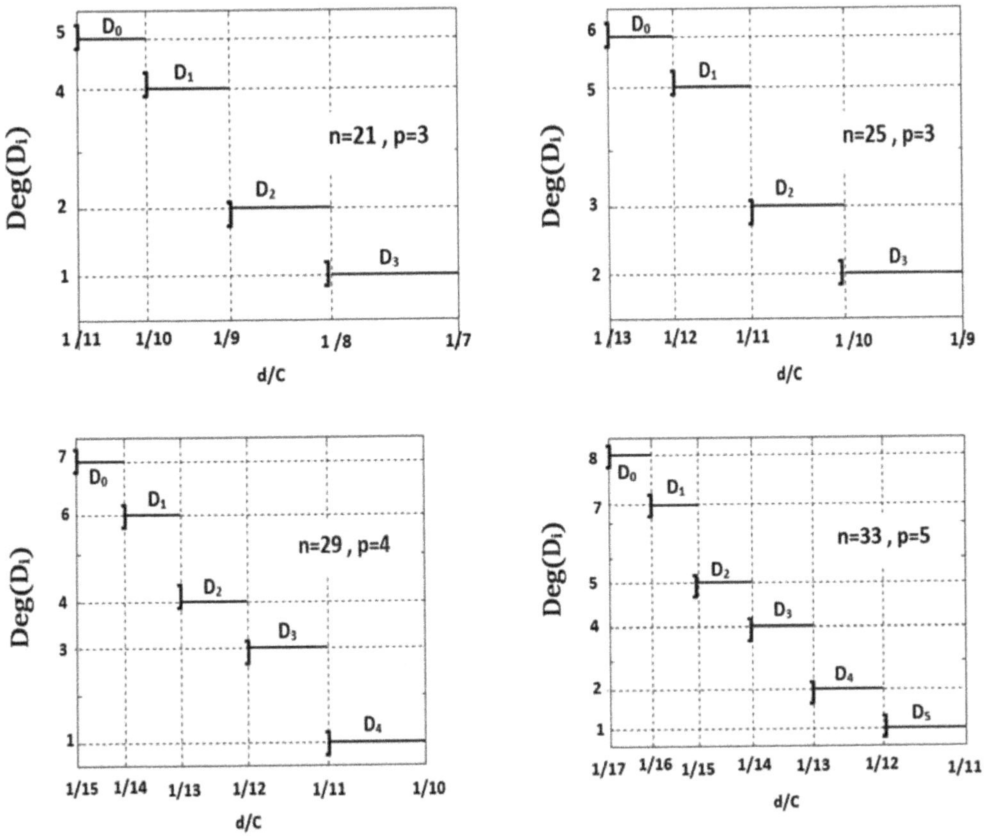

Figure A2. The variation of domain degeneracy as a function of vaccination centre demands «site needs» for selected odd values of n.

Appendix C

For n fixe ∈ {6+4k/k∈N}, q = E(n/6)

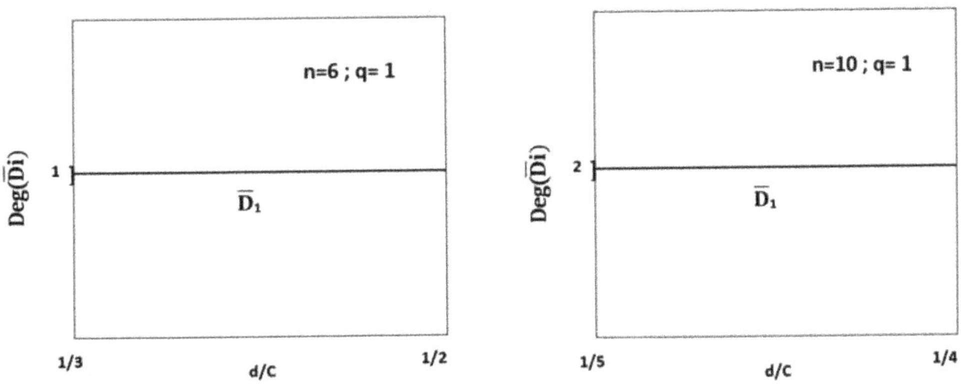

Figure A3. *Cont.*

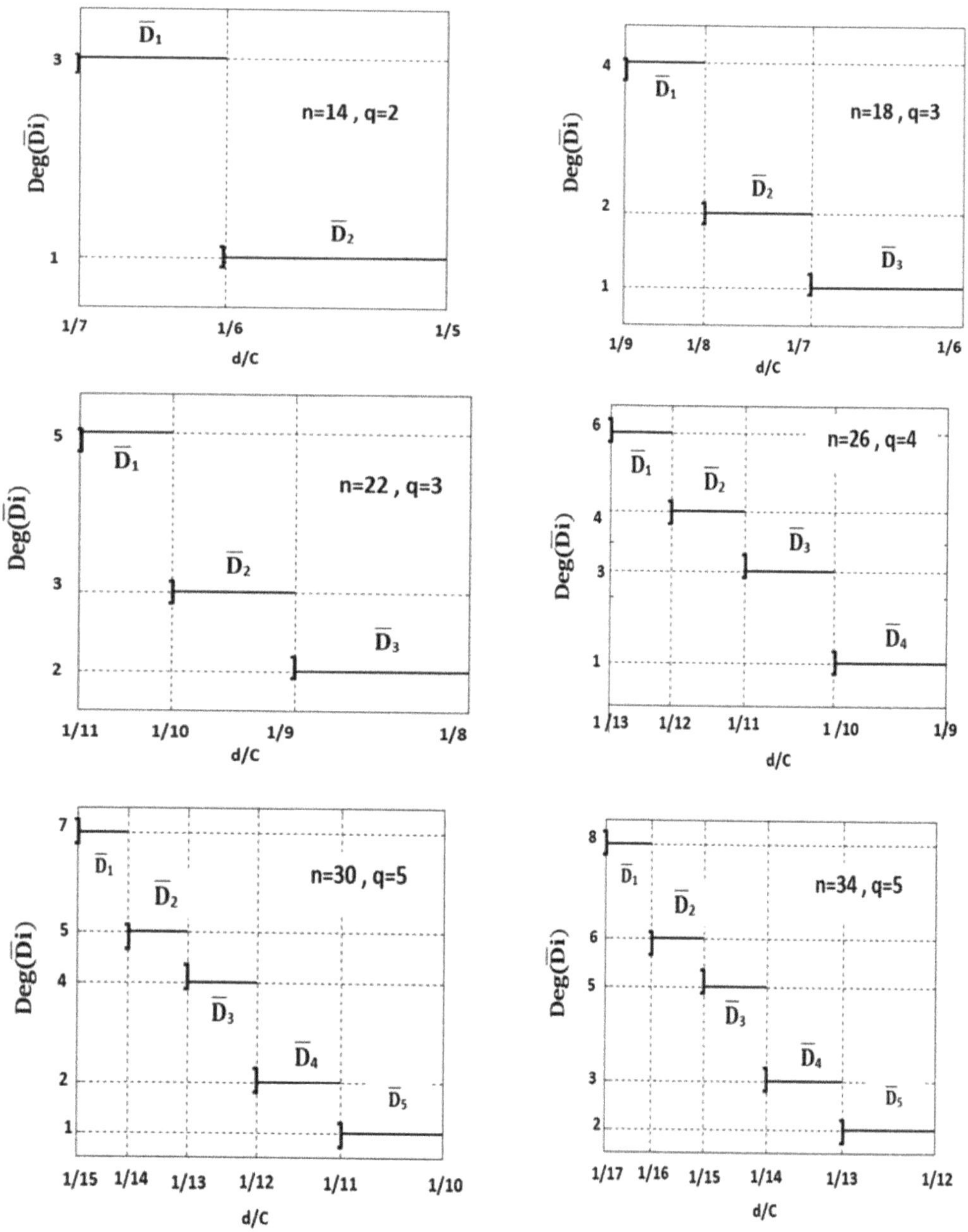

Figure A3. *Cont.*

For n fixe ∈ {8 + 4k/k ∈ N}, q = E(n/6)

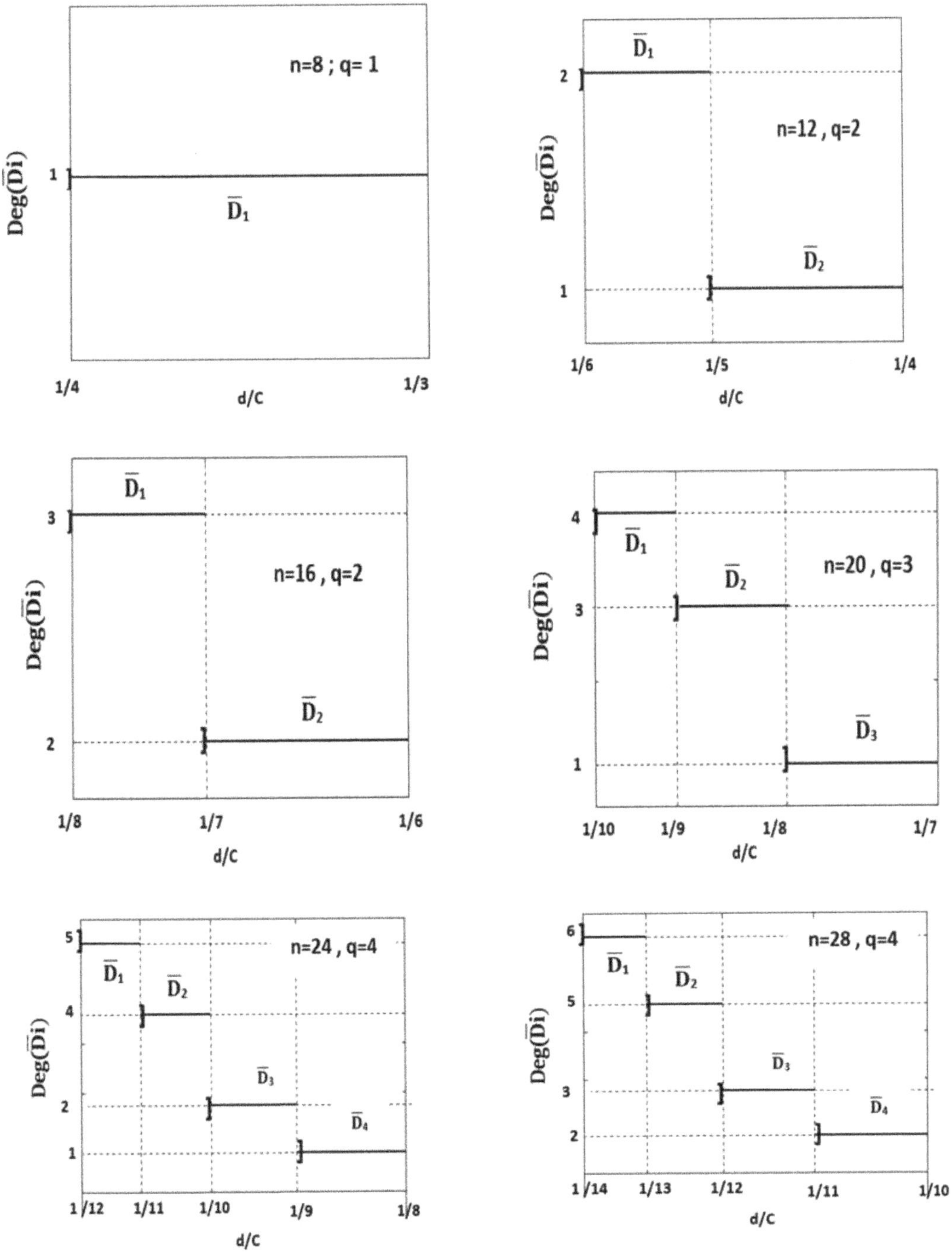

Figure A3. *Cont.*

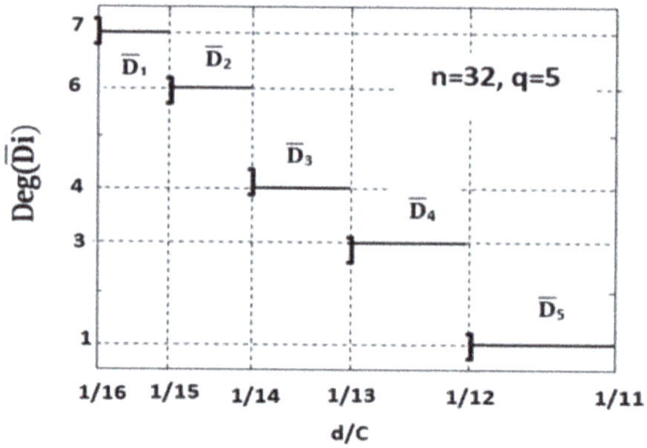

Figure A3. The variation of domain degeneracy as a function of the vaccination centres demands for selected even values of n.

References

1. Dorling, K.; Heinrichs, J.; Messier, G.G.; Magierowski, S. Vehicle routing problems for drone delivery. *IEEE Trans. Syst. Man Cybern. Syst.* **2017**, *47*, 70–85. [CrossRef]
2. Goodchild, A.; Toy, J. Delivery by drone: An evaluation of unmanned aerial vehicle technology in reducing CO_2 emissions in the delivery service industry. *Transport. Res. Part D Transp. Environ.* **2018**, *61*, 58–67. [CrossRef]
3. Amazon.com, Inc. Amazon Prime. 2016. Available online: http://www.amazon.com/primeair (accessed on 3 July 2022).
4. DHL International GmbH. DHL Parcelcopter Launches Initial Operations for Research Purposes. Available online: http://www.dhl.com/en/press/releases/ (accessed on 22 June 2022).
5. Stewart, J. Google Tests Drone Deliveries in Project Wing Trials. BBC. Available online: http://www.bbc.com/news/technology-28964260 (accessed on 29 June 2022).
6. Dillow, C. Meet Matternet, the Drone Delivery Startup Thats Actually Delivering. Fortune. Available online: http://fortune.com/2015/05/01/matternet-drone-delivery/ (accessed on 1 May 2022).
7. Haidari, L.A.; Brown, S.T.; Ferguson, M.; Bancroft, E.; Spiker, M.; Wilcox, A.; Ambikapathi, R.; Sampath, V.; Connor, D.L.; Lee, B.Y. The economic and operational value of using drones to transport vaccines. *Vaccine* **2016**, *34*, 4062–4067. [CrossRef] [PubMed]
8. Rosser, J.C., Jr.; Vignesh, V.; Terwilliger, B.A.; Parker, B.C. Surgical and medical applications of drones: A comprehensive review. *J. Soc. Laparoendosc. Surg.* **2018**, *22*, e2018.00018. [CrossRef]
9. Wang, D. The economics of drone delivery. *IEEE Spectr.* **2016**. Available online: https://spectrum.ieee.org/automaton/robotics/drones/the-economics-of-drone-delivery (accessed on 5 July 2022).
10. Multikopter. Transport und Logistik. 2019. Available online: http://www.multikopter.de/anwendungsgebiete/transport-und-logistik/ (accessed on 11 July 2022).
11. Syed, F.; Gupta, S.K.; Alsamhi, S.H.; Rachid, M.; Liu, X. A survey on recent optimal techniques for securing unmanned aerial vehicles applications. *Trans. Emerg. Telecommun. Technol.* **2020**, *32*, e4133. [CrossRef]
12. Ackerman, E.; Koziol, M. In the air with Zipline's medical delivery drones. *IEEE Spectr.* **2019**, *56*, 24–31. Available online: https://spectrum.ieee.org/robotics/drones/in-the-air-with-ziplines-medical-delivery-drones (accessed on 30 April 2022). [CrossRef]
13. Morgan, P. *Carbon Fibers and Their Composites*; ser. Materials Engineering; CRC Press: Boca Raton, FL, USA, 2005.
14. Reiter, C. BMW Makes Lone Shift to Carbon Fiber to Gain Auto Edge. Bloomberg. Available online: http://www.bloomberg.com/news/articles/2013-11-14/bmwmakes-lone-shift-to-carbon-fiber-to-gain-auto-edge (accessed on 15 November 2013).
15. Reddy, T. *Linden's Handbook of Batteries*, 4th ed.; McGraw-Hill Education: New York, NY, USA, 2010.
16. National Coordination Office for Space-Based Positioning, Navigation, and Timing. GPS.gov: Augmentation Systems. Available online: http://www.gps.gov/systems/augmentations/ (accessed on 24 December 2021).
17. Karpenko, S.; Konovalenko, I.; Miller, A.; Miller, B.; Nikolaev, D. UAV control on the basis of 3D landmark bearing-only observations. *Sensors* **2015**, *15*, 29802–29820. [CrossRef]
18. Merz, T.; Kendoul, F. Dependable low-altitude obstacle avoidance for robotic helicopters operating in rural areas. *J. Field Robot* **2013**, *30*, 439–471. [CrossRef]
19. Carloni, R.; Lippiello, V.; D'auria, M.; Fumagalli, M.; Mersha, A.Y.; Stramigioli, S.; Siciliano, B. Robot vision: Obstacle-avoidancetechniques for unmanned aerial vehicles. *IEEE Robot. Autom. Mag.* **2013**, *20*, 22–31. [CrossRef]
20. Bekmezci, I.; Sahingoz, O.K.; Temel, Ş. Flying ad-hoc networks (FANETs): A survey. *Ad Hoc Netw.* **2013**, *11*, 1254–1270. [CrossRef]
21. Li, J.; Zhou, Y.; Lamont, L. Communication architectures and protocols for networking unmanned aerial vehicles. In Proceedings of the 2013 IEEE Globecom Workshops (GC Wkshps), Atlanta, GA, USA, 9–13 December 2013; pp. 1415–1420.

22. Scott, J.E.; Scott, C.H. U. of Colorado Denver, U.U. of California Irvine, and USA. Drone delivery models for healthcare. In Proceedings of the 50th Hawaii International Conference on System Sciences, Honolulu, HI, USA, 4–7 January 2017.
23. Rabta, B.; Wankmuller, C.; Reiner, G. A drone fleet model for last-mile distribution in disaster relief operations. *Int. J. Disaster Risk Reduct* **2018**, *28*, 107–112. [CrossRef]
24. Manyam, S.G.; Sundar, K.; Casbeer, D.W. Cooperative Routing for an Air-Ground Vehicle Team—Exact Algorithm, Transformation Method, and Heuristics. *arXiv* **2018**, arXiv:1804.09546. [CrossRef]
25. Holzmann, P.; Wankmüller, C.; Globocnik, D.; Schwarz, E.J. Drones to the rescue? Exploring rescue workers' behavioral intention to adopt drones in mountain rescue missions. *Int. J. Phys. Distrib. Logist. Manag.* **2021**. *ahead-of-print*. [CrossRef]
26. Wen, T.; Zhang, Z.; Wong, K.K.L. Multi-objective algorithm for blood supply via unmanned aerial vehicles to the wounded in an emergency situation. *PLoS ONE* **2016**, *11*, e0155176.
27. Greaves, R.F.; Bernardini, S.; Ferrari, M.; Fortina, P.; Gouget, B.; Gruson, D.; Lang, T.; Loh, T.P.; Morris, H.A.; Park, J.Y.; et al. Key questions about the future of laboratory medicine in the next decade of the 21st century: A report from the IFCC-Emerging Technologies Division. *Clin. Chim. Acta* **2019**, *495*, 570–589. [CrossRef]
28. Otto, A.; Agatz, N.; Campbref, J.; Goklen, B.; Pesch, E. Optimization approaches for civil applications of unmanned aerial vehicles (uavx) or aerial drones: A survey. *Networks* **2018**, *72*, 411–458. [CrossRef]
29. Amukele, T.K.; Sokoll, L.J.; Pepper, D.; Howard, D.P.; Street, J. Can unmanned aerial systems (drones) be used for the routine transport of chemistry, hematology, and coagulation laboratory specimens? *PLoS ONE* **2015**, *10*, e0134020. [CrossRef]
30. Amukele, T.; Ness, P.M.; Tobian, A.A.; Boyd, J.; Street, J. Drone transportation of blood products. *Transfusion* **2017**, *57*, 582–588. [CrossRef]
31. Gavi. The Vaccine Alliance. Rwanda Launches World's First National Drone Delivery Service Powered by Zipline. 2016. Available online: https://www.gavi.org/library/news/gavi-features/2016/rwanda-launches-world-s-firstnational-drone-delivery-service-powered-by-zipline/ (accessed on 14 July 2019).
32. UNICEF. Malawi Tests First Unmanned Aerial Vehicle Flights for HIV Early Infant Diagnosis. 2016. Available online: https://www.unicef.org/media/media_90462.html (accessed on 8 February 2019).
33. Medecins Sans Fronti Eres. Innovating to Reach Remote TB Patients and Improve Access to Treatment. 2014. Available online: https://www.msf.org/papua-new-guinea-innovating-reach-remote-tb-patients-and-improveaccess-treatment (accessed on 31 December 2016).
34. Furer, F. Swiss Post Drone Takes Off again for Healthcare Services. Swiss Post. 2019. Available online: https://post-m-dien.ch/en/swiss-post-dronelost-over-lake-zurich/ (accessed on 26 July 2020).
35. Makoye, K. Buzz as World's Biggest Drone Drug Deliveries Take Off in Tanzania. Reuters. 2017. Available online: https://www.reuters.com/article/ustanzania-health-drones/buzz-as-worlds-biggest-drone-drug-deliveries-takeoff-in-tanzania-idUSKCN1B91F7 (accessed on 17 July 2019).
36. Kelland, K. Drones to Deliver Vaccines, Blood and Drugs Across Ghana. Reuters. 2019. Available online: https://af.reuters.com/article/topNews/idAFKCN1S014J-OZATP (accessed on 21 July 2020).
37. McNeil, D.G., Jr. An Island Nation's Health Experiment: Vaccines Delivered by Drone. The New York Times. 2018. Available online: https://www.nytimes.com/2018/12/17/health/vanuatu-vaccines-drones.html (accessed on 17 July 2019).
38. Paul, S.K.; Chowdhury, P. A production recovery plan in manufacturing supply chains for a high-demand item during COVID-19. *Int. J. Phys. Distrib. Logist. Manag.* **2021**, *51*, 104–125. [CrossRef]

safety

MDPI

Article

Numerical Calculation and Analysis of Water Dump Distribution Out of the Belly Tanks of Firefighting Helicopters

Tejun Zhou [1,2,*], Jiazheng Lu [1], Chuanping Wu [1] and Shilong Lan [3]

1 State Key Laboratory of Disaster Prevention and Reduction for Power Grid Transmission and Distribution Equipment, Changsha 410029, China
2 School of Electrical & Information Engineering, Changsha University of Science & Technology, Changsha 410205, China
3 School of Aeronautical Science and Engineering, Beijing University of Aeronautics and Astronautics, Beijing 100190, China
* Correspondence: zhoutejun1988@126.com; Tel.: +86-189-7310-2024

Abstract: Helicopters are more and more widely used for water dumping in fire extinguishing operations nowadays. Increasing attention is being paid to improving helicopter firefighting efficiency. Water distribution onto the ground from the helicopter tank is a key reference target to evaluate firefighting efficiency. Numerical simulations and calculations were carried out concerning water dumping out of the belly tank of a helicopter using the VOF (Volume of Fluent Model) model and mesh adaptation in ANSYS Fluent, and the effects of two parameters, the height of the tank above the ground and the wind speed, on the wake flow and water distribution were discussed. The results showed that for forward flight, the higher the forward flight speed, the less the average water depth on the ground. Similar results were obtained for flight height. The average water depth was one order of magnitude less than in the cases of the corresponding hovering helicopter for a given wind speed. As for hovering flight, the higher the wind speed, the less the average water depth on the ground. The simulation results were basically consistent with the conclusions of water dump tests of fire-fighting equipment carried by helicopters. For example, when the helicopter flew at a forward flight speed of 15 m/s and the tank bottom was 30 m above the ground, the area covered by the dumped water would be 337.5 m^2, and the average water depth accumulated per square meter would be 0.3 cm. This result was close to the 0.34 cm obtained under Hayden Biggs's test condition with a forward flight speed of 70 km/h and a height above the ground of 24 m.

Keywords: helicopter; tank; water dump; wind speed; numerical calculation

Citation: Zhou, T.; Lu, J.; Wu, C.; Lan, S. Numerical Calculation and Analysis of Water Dump Distribution Out of the Belly Tanks of Firefighting Helicopters. *Safety* **2022**, *8*, 69. https://doi.org/10.3390/safety8040069

Academic Editor: Raphael Grzebieta

Received: 25 February 2022
Accepted: 28 May 2022
Published: 3 October 2022

1. Introduction

Forests in China cover an area of nearly two million square kilometers, accounting for nearly 20% of the country's land area. Forest fires occur frequently every year, causing extensive damage to natural resources, the ecological environment, and production facilities [1–3], and even sometimes causing heavy casualties. Therefore, it is very important to carry out proper monitoring, early warning, and forest fire suppression. During forest fire suppression, helicopters can rapidly reach the forest, where it is difficult for people to enter to extinguish the fire. The suppression achieved by the helicopter's water dumping on the fire line and the fire head reduces the intensity of effort by ground personnel against the fire and reduces the casualty rate. At present, firefighting departments in the United States, Canada, Russia, Japan, and other countries are equipped with many firefighting helicopters to execute tasks such as forest fire suppression and high-rise building firefighting [4,5]. Because the aviation industry in China started late, it has lagged behind the developed countries just mentioned in both research and development and the quantity of firefighting helicopters. Moreover, technology and applications related to helicopter firefighting are also in need of development. Helicopter firefighting mainly includes onboard tank (belly/under-deck) water dumping, bucket/capsule water dump firefighting, fire water-monitor firefighting, and fire water-bomb drop firefighting. The firefighting effect is closely related to the water distribution in the target region [6,7]. Studies on water distribution in onboard tanks and bucket/capsule water dump firefighting mainly came from flight tests. The following is a review of studies on water distribution in onboard tank firefighting and bucket /capsule water dump firefighting [8–15].

Experimental data from the studies just described are as follows, where the water depth accumulated was an average, whereas the data from Xie Yingmin et al. [12] were merely the results on flat ground. The results of Wu Zepeng et al. [8] show that if the bucket was more than 30 m above the fire scene, the water dumped would be atomized completely, whereas the results of both Xie Yingmin et al. [12] and Zhou Tejun et al. [13] showed that, at a height of 30 m, the water depth accumulated was still 0.1–0.2 cm. The results of Chen Zhaopeng et al. [10] and Zhou Wanshu [11] showed that at a height of 50 m, the water depth accumulated could reach 0.2 cm, and could even reach 1.25 cm under the no-wind circumstance, as proved by Chen Zhaopeng et al. [10]. These results were obviously inconsistent with each other. Such an inconsistency might have been due to several aspects, for example, whether foaming agent and other surface-active materials had been added to the water. If so, the materials could reduce the formation of small water droplets. In addition, the bucket bottom valves might have been of different sizes and shapes, which would have an impact on water flow and pattern, thus resulting in differences in water dump coverage areas and the average water depth on the ground.

Because renting helicopters is expensive, the firefighting tests involve both great material consumption and high cost, and fine data cannot be obtained through conventional test techniques. Therefore, the helicopter firefighting test is restricted; however, as one of the study objectives, numerical simulation can either supplement or even replace such tests. With current physical firefighting process knowledge of water dumping out of helicopters, the application of relevant models, and constant development of numerical simulation software and computer performance, numerical simulation of firefighting by water dumping out of helicopters has developed gradually from nothing. However, its technical level has not yet reached maturity, and there are few simulation studies of firefighting by water dumping out of helicopters. Two such studies will be briefly introduced in the following.

In the calculation model of X. Zhao et al. [16], the fact or principle used to set the diameter of the water droplets was not specified, nor were the calculation results verified by experiment. If the distribution rule of water droplet diameters were known beforehand, the calculation scheme of X. Zhao et al. would be feasible. In the study of Satoh et al. [17], the actual rotor wings of the helicopter were not simulated in the numerical simulation, and the downwash velocity field generated from the rotor wings was approximated by setting a downward air velocity of 30 m/s at the upper boundary of the computational domain, an approach that greatly reduced computational effort. Borisov et al. [18] performed a relatively complete study on water dump firefighting simulation. The blades were not simulated; instead, a downward speed was imparted to the plane of the lower blade by means of a virtual blade, in accordance with the measured velocity distribution, and a corresponding velocity was imparted to the plane of the upper blade.

The above discussion confirms that when a model with low degree of approximation was used to simulate a tank or bucket water dump process, a relatively accurate water distribution was not provided, and the accuracy of firefighting effect evaluation was affected. In addition, regarding the influence of the height of the tank or bucket above the ground on water distribution over the ground, there were also inconsistent conclusions in these articles. Evaluation of firefighting effect can be expressed by the water volume arriving at the ground fire source, where height above the ground is an important parameter influencing ground water distribution. In addition, because natural wind speed is hard to control, there were few reports in the literature concerning the influence of wind speed on water distribution.

2. Helicopter and Tank Models

In the present paper, simulation calculation of helicopter tank water dumping was performed using two parameters: the height of the helicopter tank bottom above the ground and the wind speed. The volume-of-fluid model (VOF model) was used to calculate the air-water interface, and dynamic mesh adaptation was used to better differentiate the air-water interface. The rule of influence of the height of the helicopter tank bottom above the ground (H = 10 m, 20 m, and 30 m) and the wind speed (U = 0 m/s, 5 m/s, 10 m/s, and 15 m/s) on the distribution of a water dump was given to provide theoretical guidance for a helicopter firefighting operation scheme. In this approach, to calculate the rotor wake, the acting disc theory of a helicopter was used instead of a simulated blade. This was more convenient to use than the virtual screw disk of Borisov et al. [18], which yields basically the same accuracy, and was more accurate than the jet model of Satoh et al. [17]. To calculate the water dump, this paper simulated the water discharge process of real water tank directly, while Satoh et al. [17] and Borisov et al. [18] did not simulate the water dump process. For the two-phase, water–air flow, this paper adopted the volume-fraction model for calculations, which is superior to the virtual gas model of Satoh et al. [17]. However, as this model is restricted by the extremely numerous calculations required, we did not calculate the breakup of drops; we note that the drops calculated by Borisov et al. [18] were also not real fluid drops, but water drop test particles representing many fluid drops.

An H125 helicopter equipped with an Isolair Eliminator II belly firefighting tank (https://www.fs.fed.us/t-d/pubs/html/95571307/95571307.html, accessed on 2 May 2022) was taken as the simulation prototype in this paper. Figure 1 shows a water dump out of an H125 helicopter equipped with the Isolair Eliminator II belly firefighting tank. Modeling was performed in accordance with the geometrical parameters of the H125 helicopter and the tank (ANSYS Design Modeler), neglecting some parts and configuration details such as the aero-engine case, the bracket under the fuselage, and the tail rotor. In this way, the helicopter and tank models used for simulation were obtained, as shown in Figure 2. The action of the blade on air was viewed as a pressure difference acting above and below a disc, specifically the *Fan* model in Fluent, which was more accurate than the jet flow approximation used by Satoh et al. [17]. If the geometrical parameters and operating parameters of the blade were known, the momentum source method [19] could also have been used to simulate the action of the blade on air, which would have been more accurate than the acting disc theory, and there is also a momentum source model in Fluent. Both the *Fan* model and the momentum source model eliminate the large numbers of mesh cells required to simulate actual blades, while still obtaining a relatively accurate time-mean wake flow field.

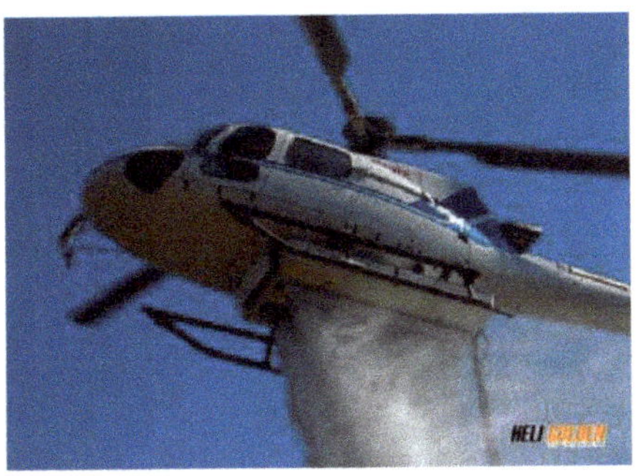

Figure 1. H125 firefighting helicopter and Isolair Eliminator II belly firefighting tank (from http://www.isolairinc.com/_gallery/4600-350A.jpg, accessed on 2 May 2022).

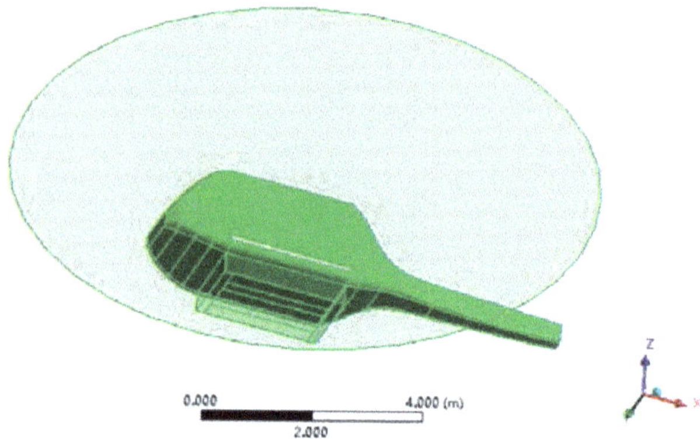

Figure 2. Helicopter and tank model in the simulation.

The tank used in the calculation was 2.32 m long, 1.38 m wide, and 0.4 m high, with two long narrow valves, each 2 m long and 0.23 m wide with a gap of 0.3 m. The tank had a maximum capacity of 1280.64 L. To maintain consistent air pressure inside and outside the tank at the time of water dumping, a long narrow ventilation opening was designed over the rear of the tank (see Figure 3) with dimensions of 1.38 m × 0.05 m.

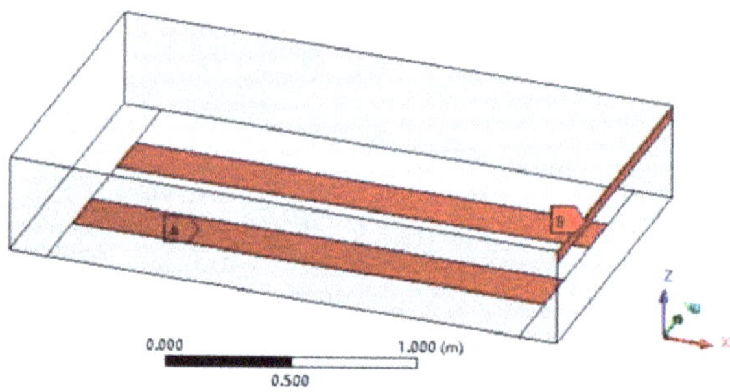

Figure 3. Details of the tank model (A is the water-dump valve, and B is the ventilation opening, for the dimensions of the tank and valve, see the description given in the main text).

3. Water Dump Simulation Model of Helicopter Belly Firefighting Tank

A parametric study was carried out in this paper regarding two key parameters that influence the distribution of the water dump: the height (H) from the tank bottom to the ground and the wind speed (U). Several examples for different heights (H = 10 m, 20 m, and 30 m) and wind speeds (U = 0 m/s, 5 m/s, 10 m/s, and 15 m/s) were calculated. The results of a calculated example are given in detail below (the height (H) from the tank bottom to the ground = 20 m, and the headwind speed U = 15 m/s), including mesh independence verification, the calculation format, and calculation scheme. This example was selected for a detailed analysis for the reason that, in this example, the height was moderate while the wind speed was relatively big, which caused very significant changes in the trajectory and shape of the water masses. Other calculated examples are given in Section 4, where the results of different heights above the ground and different wind speeds were investigated, and the rule of water distribution on the ground was generalized.

When the helicopter flew above the fire scene to prepare for a water dump, the airflow was generally stable surrounding the helicopter (the fire scene model was temporarily left out of consideration in this study). Therefore, before the water dump is calculated, the stable airflow field should be calculated first. This was then taken as the initial scenario to start transient calculations of the water dump.

3.1. Mesh Independence Verification

This section discusses the influence of mesh cell size on flow field results and especially on the resolution of the water–air phase interface. Two sets of meshes were used; namely, one set consisting of a basic mesh, and another with a fine grid. The verification was divided in two steps, where the first step compared the calculation results of the rotor flow field before water dump in the two sets of meshes, and the second step compared the calculation results of the two-phase, water–air flow after water dump in the two sets of meshes.

Figure 4 shows the simulation field of the helicopter dumping firefighting water. The blade disc diameter of the H125 helicopter (D) was 10.69 m, the distance from the front of the disc to the entry plane of the computational domain was 6D, the distance from the rear of the disc to the exit plane of the computational domain was 8D, the distance from the disc to both boundaries of the computational domain was 6D, and the distance from the disc to the upper boundary of the computational domain was 7D.

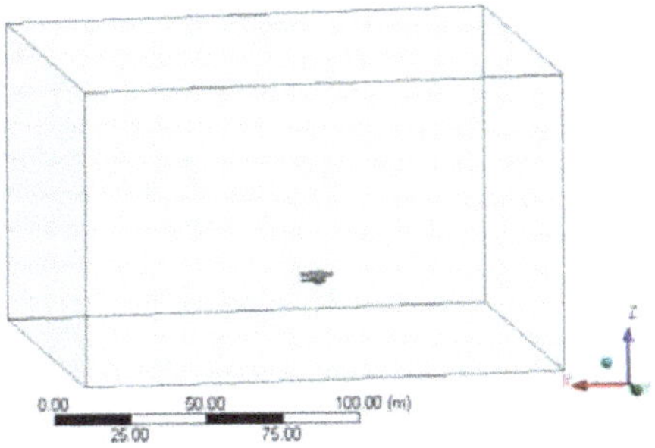

Figure 4. Computational domain of the helicopter.

For example, when the tank was 20 m from the ground, meshes generated by ANSYS Meshing, there were a total of 695,114 mesh cells (tetrahedrons and triangular prisms). The maximum mesh cell size inside and outside the tank was 0.05 m, the maximum size on the fuselage and on the disc of the rotor wings was 0.1 m, the maximum size on the external boundary plane of the computational domain was 5 m, and there were boundary-layer meshes (triangular-prism cells) on the disc of the rotor wings, the fuselage surface, the tank wall surface, and the ground. The thickness of the boundary layer was set to 0.05 m, there were 10 layers of mesh cells inside the boundary layer, and the mesh growth rate was 1.2; this mesh is referred to as the basic mesh in what follows. In Figure 5, the meshes near the helicopter and the tank on the longitudinal symmetry plan of the computational domain are given; the mesh cells in the tank can also be seen.

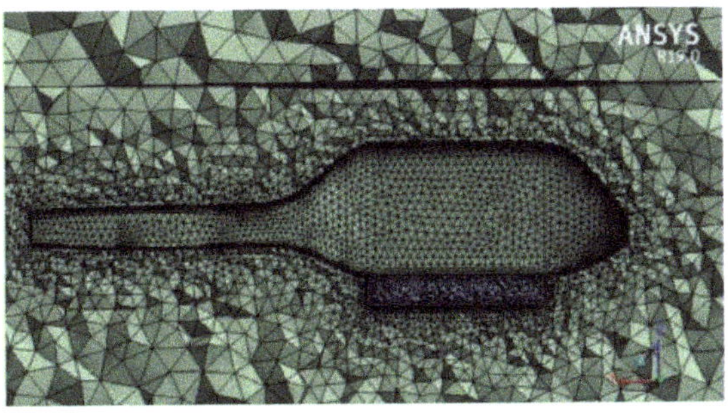

Figure 5. Meshes near the helicopter and tank on a longitudinal symmetric plan of the computational domain (there are boundary-layer meshes on the fuselage surface, the external tank surface, and both sides of the blade disc).

These new mesh cells are hereinafter referred to as fine meshes. They covered the spatial region from the bottom of the helicopter belly firefighting tank to the ground, which was 6.7 m long, 7 m wide, and 20 m high (as shown in the left side of Figure 6, the "body of influence" in ANSYS Workbench meshing was used), the maximum mesh cell size was set to 0.2 m. There were a total of 2,061,091 mesh cells, about three times the number (695,114) in the basic mesh cells described earlier. As will be seen later, the total number of mesh cells calculated up to 1.9 s reached 2,460,231 due to adaptive refinement of meshes.

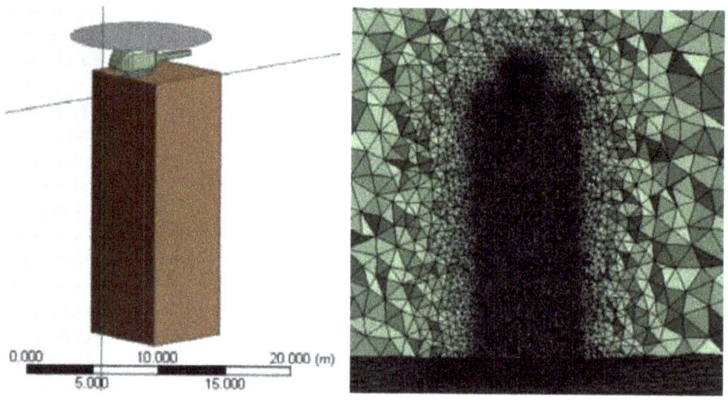

Figure 6. Fine mesh space region and mesh distribution.

The calculation method, format parameters, and self-adaptive mesh parameters were all set the same in the two sets of meshes. Results from the fine meshes are given below and are compared with the results of the basic meshes. Figure 7 shows the pressure distribution on the longitudinal symmetry cross section of the initial scenario as calculated with fine meshes. There was almost no difference compared with the results of the basic mesh. In fact, the place where mesh refinement was performed was the space below the helicopter belly, and compared with the pressure gradients near the helicopter rotor wings and near the fuselage surface, the pressure gradient in this space was relatively gentle, and the basic meshes were sufficient to calculate the pressure field accurately.

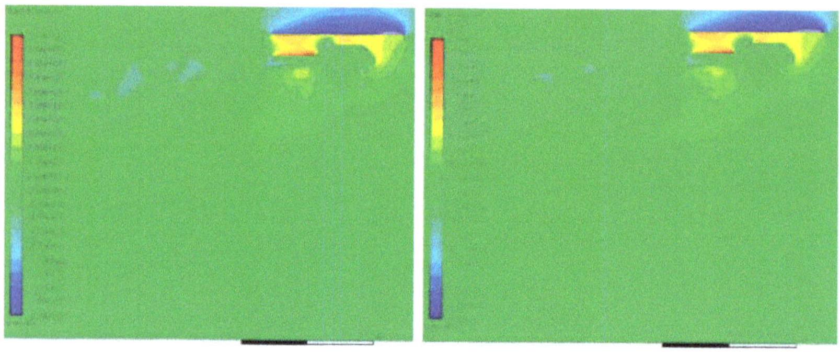

Figure 7. Pressure distributions on a longitudinal symmetry cross section of the initial scenario calculated with fine meshes (the ground is at the ruler in the figure, the left picture is the basic mesh, and the right picture is the fine mesh).

Next, we compared the calculation results of two-phase, gas–fluid flow in the two sets of meshes. Figure 8 gives contour surface diagrams for water–air phase volume fractions of 0.01, 0.1, and 0.5 calculated with fine meshes at t = 1.9 s (i.e., the water mass touched the ground just at this time). It is obvious that the fine mesh could yield a finer water–air interface and smaller water mass, but the physical quantity of interest in this paper is the average water depth (i.e., the average water depth that is equal to the result of water-dump quantity divided by the water coverage area). The longitudinal and transverse dimensions of the water mass near the ground in Figure 8 were about 3 m × 4 m, and the calculation result of the base grid was about 4 m × 7 m, which shows that a more accurate water distribution could be obtained using the basic meshes. In Section 4.4 below, the average water depth accumulated as calculated in this paper was basically consistent with that under the corresponding condition by Xie Yingmin et al. [12], which showed that it was suitable to use the basic meshes to calculate the region covered by water and the average water depth. In addition, a third finer mesh was not taken into consideration in this paper since the calculation quantity of the fine mesh was sufficient.

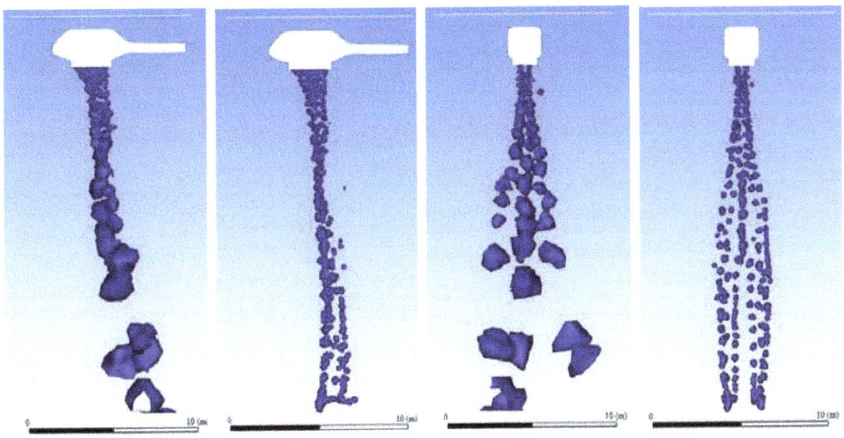

Figure 8. Contour surface of the side view and front view for a two-phase, water–air volume fraction of 0.01 at t = 1.9 s.

3.2. *Analysis of Initial Scenario Results before Water Dump*

This section first gives the calculation results of the initial flow field before the water dump. VOF can be either enabled or disabled at the time of initial scenario calculation, and VOF was disabled in this study. The internal space of the tank was set to air, and the valves and the ventilation opening were set as solid wall surfaces. The calculation was performed by a steady-state algorithm, using the k-omega SST turbulence model [20]. Since complex separation only existed near the helicopter and water tank, the wake flow with which we were concerned under the water tank was not so complexed, and to which common turbulence models were applied; hence, the equation calculation format was SIMPLE, and basic meshes were used.

Figure 9 shows the calculated residual change curve. When the number of iterations was greater than 200, the residue remained basically unchanged. The velocity field (Figure 10) and the pressure field (Figure 11) on the longitudinal symmetry plane of the fuselage at 1000 and 2000 iterations were taken, respectively, as their simulated values, and the pressure shown in Figure 11 was gauge pressure. The velocity and pressure fields at 1000 and 2000 iterations were very consistent, showing that the calculation had reached steady state. Flow field data at 2000 iterations were selected as the initial scenario for subsequent calculations of the water dump.

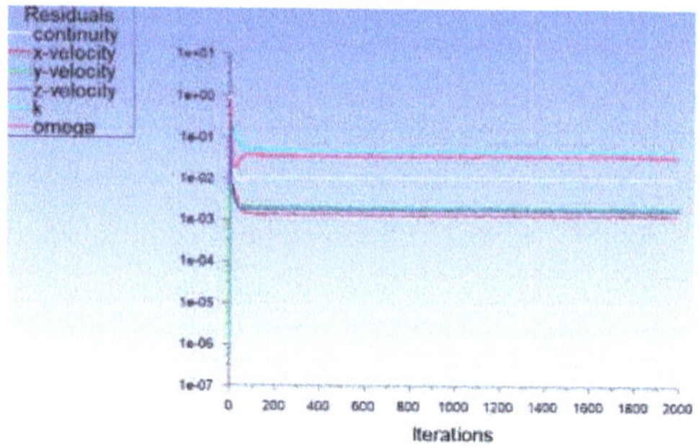

Figure 9. Residual change curve of the steady-state calculations.

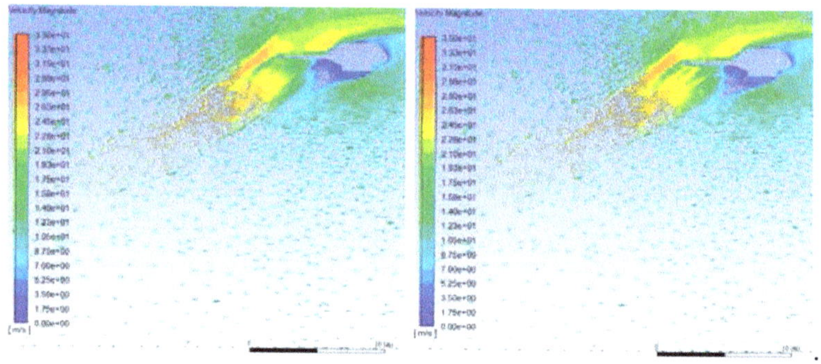

Figure 10. Velocity vector on the longitudinal symmetry plane of the fuselage in the initial scenario (1000 iterations on the (**left**), 2000 iterations on the (**right**)).

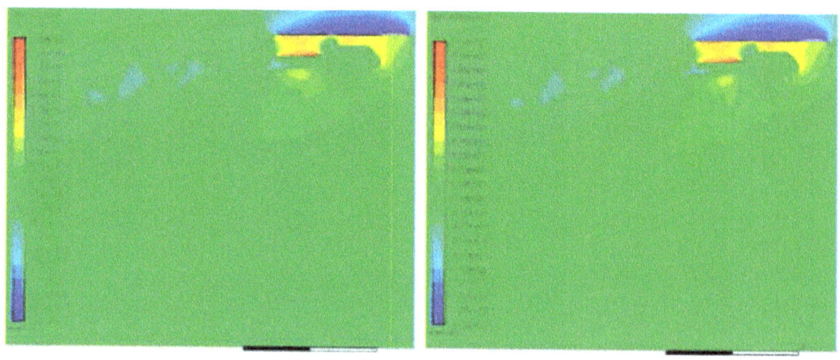

Figure 11. Pressure distribution on the longitudinal symmetry plane of the fuselage in the initial scenario (1000 iterations on the (**left**), 2000 iterations on the (**right**)).

3.3. Transient Result Analysis of Water Dump

When the transient calculations of the water dump were enabled, steady-state (1600 iterations) data were read in, and the valves and ventilation opening were set as internal boundaries. Most of the space inside the tank, 2.32 m × 1.38 m × 0.35 m (length × width × height), was defined as a region called *Region0* using cell registers in Fluent, and the initial value of this region was adjusted by *Patch* when Fluent was initialized. Specifically, the phase in this region was adjusted to water, and therefore there was initially 1.12 m^3 of water in the tank. Note that there was still air inside the tank at a height of 0.35–0.4 m, which connected with the air outside the tank through the ventilation opening. Data for other spaces required no initialization and were maintained at the input steady-state values. The turbulence model and the spatial calculation format were kept the same as for the steady-state calculation.

Time was advanced by a first-order implicit method with a fixed time step of 0.001 s, corresponding to the rapidest water mass movement at approximately 1–2 cm. This ensured that there was sufficient time resolution, and the maximum number of iterations per time step was set to 50, so as to ensure residuals below 10^{-5}. Transient calculation was enabled to t = 0.01 s, and the residual change was as shown in Figure 12. It is apparent that the residuals were significantly reduced by two or three orders of magnitude after bridging the transient calculation. If the transient calculations were continued, the residual of each equation could be maintained at 10^{-5} to 10^{-6} until the calculation ended at 1–2 s (as was the case with all transient calculation examples in this paper). When t = 0.01 s, the VOF distribution of water and air inside the tank and at the valve was as shown in Figure 13. If a cross section were taken in the middle of the tank vertical to the x-axis, meshes inside and below the tank could be seen (Figure 14), there were some flat triangular cells, which were formed by cutting off tetrahedral cells in cross section, and most of the mesh cells were near-regular tetrahedra (Figure 5).

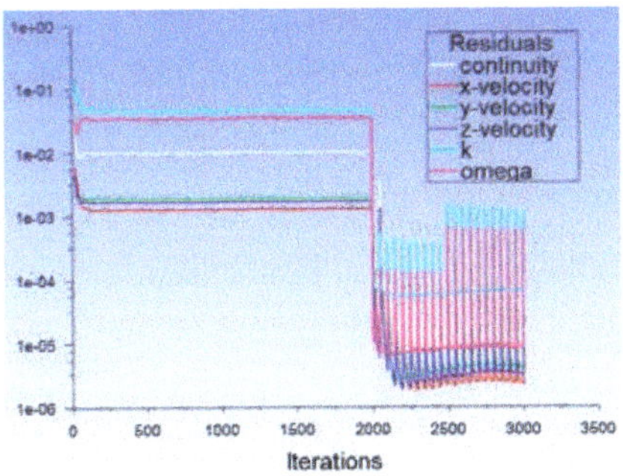

Figure 12. Residual change curve of steady-state calculations bridging to transient calculations (until t = 0.02 s).

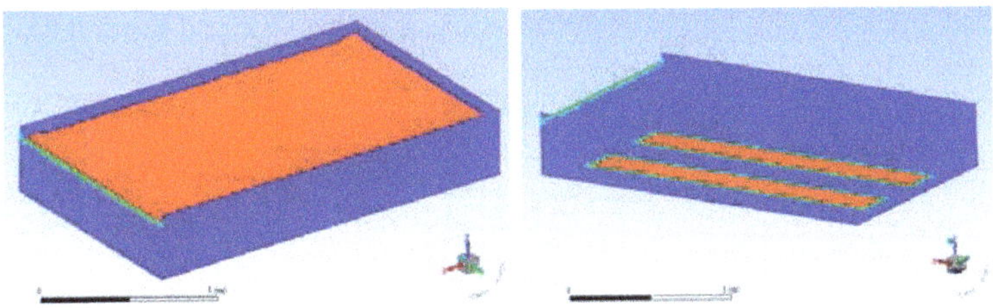

Figure 13. VOF distribution of water and air inside the tank (**left**) and at two values at the tank bottom (**right**) when t = 0.01 s (red indicates water).

Dynamic mesh adaptation (based on the curvature of the water–air interface) was enabled after the tank water dump had been enabled for 0.01 s. Meanwhile, mesh adaptation was set at one per time step, with the time step still being 0.001 s, and for each time step, mesh adaptation, the coarsening threshold (10^{-8}) and the refining threshold (10^{-2}) were implemented. In addition, dynamic self-adaptation was enabled, the maximum level of refinement was set to 2, the minimum cell volume was set to 1.25×10^{-4} m^3 (the corresponding mesh cell was 0.05 m), and mesh adaptation load balancing was used to improve parallel efficiency. The calculation lasted from t = 0.01 s to t = 0.45 s. The VOF distribution and the meshes of water and air on the same cross section are shown in Figure 12. The meshes near the water–air interface were encrypted to a certain extent so that the water–air interface could be better distinguished.

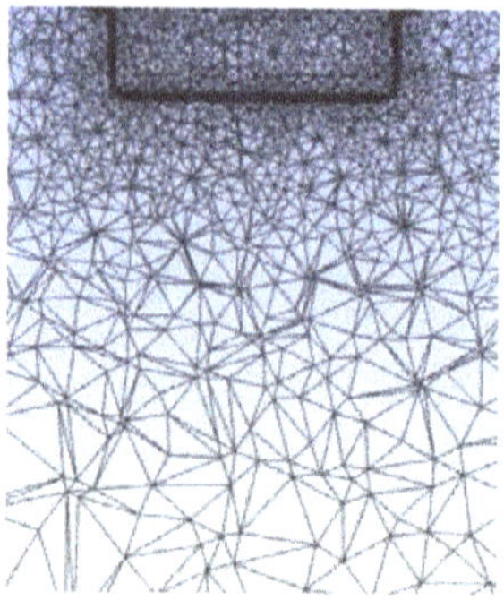

Figure 14. Mesh distributions inside and below the tank in cross section.

Figure 15 shows the water in the tank and nearby meshes at t = 1.9 s of the water dump. At this time, most of the water in the tank has been dumped. Figure 8 shows the contour surface with a water–air volume fraction = 0.01 in space (the ground is at the ruler in the figure). The side view in Figure 8 shows that large water masses have been subjected to a certain influence by Level-3 wind, the dumped water has been deflected in the wind direction, the water mass near the ground has been deflected in the wind direction by 3–4 m, and the longitudinal dimension of the water mass has reached about 4 m. The front view in Figure 8 shows that under the action of wind, the water flow has developed laterally, and that the sideways deflection of the water mass near the ground is about 7 m. This means that the area covered by the water dump on the ground is approximately 4 m $\times$ 7 m = 28 m^2, under the assumption that all 1.12 m^3 of the water in the tank was dumped to this region. The average water depth accumulated in this region would then be approximately 0.04 m. Although in fact small water droplets would be created and would fly away with the wind, thus causing the region covered by water to be larger than the value calculated above, in the dense mesh calculation (Figure 8), the area covered by the water dump on the ground was approximately 3 m $\times$ 4 m = 12 m^2. Therefore, taking the two circumstances causing contrary results into full consideration, the region covered by water might not have been underestimated in the calculation using basic meshes. Hence, the region covered by water and the average water depth accumulated from the above basic mesh calculations were used as important data for drawing conclusions.

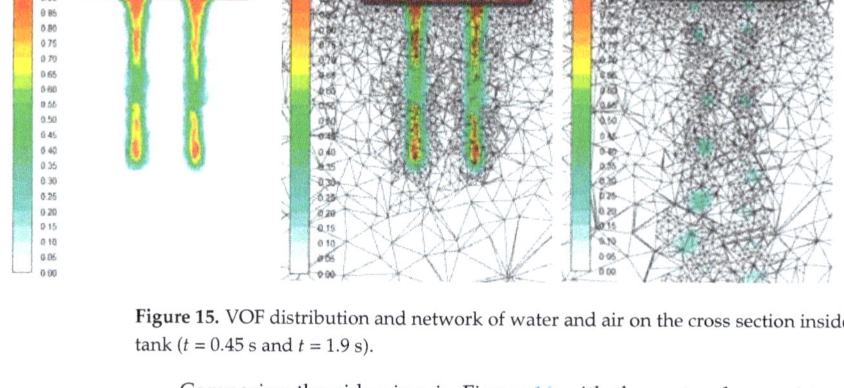

Figure 15. VOF distribution and network of water and air on the cross section inside and under the tank (t = 0.45 s and t = 1.9 s).

Comparing the side view in Figure 16 with the water dump picture in Figure 17 reveals a similar important phenomenon: the water flow was not smooth or continuous, but experienced many interruptions. Only a rough qualitative comparison could be performed because the forward flight speed of the helicopter in the picture and the wind speed were unknown. Except for the fact that small water droplets could not be differentiated in the calculations, the water masses were of similar qualitative distribution, showing that the calculated results were qualitatively correct. Figure 18 gives a local panoramic view of the two-phase, water–air volume fraction contour surface below the helicopter belly at two moments, t = 0.9 s and t = 1.9 s. The water-air interface at t = 0.9 s was relatively more continuous than that at t = 1.9 s, because the water dump flow was greater at the former. These images resemble the photograph of the helicopter belly firefighting tank water dump in Figure 1. Because of the lack of quantitative experimental data in the literature, the results calculated here were only qualitatively compared with the actual pictures.

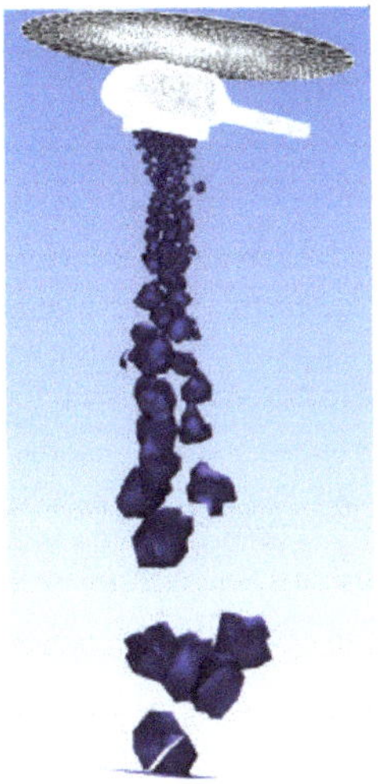

Figure 16. Panoramic view of the contour surface for a volume fraction = 0.01 in space at t = 1.9 s (the side and front views are shown in Figure 8).

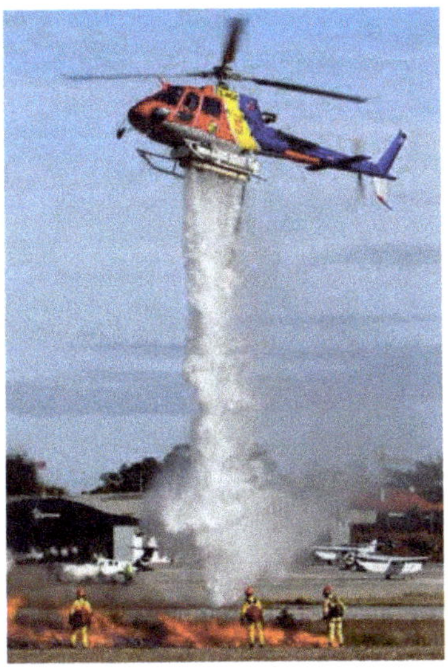

Figure 17. AS350B2 firefighting tank used for water dump firefighting (found online at http://www.isolairinc.com/_gallery/4600-350D.jpg, accessed on 2 September 2021).

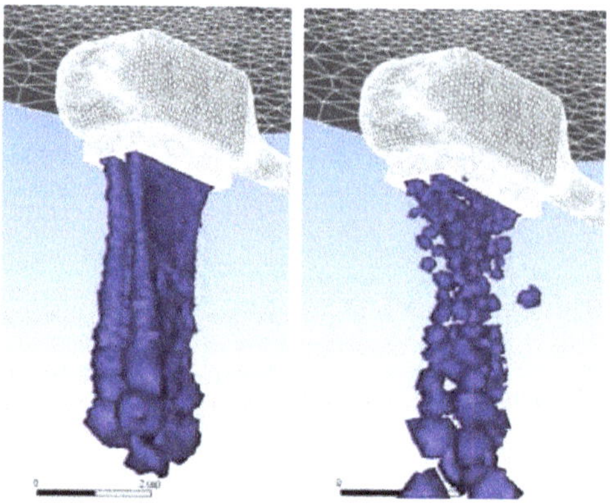

Figure 18. Local panorama of contour surface when the volume fraction of the water–air phase below the helicopter belly was 0.01 ((**left**), $t = 0.9$ s; (**right**), $t = 1.9$ s).

In fact, it is very difficult to simulate the movement of real water masses and water drops after water dump, regarding which a discussion is made below. The main force on the water mass by the airflow was in direct proportion to $\rho_{air}U^2D^2$, and the force of gravity on the water mass was in direct proportion to $\rho_{water}D^3g$, where D was the equivalent diameter of the water mass, U was the velocity of the water mass relative to the airflow, and g was the acceleration of gravity. When the force exerted on the water mass by the airflow was comparable to that of gravity, the water mass could significantly move along with the airflow. However, it can be inferred that only water droplets with diameter less than 1 cm could move significantly with the airflow, and the smaller the water droplets, the more closely they moved with the airflow. In our calculations, the minimum mesh cell scale was about 0.05 m, and it was impossible to distinguish water droplets less than 0.01 m in diameter. The equivalent diameters of the water masses of VOF-to-DPM [21] conversion in ANSYS Fluent were set to 0.01 m; therefore, the conversion was not activated. If a smaller mesh cell size and a smaller equivalent diameter of VOF-to-DPM water mass were adopted, the movement of small water droplets with the airflow could be calculated.

Interruption of the water–air interface occurred because of instability on the interface between the falling water flow and the air at greater Weber number. The interface then formed a complex curved surface, which was then broken into large water droplets, which would also experience instability with the air interface, leading to secondary breakage and creating still smaller water droplets. The water distribution of the water dump out of the helicopter involved a distance of dozens of meters from the tank to the ground and the passage of several seconds. The instability and breaking of the water flow and the secondary breakage of large water droplets occurred at a smaller space and time scale [22–25], which was nearly impossible to consider simultaneously in the simulation calculations. A water droplet breakage model would generally be used (many breakage models are available in ANSYS Fluent).

If sufficient calculation resources can be obtained, the mesh should be finer as much as possible, which can make the simulation of the water–air interface finer, and, if possible, one should adopt the breaking-drop model. A further analysis of the calculation results produced by the fine mesh is provided below. Figure 19 gives contour surface diagrams when the water–air phase volume fraction calculated with fine meshes at $t = 1.9$ s was 0.01, 0.1, and 0.5. The three contour surfaces were of relatively similar form, showing that the two-phase, water–air interface was reconstructed with reasonable accuracy under this fine mesh and with the mesh adaptation calculations. Figure 20 shows a local enlargement of the results near the ground in Figure 19, with the contour surface with volume fractions of 0.01 and 0.5, and in addition shows the mesh cells at that location on the contour surface. The maximum mesh cell size of the refined meshes near the ground was 0.2 m, and the minimum cell size of the mesh adaptation was 0.05 m. Therefore, the maximum mesh cell size was 0.05 m, which meant that water droplets smaller than 0.05 m could not be distinguished. Due to insufficient mesh refinement in the present calculations, the "VOF-to-DPM" model in ANSYS Fluent was not activated, and therefore the water droplet breakage model was not used.

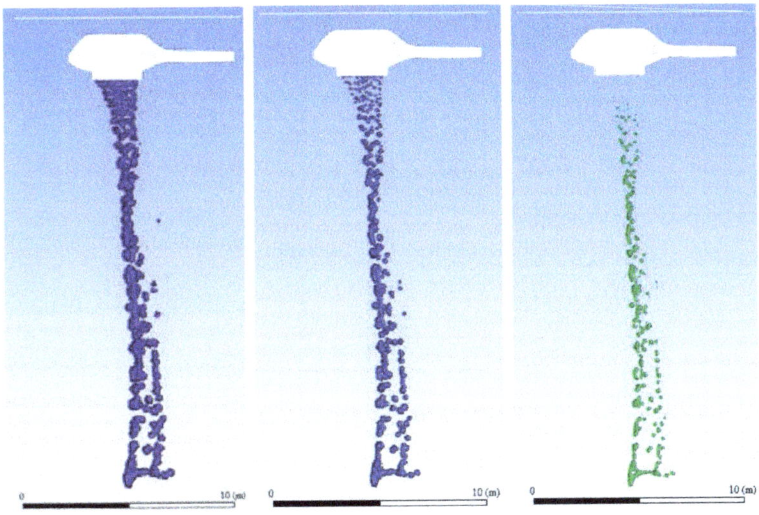

(a)

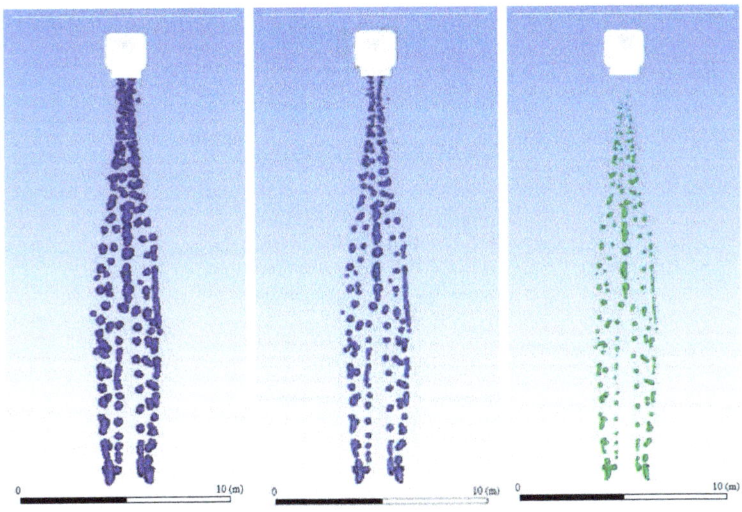

(b)

Figure 19. Contour surface of the two-phase, water–air volume fraction with fine meshes (the ground is at the ruler). (**a**) Contour surface and side view when the two-phase, water–air volume fraction was 0.01, 0.1, and 0.5, respectively, at t = 1.9 s. (**b**) Contour surface and front view when the two-phase, water–air volume fraction was 0.01, 0.1, and 0.5, respectively, at t = 1.9 s.

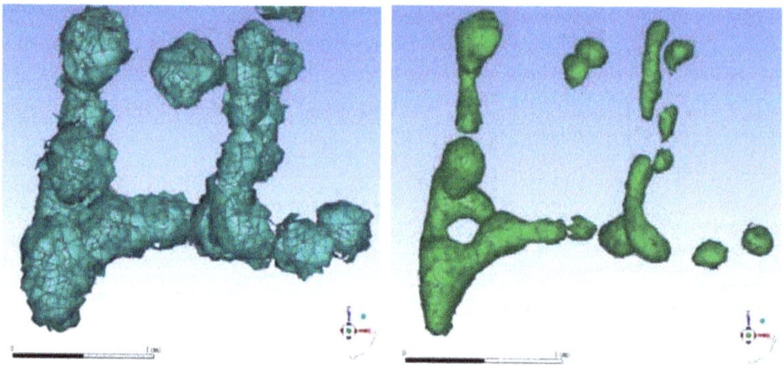

Figure 20. Contour surface of volume fraction near the ground and mesh cells in this region (the volume fraction was 0.01 in the (**left**) figure and 0.5 in the (**right**) figure).

It was calculated in the above example that, at t = 1.9 s, the water was close to the ground. If the calculation had continued, it would quickly have become unstable, because in the very short time when the water masses or large droplets hit the ground, the water mass is deformed and broken, and bouncing motions and other complex deformation and motion phenomena occur. The current mesh cell size and time step cannot distinguish such rapid and drastic changes, leading to instability in the calculations. Assuming that the main flow characteristics and the water–air distribution were obtained when the water was close to the ground, and assuming that the water in the air fell to the ground according to its existing trajectory for the rest of its time airborne, the case that the water continued to fall to the ground was not considered in this paper. If the complex process of water hitting the ground is ignored and the ground is considered as a porous media model that allows only water to pass through, or if the ground is set as a pressure outlet boundary, the problem of unstable calculations can be avoided, and an approximate distribution of accumulated water on the ground can be obtained.

4. Simulation Conclusion Analysis and Rule of Water Dumping Out of Helicopter Belly Firefighting Tank

To provide theoretical guidance for helicopter firefighting practices, a study on parameters influencing the water dump distribution was performed in this section regarding two key parameters: the height of the tank bottom above the ground (H) and the wind speed (U). A total of 12 calculation examples were considered, with H = 10 m, 20 m, and 30 m, and U = 0 m/s, 5 m/s (Level 3), 10 m/s (Level 5), and 15 m/s (Level 7). The wind direction pointed to the rear of the helicopter, or in other words, the helicopter flew into the wind. The settings of the basic meshes, computational domain, mesh dissolution, and the calculation model and method in this section were the same as those used in the examples in Section 3.

4.1. Result Analysis and Summary of Initial Scenario before Water Dump

The influence of the height of the helicopter tank bottom above the ground and of wind speed on the distribution scope of wake flow was analyzed and is summarized as follows. Figure 21 shows the distribution of wake flow when the helicopter tank bottom was 10 m above the ground and the wind speed was 0 m/s, 5 m/s, 10 m/s, and 15 m/s. Figure 22 shows the distribution of wake flow when the helicopter tank bottom was 20 m above the ground, for the same values of wind speed. Figure 23 shows the distribution of wake flow when the helicopter tank bottom was 30 m above the ground, for the same values of wind speed. These figures show that wind speed had a very significant influence on the wake flow direction of the helicopter, and when the height above the ground was between 10 and 30 m, the wake flow could be deviated by nearly 30 degrees from the straight rearward direction (the wind direction) by a wind speed of 5 m/s. The deviation increased to around 45 degrees at a wind speed of 10 m/s and around 60 degrees at a wind speed of 15 m/s. Wake flow was also influenced by the height above the ground: the higher the helicopter was above the ground, the lower the wake flow speed near the ground. When the helicopter hovered in a wind at 30 m/s, the wake flow speed near the ground was around 8 m/s. The ground in Figures 21–23 is near the ruler.

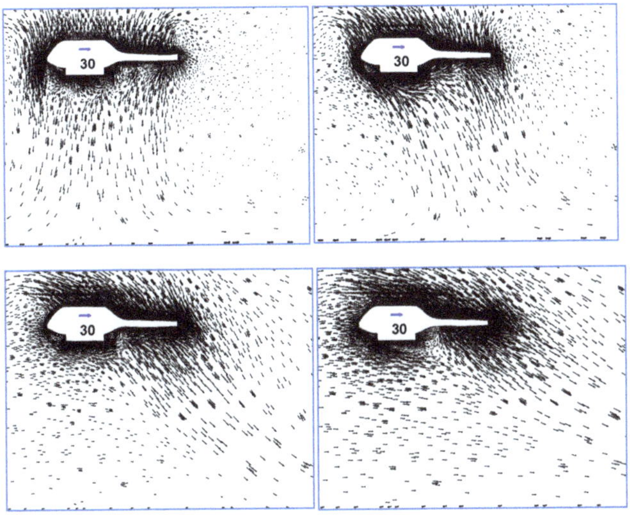

Figure 21. Distribution of wake flow when the helicopter tank bottom was 10 m above the ground (wind speed was 0 m/s, 5 m/s, 10 m/s, and 15 m/s; reference speed marked on the fuselage, indicated by a blue arrow, and the reference speed is 30 m/s).

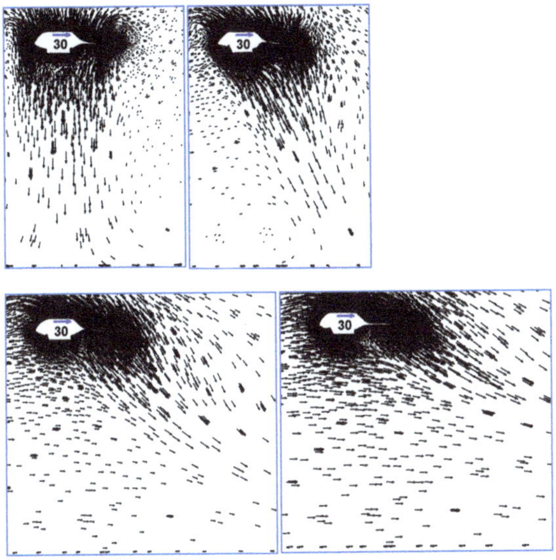

Figure 22. Distribution of wake flow when the helicopter tank bottom was 20 m above the ground (wind speed was 0 m/s, 5 m/s, 10 m/s, and 15 m/s; reference speed marked on the fuselage, indicated by a blue arrow, and the reference speed is 30 m/s).

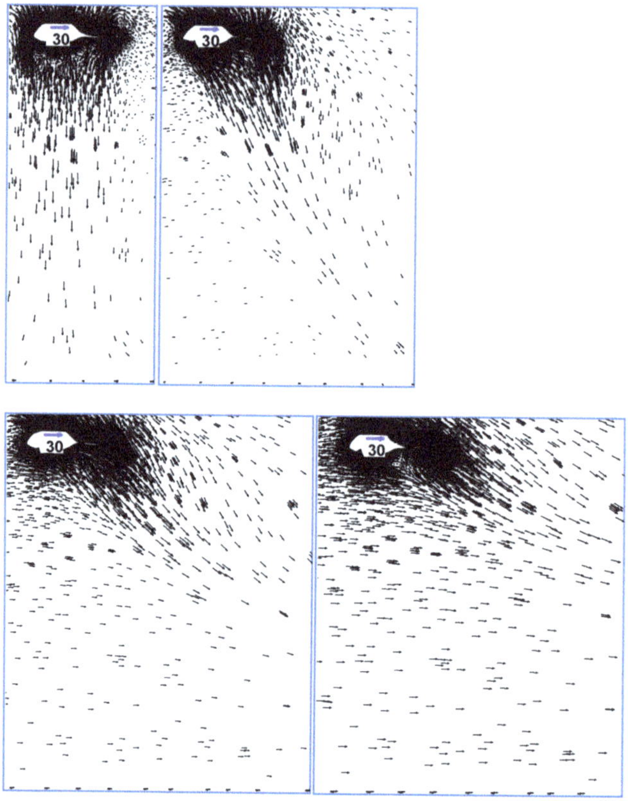

Figure 23. Distribution of wake flow when the helicopter tank bottom was 30 m above the ground (wind speed was 0 m/s, 5 m/s, 10 m/s, and 15 m/s; reference speed marked on the fuselage, indicated by a blue arrow, and the reference speed is 30 m/s).

4.2. Transient Result Analysis and Summary of Water Dump

Figure 24 shows the contour surface of the two-phase, water–air interface at a volume fraction of 0.01 when the helicopter tank bottom was 10 m above the ground and the wind speed was 0 m/s, 5 m/s, 10 m/s, and 15 m/s (t = 1.2 s, when the water mass was close to the ground). The figure shows that the motion trajectory of large water masses was basically not influenced at a wind speed of 5–10 m/s when the helicopter was 10 m above the ground, but at a wind speed of 15 m/s, the water masses moved slightly in the wind direction. The front view reveals that the water masses expanded significantly in the horizontal direction, with a horizontal expansion of nearly 50% compared with their size at a wind speed of 0 m/s.

Figure 25 shows the contour surface of the two-phase, water–air interface at a volume fraction of 0.01 when the helicopter tank bottom was 20 m above the ground and the wind speed was 0 m/s, 5 m/s, 10 m/s, and 15 m/s (t = 1.8 s, when the water mass was almost reaching the ground). Large water masses were basically not influenced at a wind speed of 5–10 m/s, but when the wind speed was 15 m/s, the water masses deviated significantly in the wind direction, with a deviation of 2–3 m compared with that at a wind speed of 0 m/s. The front view shows that the water masses also expanded significantly in the horizontal direction, with a horizontal expansion of around 7 m, which was around three times its horizontal extent at a wind speed of 0 m/s.

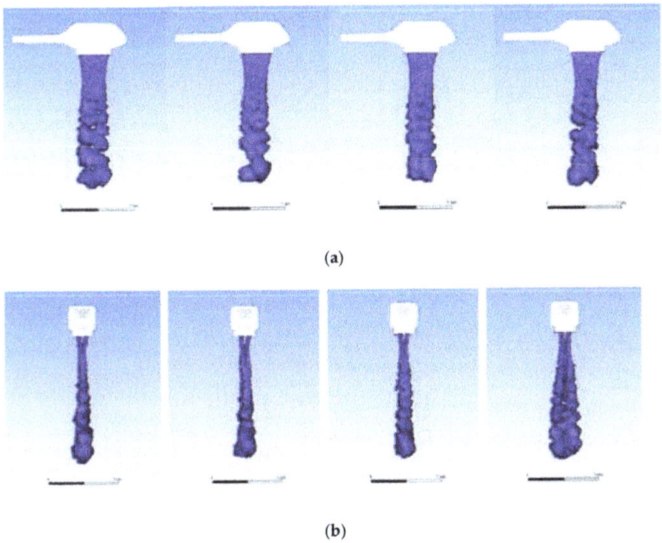

Figure 24. Contour surface of the two-phase, water–air interface at a volume fraction of 0.01 under different wind speeds (H = 10 m; the ground is at the ruler in the figure; t = 1.2 s). (**a**) Side view, showing U = 0 m/s, 5 m/s, 10 m/s, and 15 m/s, respectively, from left to right. (**b**) Front view, displaying U = 0 m/s, 5 m/s, 10 m/s, and 15 m/s, respectively, from left to right.

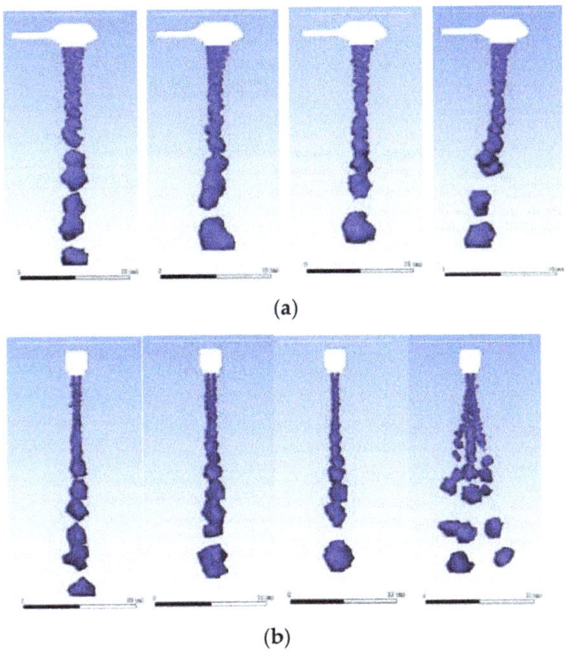

Figure 25. Contour surface of the two-phase, water–air interface at a volume fraction of 0.01 under different wind speeds (H = 20 m; the ground is at the ruler in the figure; t = 1.8 s). (**a**) Side view, displaying U = 0 m/s, 5 m/s, 10 m/s, and 15 m/s, respectively, from left to right. (**b**) Front view, showing U = 0 m/s, 5 m/s, 10 m/s, and 15 m/s, respectively, from left to right.

Figure 26 shows the contour surface of the two-phase, water–air interface at a volume fraction of 0.01 when the helicopter tank bottom was 30 m above the ground and the wind speed was 0 m/s, 5 m/s, 10 m/s, and 15 m/s, at around t = 2 s. In a similar manner, at a wind speed of 15 m/s, the water masses deviated significantly in the wind direction, and the water masses also expanded significantly in the horizontal direction, reaching around 9 m.

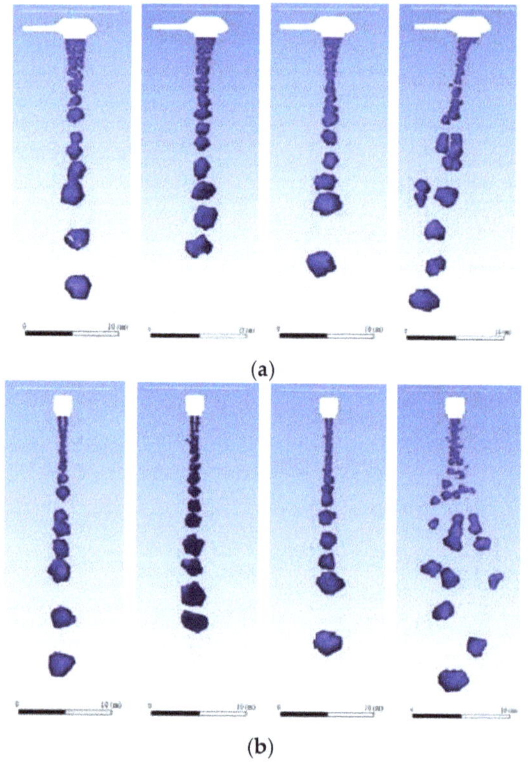

Figure 26. Contour surface of the two-phase, water–air interface at a volume fraction of 0.01 under different wind speeds (H = 30 m; the ground is at the ruler in the figure; t = 2.1 s). (**a**) Front view, showing U = 0 m/s, 5 m/s, 10 m/s, and 15 m/s, respectively, from left to right. (**b**) Front view, portraying U = 0 m/s, 5 m/s, 10 m/s, and 15 m/s, respectively, from left to right.

These observations inform us that wind speed had a very significant influence on the helicopter wake flow direction. When the height above the ground was 10–30 m, the wake flow could be deviated for nearly 30 degrees from the straight rearward direction (the wind direction) when the wind speed was 5 m/s. The deviation was around 45 degrees at a wind speed of 10 m/s and around 60 degrees at a wind speed of 15 m/s. The wake flow was also influenced by the height above the ground; the higher the helicopter, the lower the wake flow speed near the ground, and when the helicopter hovered at 30 m/s, the wake flow speed near the ground was around 8 m/s.

Large water masses were basically not influenced at wind speeds of 5–10 m/s, but when the wind speed was 15 m/s, the water masses deviated significantly in the wind direction and expanded significantly in the horizontal direction. The higher the water dump tank was above the ground, the greater the influence of wind speed on the water mass distribution.

4.3. Forward Helicopter Flight

In Section 4, it was assumed that the helicopter was hovering. In fact, before firefighting, the helicopter may fly forward at low speed above the targeted fire scene. For example, in the case where the forward flight speed was 10 m/s and there was no wind in the horizontal direction, this state could be approximated by the helicopter hovering in accordance with the principle of relativity of motion, with a headwind of 10 m/s. In addition, changes in the dip angle of the rotor discs were neglected in the calculation model. Regarding the problem of water dump distribution, although only the height of the helicopter tank above the ground and the wind speed were discussed in Section 4, the calculated result could be approximated by the circumstance where the helicopter was flying at a corresponding forward flight speed. The difference in the approximation came from changes in the dip angle of the rotor discs and the ground boundary layer, both of which had a small influence. Of course, if the hot air at the fire scene itself were taken into consideration, both wind speed and wind direction would have a significant influence on the hot air, and therefore the principle of relativity of motion might not be applicable. In the following discussion, the results obtained in Section 4 were applied to the circumstance of forward helicopter flight in accordance with the principle of relativity of motion.

Assuming that the helicopter tank was 20 m above the ground, the helicopter flew forward at a speed of 15 m/s (i.e., 54 km/h) and there was no wind (Figure 27b), then this would be equivalent to the case where the helicopter hovered against the wind at 15 m/s and the ground moved at 15 m/s in the wind direction (Figure 27a). Figure 27a shows that the helicopter hovered initially right above Point O on the ground, and when the headwind was 15 m/s, the water masses reached Point P on the ground at about 1.8 s, with a deviation of about 2–3 m from the wind direction. At this time, the water in the tank had run out, and most of the water dumped into the air would have fallen to the ground in approximately 1.8 s. Assuming that the ground moved leftward at a speed of 15 m/s, water fell finally at Point Q on the ground, and PQ was the region covered by most of the water, with an approximate length of $15 \times 1.8 = 27$ m. At this time, Point O had moved to Point O′.

Figure 27b shows that if the helicopter flew forward at a speed of 15 m/s, there was no wind, the ground was fixed, and initially the helicopter was right above Point O′ on the ground, it flew to be right above Point O on the ground 1.8 s later, the water dumped initially fell to Point P on the ground at this time. Similarly, around 1.8 s later, most of the water would have fallen, finally reaching Point Q on the ground. In this case, the PQ region was the region covered by most of the water, with an approximate length of $15 \times 2 = 30$ m. Figure 25 shows that the horizontal width of the region was around 7 m, the region covered an area of about $30 \times 7 = 210$ m^2, and after 1.12 m^3 of water were dumped, there would be about 5 mm of water accumulated per square meter in the covered region.

Figure 27b shows that if the intent is to dump water in the right region starting from Point P on the ground (PQ), the pilot needs to open the tank valve to dump the water when the helicopter is right above Point O′. The region covered by the water dumped depends on the height of the tank bottom above the ground, the flight speed, the wind speed, and the time required to empty the tank.

Note that in these calculations, foaming agents and other surface-active materials were not added to the water. If surface-active materials were added, formation of water droplets and the vaporization speed of water could be reduced, thus reducing the area covered by water on the ground and increasing the amount of water distributed per unit area.

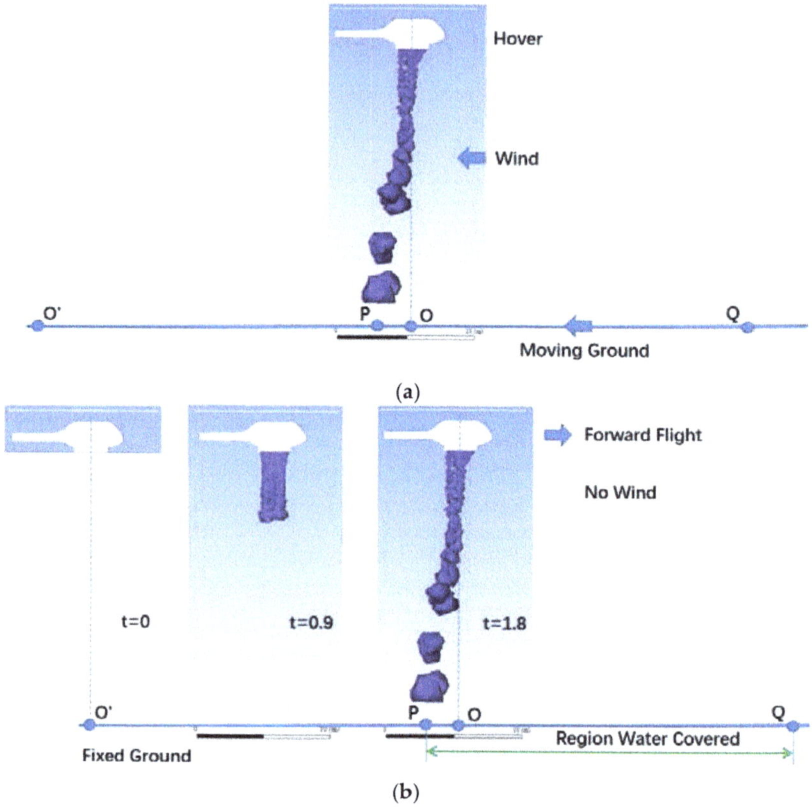

Figure 27. Water being dumped out of a helicopter tank and the distribution interval of water on the ground. (**a**) Helicopter hovering against the wind with the ground moving in the wind direction at wind speed. (**b**) Helicopter flying forward (forward flight speed = wind speed in a) with no wind and the ground fixed.

4.4. Rule of Water Distribution on the Ground

In accordance with the preceding data and calculation method, the region covered by water on the ground (also referred to as the water band in the literature) and average amount of water per unit area were given. Please note that, when calculating the average water amount per ground area, the accumulated water amount was considered in this paper instead of the water flow on the ground. However, in ANSYS FLUENT, the ground was set to have a non-slipping, fixed-wall condition, which, in this way, the water mass could flow all around after touching the ground; therefore, the accumulated water amount cannot be calculated automatically by this software. In order to calculate the accumulated water amount, the distribution of water mass just before touching the ground was taken into consideration in this paper, from which the water coverage area was given. Due to spatial–temporal changes in the water mass touching the ground, it is very complex to calculate the distribution of the water depth on the ground. Moreover, the breakup of drops and other phenomena were not taken into consideration in this paper; therefore, the average water depth was calculated in this paper only. Data on the hovering status of the helicopter, different wind speeds, the height of the tank bottom above the ground, the region covered by water on the ground, and the average amount of water were first provided, as shown in Table 1. The region covered by the water dump was approximated as a rectangle with area = longitudinal length × horizontal length. Table 1 shows that at wind speeds below 10 m/s, the region covered by water on the ground was basically not influenced by the wind, but when the wind speed reached 15 m/s, the longitudinal dimension of the region covered by water on the ground decreased slightly, whereas the horizontal dimension increased greatly. Therefore, the area covered increased greatly, and under the premise of an unchanged total amount of water, the average water depth accumulated per unit area decreased greatly. The higher the tank bottom was above the ground, the greater the area covered by water on the ground, and the less the average water depth accumulated per unit area. However, the results at a height of 10 m were significantly smaller than those at 20 m and 30 m, although the results at the latter two heights were relatively close to each other.

Table 1. Influence of wind speed and height of the tank bottom above the ground on the region covered by water and the average water amount on the ground while the helicopter was hovering.

Height of Tank bottom above the Ground/Wind Speed	0 m/s	5 m/s	10 m/s	15 m/s
10 m	2.4 m × 1.6 m = 3.84 m^2 0.29 m water depth/m^2	2.2 m × 1.7 m = 3.74 m^2 0.30 m water depth/m^2	2.1 m × 1.7 m = 3.57 m^2 0.31 m water depth/m^2	2.1 m × 2.5 m = 5.25 m^2 0.21 m water depth/m^2
20 m	3.4 m × 3.0 m = 10.2 m^2 0.11 m water depth/m^2	3.2 m × 3.0 m = 9.6 m^2 0.12 m water depth/m^2	3.2 m × 3.2 m = 10.24 m^2 0.11 m water depth/m^2	4.0 m × 7.0 m = 28.0 m^2 0.04 m water depth/m^2
30 m	2.9 m × 2.9 m = 8.41 m^2 0.13 m water depth/m^2	3.0 m × 3.0 m = 9.0 m^2 0.12 m water depth/m^2	3.0 m × 3.0 m = 9.0 m^2 0.12 m water depth/m^2	5.0 m × 9.0 m = 45.0 m^2 0.025 m water depth/m^2

As the helicopter flew forward, the region covered by water on the ground and the amount of water were also subject to the influence of forward flight speed. By the method discussed in Section 4.3, the average water distribution on the ground from the water dump when the helicopter flew forward (no wind) was as shown in Table 2. For forward flight, the higher the forward flight speed, the less the average water depth; a similar relation held for flight height. The average water depth per unit area was one order of magnitude less than in the cases of the corresponding hovering helicopter and wind speeds. For example, with a helicopter at a forward flight speed of 15 m/s and the tank bottom 30 m above the ground, the dumped water was distributed within a region of approximately 337.5 m^2, and the average water depth accumulated in this region per square meter was 0.3 cm. There were two working conditions having similar premises. The working condition of Hayden Biggs [15] was the most similar, with a forward flight speed of 70 km/h, a tank water-carrying capacity of 1.4 t, and a height above the ground of 24 m. The range of the water band on the ground was 120 m × 21 m, and the average water depth was 0.34 cm. The average water depth under similar working conditions in the present study was 0.3 cm, showing good agreement. Another similar working condition was that of Xie Yingmin [12]. In this case, the flight speed was 60 km/h (equivalent to 16.67 m/s), the height was 30 m, and the wind speed was 3 m/s. Their results showed that the maximum water belt on the ground was 110 × 25 m, the effective water belt was 65 × 15 m, and average water depth was 0.1–0.3 cm. The water-carrying capacity of the tank in the study by Xie Yingmin et al. [12] was 3 t, which was almost three times that in the present study, and assuming that the outlet flow was the same, its corresponding water belt area was also about three times that in this study. Therefore, the results of this study were basically consistent with the working conditions in Xie Yingmin et al. [12].

Table 2. Average water distribution on the ground with the helicopter flying forward when making a water dump (no wind).

Height of the Tank bottom above the Ground/Forward Flight Speed	5 m/s	10 m/s	15 m/s
10 m	$5 \times 1.2 \times 1.7 = 10.2$ m^2 0.11 m water depth/m^2	$10 \times 1.2 \times 1.7 = 20.4$ m^2 0.055 m water depth/m^2	$15 \times 1.2 \times 2.5 = 45$ m^2 0.025 m water depth/m^2
20 m	$5 \times 2.0 \times 3.0 = 30$ m^2 0.037 m water depth/m^2	$10 \times 2.0 \times 3.2 = 64$ m^2 0.0175 m water depth/m^2	$15 \times 2.0 \times 7.0 = 210$ m^2 0.005 m water depth/m^2
30 m	$5 \times 2.5 \times 3.0 = 37.5$ m^2 0.03 m water depth/m^2	$10 \times 2.5 \times 3.2 = 80$ m^2 0.014 m water depth/m^2	$15 \times 2.5 \times 9.0 = 337.5$ m^2 0.003 m water depth/m^2

5. Conclusions

This study looked at two key parameters in firefighting helicopter operation: the height of the helicopter tank (H125/Isolair Eliminator II) above the ground (H) and the wind speed (U). After considering the relevant physical processes, such as the movement of water mass in the air, changes in the shape of the water mass, and the breakup of drops after water dump from the tank we decided to calculate the accumulated water amount on the ground. The height of the helicopter from the ground and the wind speed (or forward speed of the helicopter) are also important parameters influencing these physical processes, and hence were also considered in this work. The VOF model and adaptive mesh in ANSYS FLUENT were applied in this paper, which yielded the average water amount distributed on the ground after water dump from the helicopter. A study of the parameters influencing the water dump distribution was performed, considering $H = 10$ m, 20 m, and 30 m and $U = 0$ m/s, 5 m/s (Level 3), 10 m/s (Level 5), and 15 m/s (Level 7). The main conclusions were as follows:

(1) Wind speed had a significant influence on the direction of wake flow when the helicopter was hovering. The wake flow could by deviated by nearly 30, 45, and 60 degrees by wind speeds of 5 m/s, 10 m/s, and 15 m/s, respectively;
(2) The height above the ground also influenced the wake flow speed. The higher the helicopter was above the ground, the lower the wake flow speed near the ground. When the H125 helicopter hovered 30 m above the ground, the wake flow speed near the ground was about 8 m/s;
(3) There was no significant change in water mass distribution at wind speeds below 10 m/s, but when the wind speed rose to 15 m/s, the water masses deviated significantly in the wind direction and expanded significantly in the horizontal direction. Hence, the area covered by water on the ground increased significantly, and the average depth of water accumulated per unit area decreased significantly;
(4) The higher the tank was above the ground, the greater the area covered by water on the ground, and the less the average depth of water accumulated per unit area. However, the results at a height of 10 m are significantly less pronounced than those at 20 m and 30 m, although the results at the latter two heights are relatively close to each other;
(5) For forward flight, the higher the forward flight speed, the less the average depth of water on the ground; a similar relation held for flight height. The average depth of water was one order of magnitude less than in the cases of the corresponding hovering helicopter and the various wind speeds.

The following suggestions can be drawn from our results: if only the depth of water accumulated per unit area on the ground is considered when performing water dump firefighting, the helicopter should have the lowest possible forward flight speed and flight height and should perform firefighting under low wind speed conditions.

6. Future Work

The results calculated in this study show that the model developed here could be used to study the distribution of a water dump out of a helicopter tank, which has basically met the engineering requirements for firefighting with water dumps out of helicopters. To distinguish the water and air phase interfaces more meticulously and accurately, finer meshes and a smaller mesh adaptation cell scale would be required. In the meantime, in combination with "VOF-to-DPM" and the turbulent SAS model, small water droplets at mm level could be traced. For the fine meshes used in this study, the maximum mesh cell under the helicopter tank was 0.2 m in size, and the minimum mesh adaptation cell was 0.05 m, with total numbers of mesh cells up to 2 million. Using 84 CPU of the three calculation nodes of "Milky Way One", for example, it would take 17 h to calculate 1900 time steps (1.9 s). To distinguish water droplets at 0.01 m level (small water droplets at mm level required no distinction and were realized with the VOF-to-DPM model), the number of mesh cells would have to be increased by 125 times approximately, to 200–300 million mesh cells. If 840 CPU of "Milky Way One" were used, it would take about 10 days to calculate 1900 time steps, or about 200,000 CPU hours. Therefore, such calculation could be realized, but at an enormous cost.

This paper is merely a preliminary study on belly firefighting tank water dumping by helicopter and ground water distribution, and a coupling fire-field model must also be investigated. In the complete process of helicopter water dump firefighting, the wake flow of the rotor wings, the water–air flow and droplet dynamics, and combustion and the heat and smoke generated are all involved, making this still a very challenging problem of how to use the above models to establish an effective numerical calculation scheme.

Author Contributions: Conceptualization, J.L.; methodology, T.Z., S.L.; validation, T.Z. and C.W.; formal analysis, T.Z.; investigation, S.L.; data curation, T.Z.; writing—original draft preparation, T.Z.; writing—review and editing, T.Z. and S.L.; visualization, T.Z.; supervision, T.Z.; funding acquisition, J.L. All authors have read and agreed to the published version of the manuscript.

Funding: This work was funded by State Grid Corporation of China Science and Technology Project (5216A0210041) and the National Key Research and Development Plan (No. 2016YFC0800104).

Institutional Review Board Statement: Not applicable.

Informed Consent Statement: Not applicable.

Data Availability Statement: All data generated or analyzed are available on request through the author, Zhou Tejun, whose email address is zhoutejun1988@126.com.

Acknowledgments: The authors would like to thank the Editor and the reviewers for their comments and suggestions, which have been very helpful in improving the quality of this paper.

Conflicts of Interest: The authors declared that they have no conflicts of interest in this work.

References

1. Tymstra, C.; Stocks, B.J.; Cai, X.; Flannigan, M.D. Wildfire management in Canada: Review, challenges and opportunities. *Prog. Disaster Sci.* **2020**, *5*, 100045. [CrossRef]
2. McWethy, D.B.; Schoennagel, T.; Higuera, P.E.; Krawchuk, M.; Harvey, B.J.; Metcalf, E.C.; Schultz, C.; Miller, C.; Metcalf, A.L.; Buma, B.; et al. Rethinking resilience to wildfire. *Nat. Sustain.* **2019**, *2*, 797–804. [CrossRef]
3. Hessburg, P.F.; Prichard, S.J.; Hagmann, R.K.; Povak, N.A.; Lake, F.K. Wildfire and climate change adaptation of western North American forests: A case for intentional management. *Ecol. Appl.* **2021**, *31*, e02432. [CrossRef] [PubMed]
4. Marchi, E.; Neri, F.; Tesi, E.; Fabiano, F.; Brachetti Montorselli, N. Analysis of helicopter activities in forest fire-fighting. *Croat. J. For. Eng. J. Theory Appl. For. Eng.* **2014**, *35*, 233–243.
5. Kal'avský, P.; Petríček, P.; Kelemen, M.; Rozenberg, R.; Jevčák, J.; Tomaško, R.; Mikula, B. The efficiency of aerial firefighting in varying flying conditions. In Proceedings of the 2019 International Conference on Military Technologies (ICMT), Brno, Czech Republic, 30–31 May 2019; pp. 1–5.
6. Hnilica, R.; Ťavodová, M.; Hnilicová, M.; Matej, J.; Messingerová, V. The Innovative Design of the Fire-Fighting Adapter for Forest Machinery. *Forests* **2020**, *11*, 843. [CrossRef]
7. Legendre, D.; Becker, R.; Alméras, E.; Chassagne, A. Air tanker drop patterns. *Int. J. Wildland Fire* **2014**, *23*, 272–280. [CrossRef]

8. Wu, Z.; Zhou, Y.; Zhen, X.; Li, X.; Zhang, Z.; Liu, J.; Jiang, X.; Wang, Z.; Guo, T.; Wu, Y.; et al. Research on efficiency of bucket water dump firefighting—Take K-32 helicopter for instance. *Forest Fire Prev.* **2017**, *1*, 4. (In Chinese)
9. Ma, Y.; Ma, D. Application analysis of helicopter bucket firefighting in China forests. *For. Labor Saf.* **2013**, *26*, 4. (In Chinese)
10. Chen, Z.; Wu, T. Comparison empirical analysis of helicopter forest firefighting methods. In Proceedings of the 2010 Transportation Graduate Academic Forum & Science and Technology Innovation Proceedings, Tianjin, China, 21 May 2010.
11. Zhou, W. Applicability analysis of MI-26T helicopter in fighting against forest fire in southwest forest region. *For. Fire Prev.* **2007**, *1*. (In Chinese)
12. Xie, Y.; Zhang, H.; Hu, M. Significance of introduction of K-32A helicopter and its application in forest fire prevention. *For. Fire Prev.* **2009**, *1*, 56–59. (In Chinese)
13. Zhou, T.; Lu, J.; Wu, C.; Li, B.; Tan, Y.; Liu, L. Test and application of helicopter water dump firefighting of mountain fires on power transmission lines. *High Volt. Eng.* **2021**, *47*, 2811–2819. (In Chinese) [CrossRef]
14. Solarz, P.; Jordan, C. *Ground Pattern Performance of the LA County Bell S205 Helicopter with Sheetcraft Fixed Tank*; United States Department of Agriculture Forest Service, Technology & Development Program, USDA Forest Service Missoula Technology and Development Center: Missoula, MT, USA, 2000; 0057-2863-MTDC.
15. Biggs, H. *An Evaluation of the Performance of the Simplex 304 Helicopter Belly-Tank*; Research Report no. 71; Fire Management Division Department of Sustainability and Environment: Melbourne, Australia, 2004.
16. Zhao, X.; Zhou, P.; Yan, X.; Weng, Y.; Yang, X.L. Numerical simulation of the aerial drop of water for fixed wing airtankers. In Proceedings of the 31st Congress of the International Council of the Aeronautic Sciences, Belo Horizonte, Brazil, 9–14 September 2018.
17. Satoh, K.; Maeda, I.; Kuwahara, K.; Yang, K.T. A numerical study of water dump in aerial fire fighting. *Fire Saf. Sci.* **2005**, *8*, 777–787. [CrossRef]
18. Borisov, I.V.; Tsipenko, A.V. Computing simulation for firefighting helicopter operation analysis. In Proceedings of the 29th Congress of the International Council of the Aeronautical Sciences, St. Petersburg, Russia, 7–12 September 2014.
19. Kim, Y.-H.; Park, S.-O. Navier-Stokes simulation of unsteady rotor-airframe interaction with momentum source method. *Int. J. Aeronaut. Space Sci.* **2009**, *10*, 125–133. [CrossRef]
20. Lacombe, F.; Pelletier, D.; Garon, A. Compatible wall functions and adaptive remeshing for the k-omega SST model. In Proceedings of the AIAA Scitech 2019 Forum, San Diego, CA, USA, 7–11 January 2019; p. 2329, AIAA 2020-2284.
21. Balasubramanian, A.K.; Kumar, V.; Nakod, P.; Schütze, J.; Rajan, A. Multiscale modelling of a doublet injector using hybrid VOF-DPM method. In Proceedings of the AIAA Scitech 2020 Forum, Orlando, FL, USA, 6–10 January 2020.
22. Sullivan, P.P.; McWilliams, J.C. Frontogenesis and frontal arrest of a dense filament in the oceanic surface boundary layer. *J. Fluid Mech.* **2018**, *837*, 341–380. [CrossRef]
23. Eggers, J. Nonlinear dynamics and breakup of free-surface flows. *Rev. Mod. Phys.* **1997**, *69*, 865–930. [CrossRef]
24. Sula, C.; Grosshans, H.; Papalexandris, M.V. Assessment of droplet breakup models for spray flow simulations. *Flow Turbul. Combust.* **2020**, *105*, 889–914. [CrossRef]
25. Sazhin, S.S. *Droplets and Sprays*; Springer: London, UK, 2014.

MDPI
St. Alban-Anlage 66
4052 Basel
Switzerland
Tel. +41 61 683 77 34
Fax +41 61 302 89 18
www.mdpi.com

MDPI Books Editorial Office
E-mail: books@mdpi.com
www.mdpi.com/books

www.ingramcontent.com/pod-product-compliance
Lightning Source LLC
Chambersburg PA
CBHW061806210926
51850CB00006B/630
9783036577067